Neuropsychology, Neuropsychiatry, and Behavioral Neurology

Critical Issues in Neuropsychology

Series Editors

Antonio E. Puente
University of North Carolina, Wilmington

Cecil R. Reynolds
Texas A&M University

A Continuation Order Plan is available for this series. A continuation order will bring delivery of each new volume immediately upon publication. Volumes are billed only upon actual shipment. For further information please contact the publisher.

Neuropsychology, Neuropsychiatry, and Behavioral Neurology

Rhawn Joseph

Neurobehavioral Center
Santa Clara, California

Plenum Press • New York and London

Library of Congress Cataloging in Publication Data

Joseph, Rhawn.
  Neuropsychology, neuropsychiatry, and behavioral neurology / Rhawn Joseph.
    p.   cm. — (Critical issues in neuropsychology)
  Includes bibliographical references.
  ISBN 0-306-43136-X
  1. Neuropsychiatry. 2. Neuropsychology. I. Title. II. Series. [DNLM: 1. Neuro-
physiology. 2. Neuropsychology. 3. Psychiatry. WL 103 J83n]
  RC341.J67   1989
  616.8 — dc20   ·
  DNLM/DLC   89-16319
  for Library of Congress   CIP

© 1990 Plenum Press, New York
A Division of Plenum Publishing Corporation
233 Spring Street, New York, N.Y. 10013

Printed in the United States of America

To those who say
"NO!"
I say
"YES!"

Preface

This book is written for the clinician, students, and practitioners of neuropsychology, neuropsychiatry, and behavioral neurology. It has been my intent throughout to present a synthesis of ideas and research findings. I have reviewed thousands of articles and research reports and have drawn extensively from diverse sources in philosophy, psychology, neurology, neurosurgery, neuropsychiatry, physiology, and neuroanatomy in order to produce this text. Of course I have also drawn from my own experience as a clinician and research scientist in preparing this work and in this regard some of my own biases and interests are represented.

I have long sought to understand the human mind and the phenomena we experience as conscious awareness. After many years of studying a variety of Western and Eastern psychologists and philosophers, including the Buddhist, Taoist, and Hindu philosophical systems, I began, while still an undergraduate student, to formulate my own theory of the mind. I felt, though, that what I had come upon were only pieces of half the puzzle. What I knew of the brain was minimal. Indeed, it came as quite a surprise when one day I came across the journal *Brain* as I was browsing through the periodicals section of the library. I was awed. An entire journal devoted to the brain was quite a revelation. Nevertheless, although intrigued by the possibilities, I resisted. What did the brain have to do with "consciousness," emotion, or even clinical psychology? I was to find out soon thereafter, when I met and became good friends with Dr. David Duval, then a graduate student. He was both biologist and philosopher and told me about a new experimental memory and brain injury rehabilitation clinic at the Palo Alto Veterans Administration Hospital, where he had just begun to work. I was intrigued by his stories and one day accompanied him as an invited visitor. (Later I obtained a position at the clinic for a short time.) I was astounded and deeply impressed by the seemingly bizarre variety of symptoms demonstrated by many of the brain-injured vets I met that day, and I was shocked to be confronted with what appeared to be an undeniable truth: "If you damage the brain you damage consciousness." On that day I began a quest to understand the brain and the manner in which it interacts so as to produce consciousness, awareness, personality, memory, thinking, emotion, neurosis, and psychosis.

That was almost 17 years ago. Since that time, I have been very fortunate to have had a number of opportunities to test and observe over a thousand brain-injured individuals and to conduct a variety of studies in the neurosciences. These have included animal research in neurophysiology, developmental neuroanatomy, and sensory deprivation;

human neuropsychological studies conducted on children and split-brain, brain-injured, and neurosurgical patients; and research on hormonal and early environmental influences on arousal, aggression, memory, and sex differences in cognition.

In conducting these studies my knowledge and understanding of brain psychiatry and neuropsychology have greatly expanded. Nevertheless, many of the books in the neurosciences treat psychiatry, neurology, and neuropsychology as if they were separate and mutually exclusive fields. It is my belief that these areas of study are in fact one and the same. I think it is important to realize that what appears to be a "manic" disorder may in fact be a manifestation of right frontal lobe disease, or that the patient who suddenly develops "schizophrenia" may instead have suffered a stroke involving the basal ganglia or left temporal lobe. I believe it is also important to recognize not only that diverse symptoms may be indicative of localized dysfunction but also how specific abnormalities can be secondary to disconnection syndromes, disinhibition, epileptic disturbances, and/or tumors, strokes, head injury, and diffuse physiological changes. To understand and recognize these problems it is necessary to have at least some knowledge of neuroanatomy and the manner in which various nuclei and brain regions interact. These are just some of the issues detailed in the pages that follow.

Rhawn Joseph

Santa Clara, California

Acknowledgments

This book is written for the clinician. However, it draws from a number of research and theoretical perspectives as well as my own experiences in diverse neuroscience settings, including my readings in the neurosciences, existential phenomenology, and psychoanalysis. Nietzsche, Freud, Jung, Sartre, Geschwind, Luria, and many others have greatly contributed to my thought and understanding of the brain, cognition, emotion, and conscious awareness. Drs. Oakley Ray, Peter Koestenbaum, Arlene Kasprisin, Arthur Anderson, and Roberta Gallagher have contributed significantly to my philosophical and experiental growth. Drs. Oakley Ray, Vivian Casagrande, J. Kass, and J. Siegel provided me with tremendous opportunities to undertake a broad range of neuroscience research, whereas Drs. A. Kasprisin, J. Dalton, J. Gonen, R. Delaney, R. Novelly, M. Andersen, and A. Anton provided me with opportunities to examine a wide variety of brain-injured, neurosurgical, split-brain, and psychiatric patients. Others who have contributed significantly include Drs. Edith Kaplin, S. Berenbaum, D. O'Leary, Ralph Peterson, and Joe Ryan; the Psychiatry and Neurology Departments at UHS/The Chicago Medical School and the North Chicago Veterans Administration Medical Center; the Neurology and Neurosurgery staff at West Haven Veterans Administration Medical Center and Yale University Medical School; the staff at the Veterans Administration/Yale Seizure Unit; the *Journal of Clinical Psychology* for allowing me to republish portions of my 1982 monograph and a slightly expanded version of my 1988 monograph; and Fran Bernstein and the San Jose State University Library staff.

In preparing for this book I also spent more than a few hours browsing through old editions of various periodicals. I was often fascinated by what I discovered hidden away and uncited. I once read that "the only new ideas are those which have been forgotten." I would amend that to read "many new ideas...." This is certainly apparent after reading authors such as Hughlings Jackson and many of his contemporaries, who lived and wrote during the late 1800s, as well as other researchers and scholars publishing as recently as the 1940s. Although the field of neuropsychology has grown phenomenally during the last 25 years, a good deal of the groundwork was brilliantly proposed and explored long ago. Nevertheless much remains to be explored and discovered. It is my hope that this neurosynthesis of old and new will contribute to the making of many new discoveries. I very much appreciate the assistance and patience of my two editors Steve Melvin and Eliot Werner.

Contents

Chapter 4

The Frontal Lobes: Neuropsychiatry, Neuropsychology, and Behavioral

Chapter 8

Cerebral and Cranial Trauma: Anatomy and Pathophysiology of Mild, Moderate, and Severe Head Injury

Chapter 9

Stroke and Cerebrovascular Disease 319

Brain Plates

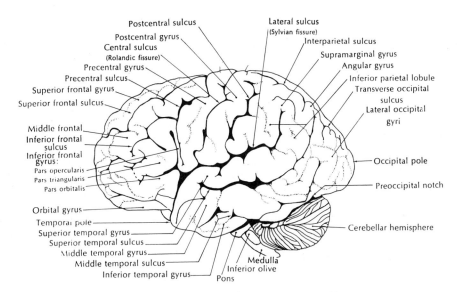

FIGURE 1. Lateral surface of the left cerebral hemisphere. From *Structure of the human brain* by S. J. DeArmond, M. M. Fusco, & M. M. Dewey, 1976. New York: Oxford University Press. Reprinted by permission.

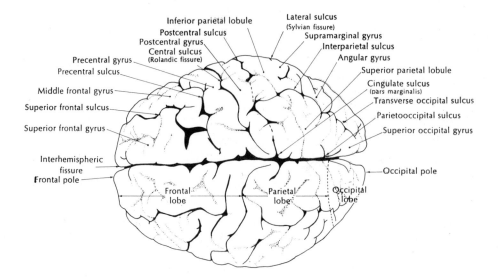

FIGURE 2. Superior surface of the brain. From *Structure of the human brain* by S. J. DeArmond, M. M. Fusco, & M. M. Dewey, 1976. New York: Oxford University Press. Reprinted by permission.

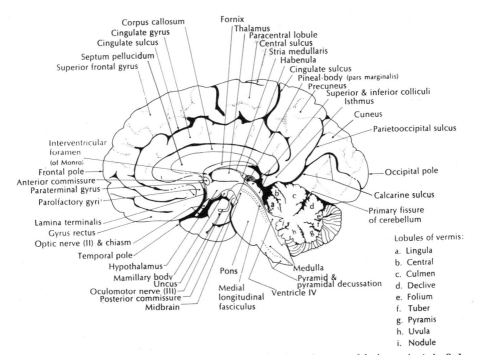

FIGURE 3. Medial (split-brain) view of the right half of the brain. From *Structure of the human brain* by S. J. DeArmond, M. M. Fusco, & M. M. Dewey, 1976. New York: Oxford University Press. Reprinted by permission.

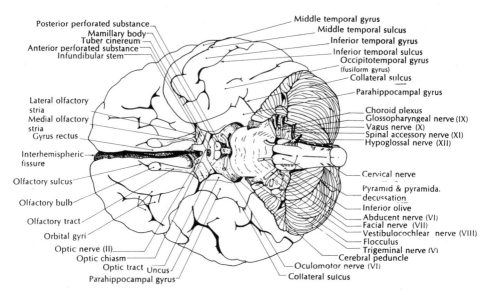

FIGURE 4. Inferior surface of the brain. From *Structure of the human brain* by S. J. DeArmond, M. M. Fusco, & M. M. Dewey, 1976. New York: Oxford University Press. Reprinted by permission.

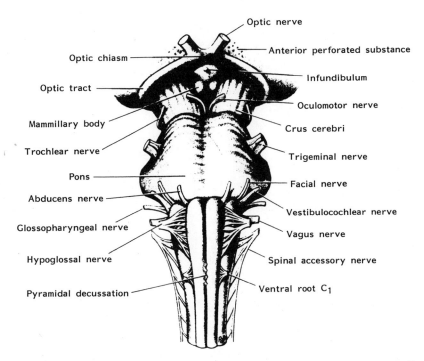

FIGURE 5. The anterior aspect of the brainstem and midbrain. From *Human neuroanatomy* by R. C. Truex &
M. B. Carpenter, 1969. Courtesy of The Williams & Wilkins Co., Baltimore, MD.

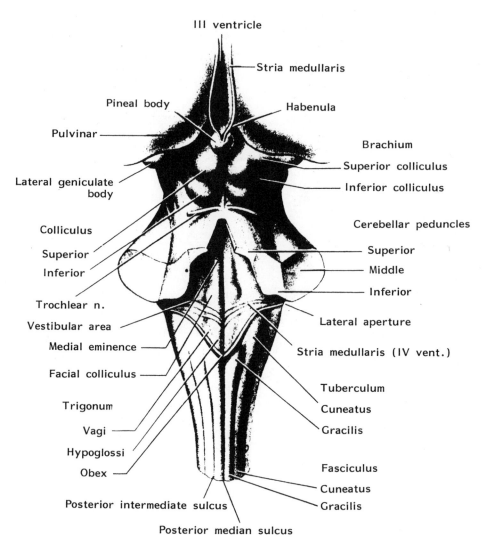

FIGURE 6. The posterior aspect of the brainstem with the cerebellum removed. From *Human neuroanatomy* by R. C. Truex & M. B. Carpenter, 1969. Courtesy of The Williams & Wilkins Co., Baltimore, MD.

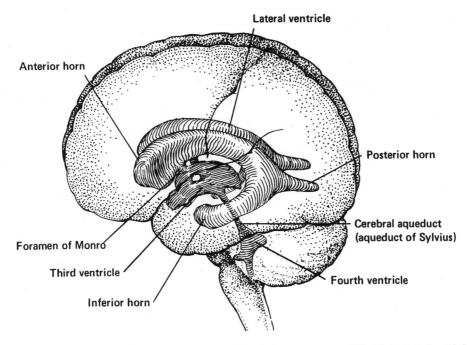

FIGURE 7. The ventricular system of the brain. From *Correlative neuroanatomy*, 20th Ed. by J. DeGroot & J. G. Chusid, 1988. Courtesy of Appleton & Lange, E. Norwalk, CT.

The Right Cerebral Hemisphere
Emotion, Music, Visual–Spatial Skills, Body Image, Dreams, and Awareness

Over the course of evolution, each half of the brain has developed its own unique strategy for perceiving, processing, and expressing information as well as specialized neuroanatomical interconnections that assist in mediating these functions. Indeed, the human brain is organized such that two potentially independent mental systems coexist, literally side by side. (cf. Gazzaniga & LeDoux, 1978; Joseph, 1982, 1988*a,b*; Levy, 1983; Sperry, 1966, 1982).

For example, expressive speech, linguistic knowledge and thought, mathematical and analytical reasoning, as well as the temporal–sequential and rhythmical aspects of consciousness, are associated with the functional integrity of the left half of the brain in most of the population. By contrast, the right cerebral hemisphere is associated with nonverbal environmental awareness; visual–spatial perceptual functioning, including analysis of depth; figure ground and stereopsis; facial recognition; and the maintenance of the body image, as well as the perception, expression, and mediation of most aspects of emotionality.

LEFT HEMISPHERE OVERVIEW

The left cerebral hemisphere is associated with the organization and categorization of information into discrete temporal units, the sequential control of finger, hand, arm, and articulatory movements (Beaumont, 1974; Heilman, Rothi, & Kertesz, 1983; Kimura, 1977; Luria, 1980; Mateer, 1983), and the perception and labeling of material that can be coded linguistically or within a linear and sequential time frame (Efron, 1963; Lenneberg, 1967; Mills & Rollman, 1980). It is also dominant in regard to most aspects of expressive and receptive linguistic functioning, including grammar, syntax, reading, writing, speaking, spelling, naming, verbal comprehension, and verbal memory (Albert, Sparks, von Strockert, & Sax, 1972; Carmazza & Zurif, 1976; DeRenzi, Zambolini, & Crisi, 1987; Efron, 1963; Goodglass & Kaplan, 1972; Hecaen & Albert, 1979; Heilman & Scholes, 1976; Kertesz, 1983*a,b;* Levine & Sweet, 1983; Luria, 1980; Milner, 1970; Vignolo,

1983; Zurif & Carson, 1970). In addition, the left hemisphere has been shown via dichotic listening tasks, to be dominant for the perception of real words, backwards speech, and consonants, as well as real and nonsense syllables (Blumstein & Cooper, 1974; Kimura, 1961; Shankweiler & Studdert-Kennedy, 1966, 1967; Studdert-Kennedy & Shankweiler, 1970).

In fact, within the left hemisphere one area largely controls the capacity to speak, and another region mediates the ability to understand speech. These regions are referred to as Broca's area (located along the left frontal convexity) and Wernicke's area (within the superior–posterior temporal lobe), respectively.

Broca's Aphasia

If a person were to sustain massive damage to the left frontal convexity, the ability to speak would be dramatically curtailed. Even if only partially damaged, disturbances that involve grammar and syntax and reductions in vocabulary and word fluency in both speech and writing result (Goodglass & Berko, 1960; Milner, 1964). However, the ability to comprehend language would remain largely, but not completely, intact. This disorder is called Broca's, or expressive, aphasia (see Goodglass & Kaplan, 1972; Levine & Sweet, 1983).

Persons with expressive aphasia, although greatly limited in their ability to speak, are nevertheless capable of making emotional statements or even singing (Gardner, 1975; Goldstein, 1942; Joseph, 1982; Smith, 1966; Smith & Burklund, 1966; Yamadori, Os-umi, Mashuara, & Okuto, 1977). In fact, they may be able to sing words they cannot say. Moreover, because persons with Broca's aphasia are able to comprehend, they are aware of their deficit and become appropriately depressed (Robinson & Szetela, 1981). Indeed, those with the smallest lesions become the most depressed (Robinson & Benson, 1981), the depression as well as the ability to sing being mediated presumably, by the intact right cerebral hemisphere (Joseph, 1982).

Wernicke's Aphasia

If, instead, the lesion were more posteriorly located along the superior temporal lobe, the patient would have great difficulty understanding spoken or written language (Good-glass & Kaplan, 1972; Hecaen & Albert, 1978; Kertesz, 1983a). This disorder is attributed in part to an impaired capacity to discern the individual units of speech and their temporal order. That is, sounds must be separated into discrete interrelated linear units, or they will be perceived as a meaningless blur (Carmon & Nachshon, 1971; Efron, 1963; Lackner & Teuber, 1973).

Wernicke's area acts to organize and separate incoming sounds into a temporal and interrelated series so as to extract linguistic meaning via the perception of the resulting sequences (Efron, 1963; Lackner & Teuber, 1973; Lenneberg, 1967). Thus, when damaged, a spoken sentence such as the "big black dog" might be perceived as "the klabgigdod." This is referred to as Wernicke's aphasia. However, comprehension is improved when the spoken words are separated by long intervals.

Patients with damage to Wernicke's area are nevertheless still capable of talking because of the preservation of Broca's area). However, because Wernicke's area also acts to code linguistic stimuli for expression, expressive speech becomes severely abnormal and is characterized by nonsequitors, paraphasic errors, sound and word-order substitutions, and the omission of pauses and sentence endings (Goodglass & Kaplan, 1972; Hecaen & Albert, 1978; Kertesz, 1983a) (Fig. 8). That is, temporal–sequential expressive linguistic encoding also becomes disrupted.

For example, one patient with severe receptive aphasia responded in the following manner: "I am a little suspicious about what the hell is the part there is one part scares, uh estate spares, Ok that has a bunch of drives in it and a bunch of good googin . . . what the hell . . . kind of a platz goasted klack. . . ." Presumably, since the coding mechanisms involved in organizing what we are planning to say are the same mechanisms that decode what they hear, expressive as well as receptive speech becomes equally disrupted.

Nevertheless, a peculiarity of this disorder is that these patients do not always realize that what they say is meaningless. Moreover, they may fail to comprehend that what they hear is meaningless as well (cf. Lebrun, 1987). This is because when this area is damaged, there is no other region left to analyze the linguistic components of speech and language. The brain cannot be alerted to the patient's disability. Such patients are at risk of being misdiagnosed as psychotic.

Presumably, as a consequence of loss of comprehension, these patients may display euphoria or paranoia because of the nonlinguistic or emotional awareness that something is not right. That is, emotional functioning and comprehension remain intact, although sometimes disrupted due to erroneously processed verbal input. Thus, aphasic patients are

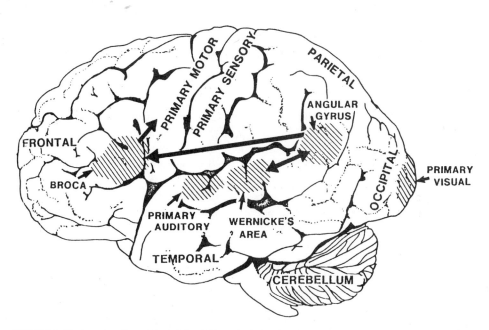

FIGURE 8. The lateral surface of the left hemisphere depicting the primary visual, auditory, motor, somesthetic (sensory) areas, and the language axis: Broca's and Wernicke's area, the angular gyrus. Heavy lines and arrows indicate probable interactive pathways involved in the formulation of language and thought. From "The Neuropsychology of Development" by R. Joseph, 1982. *Journal of Clinical Psychology, 38,* p. 23. Reprinted by permission.

often able to assess to some degree the emotional characteristic of their environment, including the prosodic (Monrad-Krohn, 1963), stress contrasts (Blumstein & Goodglass, 1972), and semantic and connotative features of what is said to them, i.e., whether they are being asked a question, given a command, or presented with a declarative sentence (Boller & Green, 1972).

For example, many people with severe receptive (Wernicke's) aphasia can understand and respond appropriately to emotional commands and questions (e.g., "Say 'shit' " or "Do you wet your bed?" (Boller, Cole, Vrtunski, Patterson, & Kim, 1979; Boller & Green, 1972). Similarly, the ability to read and write emotional words (as compared with nonemotional or abstract words) is also somewhat preserved among aphasics (Landis, Graves, & Goodglass, 1982).

Because these paralinguistic and emotional features of language are analyzed by the intact right cerebral hemisphere, the aphasic person is able to gain a general grasp of the meaning or intent of a speaker, although verbal comprehension is reduced. This, in turn, enables these patients to react in a somewhat appropriate fashion when spoken to.

For example, after I had diagnosed a patient as suffering from Wernicke's aphasia, his nurse disagreed and indicated the patient responded correctly to questions such as, "How are you this morning?" That is, the patient replied: "Fine." Later, when I re-examined the patient I used a tone of voice appropriate for "How are you today?" but instead said, "It's raining outside?" The patient replied, "Fine!" and appropriately smiled and nodded her head. Often our pets are able to determine what we mean and how we feel by analyzing similar melodic–emotional nuances.

RIGHT CEREBRAL HEMISPHERE

Comprehension and Expression of Emotional Speech

Although language is usually discussed in regard to grammar and vocabulary, there is a third major aspect to linguistic expression and comprehension by which a speaker may convey and a listener discern intent, attitude, feeling, context, and meaning. That is, language is both descriptive and emotional. A listener comprehends not only *what* is said, but *how* it is said—what a speaker *feels*.

Feeling, be it anger, happiness, sadness, sarcasm, or empathy, is often communicated by varying the rate, amplitude, pitch, inflection, timbre, melody, and stress contours of the voice. When devoid of intonational contours, language becomes monotone and bland and a listener experiences difficulty discerning attitude, context, intent, and feeling. Such conditions arise after damage to select areas of the right hemisphere or when the entire right half of the brain is anesthetized (e.g., during sodium amytal procedures).

It is now well established, based on studies of normal and brain-damaged subjects, that the right hemisphere is superior to the left in distinguishing, interpreting, and processing vocal inflectional nuances, including intensity, stress and pitch contours, timbre, cadence, emotional tone, frequency, amplitude, melody, duration, and intonation (Blumstein & Cooper, 1974; Bowers, Coslett, Bauer, Speedie, & Heilman, 1987; Carmon & Nachshon, 1973; Heilman, Scholes, & Watson, 1975; Ley & Bryden, 1979; Mahoney & Sainsbury, 1987; Ross, 1981; Safer & Leventhal, 1977; Shapiro & Danly,

1985; Tucker, Watson, & Heilman, 1977). Because of this, the right hemisphere is fully capable of determining and deducing not only *what* a persons *feels* about what he is saying, but *why* and in what *context* the person is saying it—even in the absence of vocabulary and other denotative linguistic features (Blumstein & Cooper, 1974; Dwyer & Rinn, 1981). This occurs through the analysis of tone and melody of voice.

Thus, if I were to say, "Do you want to go outside?" although both hemispheres are able to determine whether a question versus a statement has been made (Heilman, Bowers, Speedie, & Coslett, 1984; Weintraub, Mesulam, & Kramer, 1981), it is the right brain that analyzes the paralinguistic features of the voice so as to determine whether "going outside" will be fun or whether I am going to punch you in the nose. In fact, even without the aid of the actual words, on the basis of tone alone the right brain can determine context and the feelings of the speaker (Blumstein & Cooper, 1974; DeUrso, Denes, Testa, & Semenza, 1986; Dwyer & Rinn, 1981). The left hemisphere has great difficulty with such tasks.

In experiments in which verbal information was filtered and the subject was to determine the context within which a person was speaking (e.g., talking about the death of a friend, speaking to a lost child), the right hemisphere was found to be dominant (Dwyer & Rinn, 1981). It is for these and other reasons that the right half of the brain is sometimes thought to be the more intuitive half of the cerebrum.

Correspondingly, when the right hemisphere is damaged, the ability to process, recall, or even recognize these nonverbal nuances is greatly attenuated. For example, although able to comprehend individual sentences and paragraphs, such patients have difficulty understanding context and emotional connotation, drawing inferences, relating what is heard to its proper context (Brownell, Potter, & Bihrle, 1986; Foldi, Cicone, & Gardner, 1983; Wapner, Hamby, & Gardner, 1981), and recognizing discrepancies, such that they are likely to miss the point, respond to inappropriate details, and fail to appreciate fully when they are being presented with information that is incongruent or even implausible (Gardner, Brownell, Wapner, & Michelow, 1983).

These patients tend to be very concrete and literal. When presented with the statement, "He had a heavy heart," and requested to choose several interpretations, right-brain-damaged (versus aphasic) patients are more likely to choose a picture of a person staggering under a large heart as opposed to a crying person. They also have difficulty describing overall main points, morals, motives, or emotions conveyed (e.g., they lose the gestalt), although the ability to recall isolated facts and details is preserved (Delis, Robertson, & Efron, 1986; Wapner *et al.,* 1981).

Persons with right hemisphere damage sometimes have difficulty comprehending complex verbal and written statements, particularly when there are features involving spatial transformations or incongruencies. For example, when presented with the question, "Bob is taller than George. *Who is shorter?*" those with right-brain damage have difficulties, presumably due to a deficit in nonlinguistic imaginal processing or an inability to search a spatial representation of what they hear (Carmazza, Gordon, Zurif, & DeLuca, 1976).

By contrast, when presented with "Bob is taller than George. *Who is taller?*" patients with right-hemisphere damage perform similar to normals, indicating that the left brain is responsible for providing the solution (Carmazza *et al,* 1976). Because the question "Who is shorter?" does not necessarily follow the first part of the statements (i.e., incongruent), whereas ''Who is taller?'' does, these differential findings further suggest that the right brain is more involved than the left in the analysis of incongruencies.

Right Hemisphere Emotional Language Axis

Just as there are areas in the left frontal and temporal–parietal lobes that mediate the expression and comprehension of the denotative, temporal–sequential, grammatical–syntactical aspects of language, similar regions within the right hemisphere mediate emotional speech and comprehension (Gorelick & Ross, 1987; Heilman *et al.*, 1975; Ross, 1981; Shapiro & Danly, 1985; Tucker *et al.*, 1977); regions that become highly active when presented with complex nonverbal auditory stimuli (Roland, Skinhoj, & Lassen, 1981).

For example, right frontal damage has been associated with a loss of emotional speech and emotional gesturing and a significantly reduced ability to mimic various nonlinguistic vocal patterns (Ross, 1981; Shapiro & Danly, 1985) (Fig. 9). In these instances, speech can become flat and monotone or characterized by inflectional distortions.

With lesions that involve the right temporal–parietal area, the ability to comprehend or produce appropriate verbal prosody or emotional speech or to repeat emotional statements is reduced significantly (Gorelick & Ross, 1987; Heilman *et al.*, 1975; Ross, 1981; Tucker *et al.*, 1977). Indeed, when presented with neutral sentences spoken in an emo-

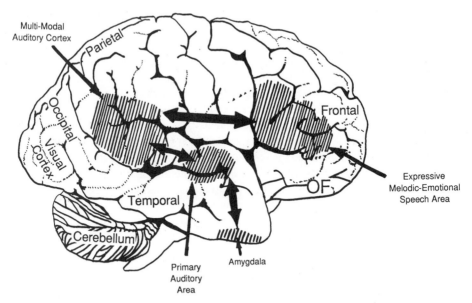

FIGURE 9. Schematic representation of melodic–emotional language areas within the right cerebral hemisphere. Auditory information is received in the primary auditory area as well as within the amygdala (and other limbic areas). Emotional and other characteristics are discerned, comprehended, and/or assigned to the sounds perceived by limbic structures as well as the multimodal auditory cortex, which extends into the inferior parietal region. When speaking in an emotional manner (or when singing, etc.), this information is transferred from the temporal–parietal and limbic areas to the right frontal convexity, which mediates its expression.

tional manner, right hemisphere damage disrupts perception (Heilman *et al.*, 1975) and the comprehension of emotional prosody (Heilman *et al.*, 1984), regardless of whether it is positive or negative in content. Moreover, the ability to differentiate between different and even oppositional emotional qualities (e.g., "love" versus "hate") can become distorted (Cicone, Wapner, & Gardner, 1980), and the capacity to appreciate and comprehend humor or mirth may be attenuated (Gardner, Ling, Flamm, & Silverman, 1975).

The semantic–contextual ability of the right hemisphere is not limited to prosodic and paralinguistic features, however, but includes the ability to process and recognize familiar, concrete, highly imaginable words (J. Day, 1977; Deloch, Serion, Scius, & Segui, 1987; Ellis & Shephard, 1975; Hines, 1976; Joseph, 1988*a,b*; Landis *et al.*, 1982; Mannhaupt, 1983), as well as emotional language in general.

The disconnected right hemisphere also can read printed words (Gazzaniga, 1970; Joseph, 1988*a;* Levy, 1983; Sperry, 1982; Zaidel, 1983), retrieve objects with the left hand in response to direct and indirect verbal commands, e.g., "a container for liquids" (Sperry, 1982), and spell simple three- and four-letter words with cut-out letters (Sperry, 1982).

Confabulation

In contrast with left frontal convexity lesions, which can result in either speech arrest (Broca's expressive aphasia) or significant reductions in verbal fluency, or both, right frontal damage has sometimes been observed to result in speech release, excessive verbosity, tangentiality, and in the extreme, confabulation (Joseph, 1986a). When secondary to frontal damage, confabulation seems to be the result of disinhibition, difficulty in monitoring responses, withholding answers, using external or internal cues to make corrections, or suppressing the flow of tangential and circumstantial ideas (Joseph, 1986*a;* Shapiro, Alexander, Gardner, & Mercer, 1981; Stuss, Alexander, Lieberman, & Levine, 1978). When this occurs, the language axis of the left hemisphere is overwhelmed and is flooded by irrelevant associations (Joseph, 1986*a*). In some cases, the content of the confabulation may border on the bizarre and fantastical as loosely associated ideas become organized and anchored around fragments of current experience.

For example, one 24-year-old patient who sustained a gunshot wound that resulted in destruction of the right inferior convexity and orbital areas attributed his hospitalization to a plot by the government to steal his inventions and ideas—the patient had been a grocery store clerk. When it was pointed out that he had undergone surgery for removal of bone fragments and the bullet, he pointed to his head and replied, "That's how they're stealing my ideas." Another patient with a degenerative disturbance that involved predominantly the right frontal lobe at times claimed to be a police officer, a doctor, or married to various members of the staff. When it was pointed out repeatedly that he was a patient, he at one point replied, "I'm a doctor. I'm here to protect people."

Gap Filling

Confabulation can also result from lesions that involve the posterior portions of the right hemisphere, immaturity or surgical section of the corpus callosum, or destruction of fiber tracts that lead to the left hemisphere (Geschwind, 1965; Joseph, 1982, 1986*a,b,*

1988*a;* Joseph, Gallagher, Holloway, & Kahn, 1984). This results in incomplete information transfer and reception. As a consequence, because the language axis of the left hemisphere is unable to gain access to needed information, it attempts to fill the gap with information that is related in some manner to the fragments received (see Joseph, 1982, 1986*a*, for review). However, because the language areas are disconnected from the source of needed information, the language axis cannot be informed that what it is saying (or, rather, making up) is erroneous, at least as far as the damaged modality is concerned.

For example, in cases presented by Redlich and Dorsey (1945), patients suffering from blindness or gross visual disturbances caused by injuries in the visual cortex continued to claim that they could see, even when they bumped into objects and tripped over furniture. Apparently, they maintained these claims because the areas of the brain that normally would alert them to their blindness (i.e., visual cortex) were no longer functioning.

Confabulation and delusional denial also often accompany neglect and body-image disturbances secondary to right cerebral damage (see Joseph, 1986*a*, for review). For example, the left hemisphere may claim that a paralyzed left leg or arm is normal or that it belongs to someone else. This occurs in many cases because somesthetic body information no longer is being processed or transferred by the damaged right hemisphere. In all these instances, however, although the damage may be in the right hemisphere, it is the speaking half of the brain that confabulates.

By contrast, there is some evidence to suggest that when information flow from the left to the right hemisphere is reduced, a visual–imaginal–hypnogic form of confabulation may result, i.e., dreaming. Dreaming is possibly one form of right hemisphere confabulation. Many other factors are involved as well (see Hobson, Lydic, & Baghdoyan, 1986). We will return to this issue.

Music and Nonverbal Environmental Sounds

Although unable to discourse fluently, persons with extensive left-hemisphere damage and/or severe forms of expressive aphasia may be capable of swearing, singing, praying, or making statements of self-pity (Gardner, 1975; Goldstein, 1942; Joseph, 1982; Smith, 1966; Smith & Burklund, 1966; Yamadori *et al.*, 1977). Even when the entire left hemisphere has been completely removed, the ability to sing familiar songs or even learn new ones may be preserved (Smith, 1966; Smith & Burklund, 1966)—although in the absence of music a patient would be unable to say the very words that he or she had just sung (Goldstein, 1942). The preservation of the ability to sing has, in fact, been used to promote linguistic recovery in aphasic patients, i.e., melodic-intonation therapy (Albert, Sparks, & Helm, 1973; Helm-Estabrooks, 1983).

Similarly, there have been reports that some musicians and composers who were suffering from either aphasia or significant left hemisphere impairment, or both, were nevertheless able to continue their work (Alajounine, 1948; Critchley, 1953; Luria, 1973). In some cases, despite severe receptive aphasia and despite the disrupted ability to read written language (alexia), the ability to read music or to continue composing was preserved (Gates & Bradshaw, 1977; Luria, 1973).

One famous example is that of Maurice Ravel, who suffered an injury to the left half of his brain in an automobile accident. This resulted in ideomotor apraxia, dysgraphia, and moderate disturbances in comprehending speech (i.e., Wernicke's aphasia). Nevertheless, Ravel had no difficulty recognizing various musical compositions, was able to detect even minor errors when compositions were played, and was able to correct those errors by playing them correctly on the piano (Alajounine, 1948).

Conversely, it has been reported that musicians suffering from right hemisphere damage (e.g., right temporal–parietal stroke) have major difficulties recognizing familiar melodies and suffer from expressive instrumental amusia (Luria, 1973; McFarland & Fortin, 1982). Even among nonmusicians, right hemisphere damage (e.g., right temporal lobectomy) disrupts time sense, rhythm, and the ability to perceive, recognize, or recall tones, loudness, timbre, and melody (Chase, 1967; Gates & Bradshaw, 1977; Milner, 1962; Yamadori et al., 1977). Right hemisphere damage also can disrupt the ability to sing or carry a tune and can cause toneless monotonous speech, as well as abolish the capacity to obtain pleasure while listening to music (Reese, 1948; Ross, 1981; Shapiro & Danly, 1985), i.e., a condition also referred to as amusia. For example, Freeman and Williams (1953) report that removal of the right amygdala in one patient resulted in a great change in the pitch and timbre of speech and that the ability to sing also was severely affected. Similarly, when the right hemisphere is anesthetized the melodic aspects of speech and singing become significantly impaired (Gordon & Bogen, 1974).

It has also been demonstrated consistently in normals (such as in dichotic listening studies) and with brain-injured persons that the right hemisphere predominates in the perception (and/or expression) of timbre, chords, tone, pitch, loudness, melody, and intensity (Breitling, Guenther, & Rondot, 1987; Curry, 1967; R. Day, Cutting, & Copeland, 1971, Gates & Bradshaw, 1977; Gordon, 1970; Gordon & Bogen, 1974; Kimura, 1964; Knox & Kimura, 1970; McFarland & Fortin, 1982; Milner, 1962; Molfese, Freeman, & Palermo, 1975; Piazza, 1980; Reese, 1948; Segalowitz & Plantery, 1985; Spellacy, 1970; Swisher, Dudley, & Doehring, 1969; Tsunoda, 1975; Zurif, 1974)—the major components (in conjunction with harmony) of a musical stimulus. In addition, Penfield and Perot (1963) report that musical hallucinations most frequently result from electrical stimulation of the superior and lateral surface of the temporal lobes, particularly the right temporal region. Such findings have added greatly to the conviction that the right cerebral hemisphere is dominant in regard to most aspects of musical perception and expression.

Environmental Sounds

In addition to music, the right hemisphere has been shown to be superior to the left in discerning and recognizing nonverbal and environmental sounds (Curry, 1967; Kimura, 1963; King & Kimura, 1972; Knox & Kimura, 1970; Nielsen, 1946; Piazza, 1980; Roland, Skinhoj, & Lassen, 1981; Spreen, Benton, & Fincham, 1965; Tsunoda, 1975). Similarly, not only may damage involving select areas within the right hemisphere disturb the capacity to discern musical and social–emotional vocal nuances, but it can disrupt the ability to perceive or recognize a diverse number of sounds that occur naturally within the environment as well (Nielsen, 1946; Spreen et al., 1965), such as water splashing, a door banging, applause, or even a typewriter; this condition also plagues the disconnected left hemisphere (Joseph, 1988b).

The possibility has been raised that music, verbal emotion, and nonverbal environmental sounds are phylogenetically linked in some manner (Joseph, 1982). For example, it is possible that right hemisphere dominance for music may be an outgrowth or strongly related to its capacity to discern and recognize environmental acoustics as well as its ability to mimic these and other nonverbal and emotional nuances. That is, it is somewhat probable that primitive man's first exposure to the sounds of music was environmentally embedded, for obviously musical sounds are heard frequently throughout nature (e.g., birds singing, the whistling of the wind, the humming of bees or insects). For example, bird songs can encompass sounds that are "flute-like, truly chime- or bell-like, violin- or guitar-like" and "some are almost as tender as a boy soprano" (Hartshorne, 1973, p. 36).

Thus, perhaps our musical nature is related to our original relationship with nature and resulted from the tendency of humans to mimic sounds that arise from the environment—such as those that conveyed certain feeling states and emotions. Perhaps this is also why certain acoustical nuances, such as those employed in classical music, can affect us emotionally and make us visualize scenes from nature (e.g., an early spring morning, a raging storm, bees in flight).

Music and Emotion

Music is related strongly to emotion and, in fact, may not only be "pleasing to the ear," but invested with emotional significance. For example, when played in a major key, music sounds happy or joyful. When played in a minor key, music is often perceived as sad or melancholic. We are all familiar with the "blues" and perhaps at one time or another have felt like "singing for joy" or have told someone, "You make my heart sing!"

Interestingly, it has been reported that music can act to accelerate pulse rate (Reese, 1948), raise or lower blood pressure, and thereby alter the rhythm of the heartbeat. Rhythm, of course, is a major component of music. Music and vocal emotional nuances also share certain features, such as melody and intonation, all of which are predominantly processed and mediated by the right brain. In addition, the right hemisphere has been found superior to the left in identifying the emotional tone of musical passages and, in fact, judges music to be more emotional as compared to the left brain (Bryden, Ley, & Sugarman, 1982).

Left Hemisphere Musical Contributions. There is some evidence to indicate that certain aspects of pitch, time sense, and rhythm are mediated to a similar degree by both cerebral hemispheres (Milner, 1962), perhaps more so by the left. Time sense and rhythm are also crucial in speech perception. These findings support the possibility of a left hemisphere contribution to music. In fact, some investigators have argued that receptive amusia is due to left hemisphere damage and that expressive amusia is due to right hemisphere dysfunction (Wertheim, 1969).

It also has been reported that some musicians tend to show a left hemisphere dominance in the perception of certain aspects of music (see Gates & Bradshaw, 1977, for review). However, these findings are based on persons with just a few years of experience and others still in training; i.e., those who are treating music as something to be analyzed. It also appears that when the sequential and rhythmical aspects of music are emphasized, the left hemisphere becomes increasingly involved (Breitling *et al,* 1987; Halperin, Nachson, & Carmon, 1973). In this regard, it seems that when music is treated as a type of language to be acquired or when its mathematical and temporal–sequential features are emphasized (Breitling *et al.*, 1987), the left cerebral hemisphere becomes heavily involved in its production and perception. Thus, just as the right hemisphere makes important contributions to the perception and expression of language, it also takes both halves of the brain to make music.

Music, Math, and Geometrical Space

Pythagoras, the great Greek mathematician, argued almost 2000 years ago that music is numerical, the expression of number is sound (Durant, 1939; McClain, 1978). In fact, long before the advent of digital recordings, the Hindu-Babylonians and then Pythagoras and his followers translated music into number and geometrical proportions (Durant, 1939). For example, by dividing a vibrating string into various ratios, they discovered that several very pleasing musical intervals could be produced. Thus, the ratio 1 : 2 was found to yield an octave, 2 : 3 a fifth, and 3 : 4 a fourth, 4 : 5 a major third, and 5 : 6 a minor third (McClain, 1978). The harmonic system used during the nineteenth century by various composers was based on these same ratios. Indeed, Bela Bartok used these ratios in his musical compositions.

The Pythagorians discovered that these same musical ratios have the capability of reproducing themselves. That is, the ratio can reproduce itself within itself and form a unique geometrical configuration that Pythagoras and the ancient Greeks referred as the golden ratio or golden rectangle. It was postulated to have devine inspirational origins. Indeed, music itself was thought by early man to be magical, whereas musicians were believed by the ancient Greeks to be "prophets favored by the Gods" (Worner, 1973) (Fig. 10).

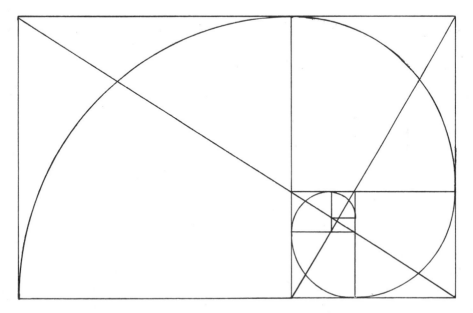

FIGURE 10. A "golden rectangle."

This same golden rectangle is found in nature, i.e., the chambered nautilus shell, the shell of a snail, and in the ear—the cochleus. The geometric proportions of the golden rectangle also were employed in designing the Parthenon in Athens and by Ptolemy in developing the tonal calender and the tonal zodiac (McCain, 1978)—the scale of ratios "bent round in a circle."

In fact, the first cosmologies, such as those developed by the ancient Egyptians, Hindus, Babylonians, and Greeks, were based on musical ratios (Durant, 1939; McClain, 1978). Pythagorus, and later Plato, applied these same musical proportions to their theory of numbers, to planetary motion, and to the science of stereometry—the gauging of solids (McClain, 1978). Indeed, Pythagorus attempted to deduce the size, speed, distance, and orbit of the planets on the basis of musical ratios as well as estimates of the sounds generated (e.g., pitch and harmony) by their movement through space, i.e., "the music of the spheres" (Durant, 1939). Interestingly, in describing his laws of planetary motion, the famous mathematician and physicist Johannes Kepler also referred to them as being based on the "music of the spheres." Thus, music seems to have certain geometrical properties, such as are expressed by the ratio. Indeed, Pythagorus, the "father" of arithmetic, geometry, and trigonometry, believed music to be geometrical. As we know, geometry is employed in the measurement of land, the demarcation of boundaries, and, thus, in the analysis of space, shape, points, lines, angles, surfaces, and configuration.

In nature, one form of musical expression, that is, the songs of most birds, is also produced for geometrical purposes. That is, a bird does not "sing for joy" but to signal others of impending threat, to attract mates, to indicate direction and location, to stake out territory, and to warn away others who might attempt to intrude on its space (Catchpole, 1979; Hartshorne, 1973).

If we may assume that long before man sang his first song, the first songs and musical compositions were created by our fine feathered friends (sounds that inspired mimicry by man), it would appear that musical production is first and foremost emotional and motivational and directly related to the geometry of space; the demarcation of one's territory. Emotion and geometry are characteristics that music still retains today.

Constructional and Spatial–Perceptual Skills

Studies of brain-injured, neurosurgical (e.g., temporal lobectomy, split-brain), and normal populations have shown the right cerebral hemisphere to be dominant over the left in the analysis of geometrical and visual space, the perception of depth, distance, direction, shape, orientation, position, perspective, and figure ground; the detection of complex and hidden figures, the performance of visual closure, and the ability to infer the total stimulus configuration from incomplete information, route finding and maze learning, localizing targets in space, the performance of reversible operations, stereopsis, and the determination of the directional orientation of the body as well as body-part positional relationships (Benton, 1979; Butters & Barton, 1970; Carmon & Bechtoldt, 1969; Fontenot, 1973; Franco & Sperry, 1977; Fried, Mateer, Ojemann, Wohns, & Fedio, 1982; Hannay *et al.*, 1987; Kimura, 1966; 1969; Landis, Cummings, Christen, Bogen, & Imhof, 1986; Lansdell, 1968, 1970; Levy, 1974; Milner, 1968; Nebes, 1971; Sperry, 1982).

In addition, the isolated right hemisphere has been found to be superior in "fitting designs into larger matrices, judging whole circle size from a small arc, discriminating and recalling nondescript shapes, making mental spatial transformations, sorting block sizes and shapes into categories, perceiving wholes from a collection of parts, and the intuitive perception and apprehension of geometric principles'' (Sperry, 1982, p. 1225).

Thus, it is the right brain that enables us to find our way in space without getting lost, to walk and run without tripping and falling, to throw and catch a football with accuracy, to drive a car without bumping into things, to draw conclusions based on partial information, and to see the forest when looking at the trees. The right brain is also superior to the left in analyzing manipulospatial problems; in drawing and copying simple and complex geometric-like figures; and in performing constructional tasks, block designs, and puzzles (Benson & Barton, 1970; Black & Strub, 1976; Critchley, 1953; DeRenzi, 1982; Gardner, 1975; Hecaen & Albert, 1978; Hier, Mondlock, & Caplan, 1983; Kertesz, 1983b; Levy, 1974; Luria, 1973, 1980; Piercy, Hecaen, & Ajuriaguerra, 1960). It is for these and other reasons that the right brain is often viewed as the artistic half of the cerebrum.

Visual–Perceptual Abnormalities

When the right hemisphere is damaged, most aspects of visual–spatial and perceptual functioning can become altered, including nonverbal memory. For example, right temporal lobe damage impairs memory for abstract designs, tonal melodies, and visual mazes (Kimura, 1963; Milner, 1968). Deficits in the ability to make judgments that involve visual–figural relationships; to detect hidden, embedded, and overlapping nonsense figures; and to recognize or recall recurring shapes, as well as problems with the appreciation of spatial wholes and achieving visual closure can result (Benton, 1979; DeRenzi, 1982; DeRenzi et al., 1969; Ettlinger, 1960; Gardner, 1975; Kimura, 1963, 1966, 1969; Landis et al., 1986; Lansdell, 1968; 1970; Levy, 1974).

One such patient with normal visual acuity could not tell which of two objects was closer; she was unable to recognize or correctly use tools, common utensils, or other objects, and her recognition was impaired further by surrounding the object with unrelated items (Levine, 1978). This patient was unable to recognize the faces of friends, her pets, or even her own face. Rather, she (i.e., her intact left hemisphere) was forced to rely on the presence of one or two details in order to make identifications, such as the presence of a mustache). Even so, her perceptions remained inaccurate. For example, she called a harmonica a comb because of the serrated partitions. Nevertheless, she had no difficulty recognizing verbal stimuli, such as letters.

In addition, such persons may misplace things, have difficulty with balance and stumble and bump into walls and furniture, become easily lost, confused, and disoriented while they are walking or driving; and have difficulty following directions or even putting on their clothes. Indeed such patients easily can get lost while they are walking down familiar streets and even in their own homes (Benton, 1979; DeRenzi, 1982; DeRenzi et al., 1969; Ettlinger, 1960; Gardner, 1975; Landis et al., 1986; Lansdell, 1968a, 1970; Levy, 1974). Right brain damage also can also result in disorientation, problems in assuming different perspectives, and even problems with dressing (Hecaen, 1962; Hier et al., 1983).

In some instances, the deficit can be quite subtle and circumscribed. For example, one patient's only complaint (3 months after suffering a circumscribed blunt head injury that resulted in a subdural hemotoma over the right posterior temporal–parietal area) was that his golf game had deteriorated significantly and he was no longer as accurate when throwing wads of paper into the trash can in his office. Formal testing, however, indicated mild constructional and manipulospatial disturbances, with most other capacities in the high average to superior range.

Drawing and Constructional Deficits

The left hemisphere also contributes to these processes such that when damaged, constructional and drawing ability can be affected, albeit in a manner different from that of the right (Mehta, Newcombe, & Damasio, 1987). For example, because the left is concerned with the analysis of parts or details and engages in temporal–sequential motor manipulations, lesions can result in oversimplification and a lack of detail in drawings although the general outline or shape may be retained (Gardner, 1975, Levy, 1974).

In contrast, the right cerebrum is more involved in the overall perceptual analysis of visual and object interrelations including visual closure and gestalt formation. Thus, patients with right brain damage have trouble with general shape and organization, although certain details may be drawn correctly.

Right-sided damage also can affect writing. When patients are asked to write cursively, writing samples may display problems with visual closure, as well as excessive segmentation due to left hemisphere release. That is, cursively the word "recognition" may be written "re co g n it ion," or letters such as "o" may be only partly formed.

Similarly, although constructional deficits are more severe after right hemisphere damage (Arrigoni & DeRenzi, 1964; Black & Strub, 1976; Benson & Barton, 1970; Critchley, 1953; Hier et al., 1983; Piercy et al., 1960), disturbances that involve constructional and manipulospatial functioning can occur with lesions to either hemisphere (Arrigoni & DeRenzi, 1964; Mehta et al., 1987; Piercy et al., 1960). However, depending on which half of the brain is damaged, the disturbance can be secondary to a problem in perceptual analysis, the transformation of the percept into a motor program or due to executive-motor difficulties with preservation of good spatial–perceptual functioning (Warrington et al., 1966). Similar deficiencies can be manifested on drawing tasks.

Nevertheless, although a patient with a visual–perceptual deficit will also show a visual–motor disturbance, the converse is not often the case (Hecaen & Assal, 1970). This is because the motor aspect may be impaired with preservation of good perceptual functioning. As such, the patient is likely to recognize that errors have been made (Fig. 11).

In general, visual–motor deficits can result from lesions in either hemisphere (Arrigoni & DeRenzi, 1964; Piercy et al., 1960). Visual–perceptual disturbances are more likely to result from right hemisphere damage. By contrast, lesions to the left half of the brain may leave the perceptual aspects undisturbed, whereas visual–motor functioning and selective organization may be compromised (Kim, Morrow, Passafiume, & Boller, 1984; Mehta et al., 1987; Poeck, Kerschensteiner, Hartje, & Orgass, 1973; Teuber & Weinstein, 1956).

In general, the size and sometimes the location of the lesion within the right hemisphere have little or no correlation with the extent of the visual–spatial or constructional deficits demonstrated, although right posterior lesions tend to be worst of all. For exam-

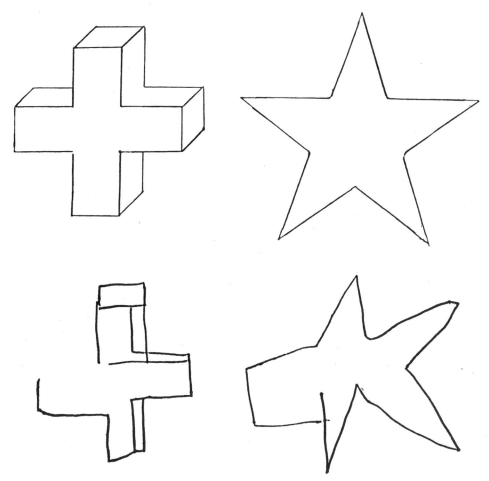

FIGURE 11. Examples of left sided neglect and distortion. Note preservation of right sided details. The patient, a 33-year-old woman with damage involved the right parietal area, was instructed to copy the "cross" and the "star."

ple, in a retrospective study of 656 patients with unilateral lesions that employed a short form of the WAIS, Warrington, James, & Maciejewski (1986), found that only those with right posterior (versus anterior or left hemisphere) damage showed lower Performance IQs and a selective impairment on block design and picture arrangement. Conversely, visual–perceptual disturbances associated with left hemisphere damage are correlated positively with lesion size, and left anterior lesions are worse than left posterior (Benson & Barton, 1970; Black & Bernard, 1984; Black & Strub, 1976; Lansdell, 1970). The larger the lesion, the more extensive the deficit. As pertaining to WAIS PIQ–VIQ differences, based on an extensive review of the literature, Bornstein and Matarazzo (1982) noted that those with left hemisphere lesions have lower VIQs, whereas those with right-sided damage have lower mean PIQs.

Reading and Math. Because of its importance in visual orientation, the functional integrity of the right brain also aids in performing such tasks as math and reading. For example, right sided lesions may cause the patient to neglect the left half of digit pairs while adding or subtracting (Hecaen & Albert, 1978; Luria, 1980).

Moreover, through analysis of position, orientation, and so forth, the right brain enables us to read the words on this page without losing our place and jumping haphazardly from line to line. Conversely, when damaged, patients may fail to attend to the left half of written words, or even the left half of the page (Critchely, 1953; Gainotti, D'Erme, Monteleone, & Silveri, 1986; Gainotti, Messerlie, & Tissot, 1972).

Because the right half of the cerebrum can draw conclusions based on partial information, e.g., closure and gestalt formation, we also need not read every or all of each word in order to know what we have read. For example, when presented with incomplete words or perceptually degraded written stimuli, there is an initial right hemisphere superiority in processing (Hellige & Webster, 1979); i.e., visual closure. Of course, we sometimes draw the wrong conclusions from incomplete perception (e.g., reading "word power" as "world power"), a problem that can become exaggerated if the right half of the brain has been damaged.

In addition, when the visual–figural characteristics of written language are emphasized, such as when large Gothic script is employed (e.g., in tachistoscopic studies), the right brain is dominant (Bryden & Allard, 1976). Moreover, when presented with unfamiliar written words or a foreign alphabet, there is an initial right hemisphere perceptual dominance (Silverberg, Bentin, Gaziel, Obler, & Albert, 1979).

. Indeed, the evolution of written language also suggests the possibility of an initial right hemisphere dominance, for much of what was written was at first depicted in a pictorial, gestalt-like fashion (Breasted, 1937). The use of images preceded the use of signs (cf. Bronowski, 1973; Jung, 1964).

Inattention and Visual–Spatial Neglect

Unilateral inattention and neglect are associated most commonly with right hemisphere (parietal, frontal, thalamic, basal ganglia) damage and, in particular lesions located in the temporal–parietal and occipital junction (Bisiach, Bulgarelli, Sterzi, & Vallar, 1983; Bisiach & Luzzatti, 1978; Brain, 1941; Calvanio, Petrone, & Levine, 1987; Critchely, 1953; De Renzi, 1982; Ferro, Kertesz, & Black, 1987; Gainotti *et al.,* 1986; Heilman, 1979; Heilman, Watson, Valenstein, & Damasio, 1983; Joseph, 1986*a;* Motomura *et al.,* 1986; Nielsen, 1937; M. Roth, 1949; N. Roth, 1944, Watson, Valenstein, & Heilman, 1981). These patients may initially fail to respond, recall, or perceive left-sided auditory, visual, or tactile stimulation; fail to comb, wash, or dress the left half of their head, face, and body; eat food only on the right half of their plate; write only on the right half of a paper; fail to read the left half of words or sentences (e.g., if presented with "toothbrush" they may see only the word "brush"); or, on drawing tasks, distort, leave out details, or fail to draw the left half of various figures (e.g., a clock or daisy) (Bisiach *et al.,* 1983; Calvanio *et al.,* 1987; Critchley, 1953; DeRenzi, 1982; Gainotti *et al.,* 1972, 1986; Hecaen & Albert, 1978). In fact, when shown their left arm or leg, such patients may deny that it is their own and claim that it belongs to the doctor or a patient in the next room (Joseph, 1986a). Indeed, "patients with severe unilateral neglect behave as

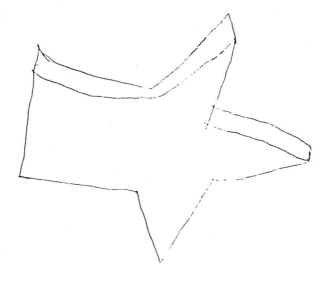

FIGURE 12. Example of left-sided neglect.

if a whole system of beliefs had vanished, as if one half of the inner model of the environment were simply deleted from their mind" (Bisiach *et al.*, 1983, p. 35). In less extreme cases, patients may seem inattentive such that when their attention is directed to the left half of the environment, they are able to respond appropriately (see Jeannerod, 1987, for a detailed review) (Figs. 12 and 13).

Imaginal and memory functioning also are disrupted such that patients may fail to attend to the left half of images recalled from memory. For example, Bisiach and Luzzatti (1978) found that when right brain-damaged patients were asked to recall and describe a familiar scene from different perspectives, regardless of perspective (e.g., imagining a

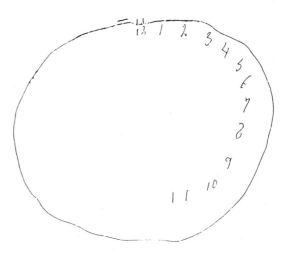

FIGURE 13. Example of left-sided neglect. The patient, a 54-year-old man who suffered a blunt head injury and damage that involved the right frontal–parietal area was instructed to "Draw the face of clock and put all the numbers in it and make it say 10 after 11."

street from one direction and then from another), patients consistently failed to report details that fell to their left—even when the same details were recalled when imagined from the opposite direction. Bisiach and Luzzatti (1978) suggest that visual images and scenes may be split into two images when conjured up, such that the right brain images the left half of space and the left brain images the right half of space. Similar results were presented by Meador, Loring, Bowers, and Heilman (1987).

Neglect also can be influenced by the task demands. When the task is performed best or typically by the damaged hemisphere (i.e., before it was damaged), the neglect will be more pronounced (Leicester, Sidman, Stoddard, & Mohr, 1969). Thus, left brain-damaged patients also may show unilateral inattention or neglect (Albert, 1973; Denny-Brown, Meyer, & Horenstein, 1952; Gainotti et al., 1986), albeit in a less severe form.

In general, there is some evidence to suggest that the right cerebral hemisphere may be more involved in attention and arousal (Beck, Dustman, & Sakai, 1969; Dimond & Beaumont, 1974; Heilman, 1979; Joseph, 1986a) such that with massive damage there results hypoarousal, bilateral reductions in reaction time and thus diminished attentional functioning (DeRenzi & Faglioni, 1965; Heilman, Schwartz, & Watson, 1978; Heilman & Van Den Abell, 1979; Howes & Boller, 1975; Joseph, 1986a; S. Weinstein, 1978). In this regard, Meador et al. (1987) found that by turning the head to the left (thereby supposedly increasing the activation at the right hemisphere), patients were still deficient but were able to recall more left-sided objects and stimuli. By contrast, with smaller lesions, particularly those that involve the right frontal area, instead of a loss of arousal, a loss of control over arousal can result and such patients can respond in a highly disin-hibited fashion (Joseph, 1986a).

Disturbances of the Body Image

In addition to nonlinguistic, prosodic, melodic, emotional, and visual–spatial domi-nance, the right cerebrum has been shown to be superior to the left in processing various forms of somesthetic and tactile–spatial–positional information, including geometrical, tactile-form, and Braille-like pattern recognition (Bradshaw, Nettleton, & Spher, 1982; Carmon & Benton, 1969; Corkin, Milner, & Rasmussen, 1970; Desmedt, 1977; Dodds, 1978; Fontenot & Benton, 1971; Franco & Sperry, 1977; Hatta, 1978a; Hermelin & O'Connor, 1971; Hom & Reitan, 1982; E. Weinstein & Sersen, 1961). The right brain is also dominant for two-point discrimination (S. Weinstein, 1978) pressure sensitivity (Semmes, Weinstein, Ghent, & Teuber, 1960; S. Weinstein, 1978; E. Weinstein & Sersen, 1961) and processing tactual–directional information (Carmon & Benton, 1969; Fontenot & Benton, 1971). There is also some evidence to suggest that the right hemi-sphere may be more involved than the left in the perception of somesthetically mediated pain (Cubelli, Caselli, & Neri, 1984; Haslam, 1970; Murray & Hagan, 1973). In addition, unlike the left, the right hemisphere is responsive to tactual stimuli that impinge on either side of the body (Desmedt, 1977). Therefore, a somesthetic image of the entire body appears to be maintained by the right half of the brain.

When the right hemisphere is damaged, somesthetic functioning can become grossly abnormal, and patients may experience peculiar disturbances involving the body image (Critchley, 1953, Hillbom, 1960; Joseph, 1986a; Miller, 1984; Nathanson, Bergman, & Gordon, 1952; M. Roth, 1949; N. Roth, 1944; Sandifer, 1946; E. Weinstein & Kahn,

1950, 1952). These patients may fail to perceive stimuli applied to the left side; wash, dress, or groom only the right side of the body, confuse body-positional and spatial relationships; misperceive left-sided stimulation as occurring on the right; fail to realize that their extremities or other body organs are in some manner compromised; and/or literally deny that their left arm or leg is truly their own (see Joseph, 1986a, for review).

When confronted with their unused or paralyzed extremities, these patients may claim that they belong to the doctor or a person in the next room or, conversely, seem indifferent to their condition and/or claim that their paralyzed limbs are normal—even when unable to comply with requests to move them (Nathanson et al., 1952):

> When asked why she could not move her hand she replied, "somebody has ahold of it." Another patient, when asked if anything was wrong with her hand, said, "I think it's the weather. I could warm it up and it would be alright." One woman, when asked whether she could walk said, "I could walk at home, but not here. It's slippery here." Another patient, when asked why he couldn't raise his arm said, "I have a shirt on." (p. 383)

One of the most striking affective aspects of this type of disturbance include indifference and/or inappropriate emotional concern with regard to the patients disability. In an extensive examination of these disturbances, E. Weinstein and Kahn (1950) found that of 22 patients (only 3 of whom were thought to have predominantly left hemisphere dysfunction), 15 were euphoric and manifested an air of serenity or bland unconcern about their condition despite the fact that they were suffering from disorders such as hemiplegia, blindness, loss of memory, and incontinence. Ten of these patients also behaved in a labile or transiently paranoid fashion. Right cerebral lesions have been reported to slow the appearance of phantom limbs on either side of the body and can result in the loss of phantom limb pain (S. Weinstein, 1978). By contrast, left-sided lesions seem to have little effect.

In general, like neglect and inattention, lesions that result in body-image disturbances tend to involve the right parietal region (Critchley, 1953; Joseph, 1986a). In this regard, the fact that lesions of the left hemisphere rarely result in neglect or body image disturbances suggests that the right hemisphere maintains a bilateral representation of the body, whereas the left cerebrum maintains a unilateral representation (Fig. 14). Hence, when the left hemisphere is damaged, the right brain continues to monitor both halves of the body and there is little or no neglect—an impression supported by findings that indicate that the right hemisphere electrophysiologically responds to stimuli that impinge on either side of the body, whereas the left hemisphere responds predominantly only to right-sided stimulation (Desmedt, 1977).

Pain and Hysteria

In addition to body-image distortions, parietal lobe injuries (particularly when secondary to tumor or seizure activity) also can give rise to sensory misperceptions such as pain (Davidson & Schick, 1935; Hernandez-Peon, Chavez-Iberra, & Aguilar-Figuerua, 1963; Ruff, 1980; Wilkinson, 1973; York, Gabor, & Dreyfus, 1979). That is, in the less extreme cases, rather than failing to perceive (i.e., neglecting) the left half of the body, patients may experience sensory distortions that concern various body parts due to abnormal activation of the right hemisphere.

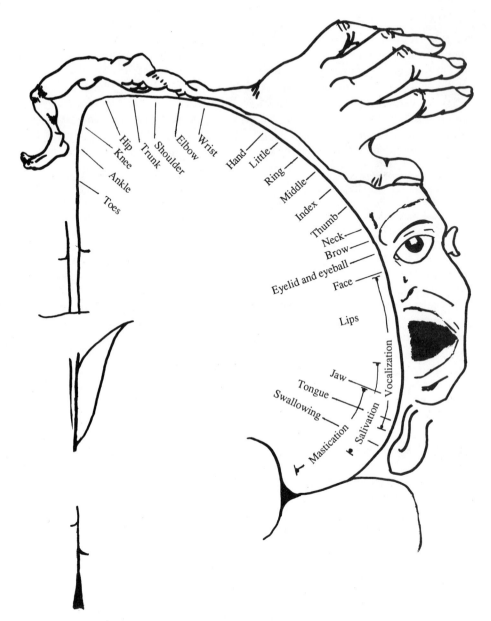

FIGURE 14. The motor homunculus of the frontal lobe.

For example, one 48-year-old housewife complained of diffuse, poorly localized (albeit intense) pain in her left leg that occurred in spasms that lasted minutes. She subsequently was found to have a large tumor in the right parietal area, which when removed, alleviated all further attacks. Head and Holmes (1911) reported a patient who suffered brief attacks of "electric shock"-like pain that radiated from his foot to the trunk; a glioma in the right parietal area subsequently was discovered. McFie and Zangwill

(1960) reported on an individual who began to experience intense, extreme pain in a phantom arm after a right posterior stroke. In another instance, reported by York *et al.* (1979), a 9-year-old boy experienced spontaneous attacks of intense scrotal and testicular pain and was found to have seizure activity in the right parietal area. Ruff (1980) reports two patients who experienced paroxsymal episodes of spontaneous and painful orgasm, secondary to right parietal seizure activity. In one patient, the episodes began with the sensation of clitoral warmth, engorgement of the breasts, tachycardia, and so forth, all of which rapidly escalated to a painful climax. Interestingly, in the normal intact individual, orgasm is associated with electrophysiological arousal predominantly within the right hemisphere (H. Cohen, Rosen, & Goldstein, 1976).

It is important to note, however, that although the predominant focus for paroxysmal pain is the right hemisphere, pain also has been reported to occur with tumors or seizures activity that involves the left parietal region (Bhaskar, 1987; McFie & Zangwill, 1960).

Unfortunately, when the patient's symptoms are not considered from a neurological perspective, their complaints with regard to pain may be viewed as psychogenic in origin. This is because the sensation of pain, stiffness, engorgement, is, indeed entirely "in their head" and based on distorted neurological perceptual functioning. Physical examination will indicate nothing wrong with the seemingly affected limb or organ. Thus, such patients may be viewed as hysterical or hypochondriacal, particularly in that right hemisphere damage also disrupts emotional functioning.

In this regard, it is noteworthy that patients suspected of suffering from hysteria are two to four times more likely to experience pain and other distortions on the left side of the body (Axelrod, Noonan, & Atanacio, 1980; Galin, Diamond, & Braff, 1977; Ley, 1980; D. Stern, 1977); findings that in turn, suggest that the source of the hysteria may be a damaged right hemisphere (cf. Miller, 1984).

This supposition is further supported by the raw MMPI data provided by Gasparrini, Satz, Heilman, and Coolidge (1978) in their study of differential effects of right versus left hemisphere damage on emotional functioning. That is, whereas depression (elevated MMPI scale 2) is more likely subsequent to left cerebral damage, a pattern suggestive of hysteria and conversion reactions (elevations on scales 1 and 3, reductions on scale 2, i.e., the Conversion V) are more likely subsequent to right hemispheric lesions.

The findings of Gasparrini *et al.* (1978) were replicated based on a retrospective case analysis of patients with long-standing right versus left hemisphere injury, verified by neuropsychological examination coupled with computed tomography (CT) scan and/or electroencephalography (EEG). In this study, the MMPI Conversion V profile was found to be associated significantly and almost exclusively with right hemisphere injuries (among males only), whereas elevated scale 2 was associated with those with left-sided damage (Joseph, unpublished data). However, not every patient demonstrated this pattern; in another case a woman patient suspected of hysteria subsequently was found to have a right frontal–parietal and midtemporal cyst. This same patient had difficulty recognizing or mimicking emotional and environmental sounds.

At least one investigator, however, reporting on psychiatric patients has attributed hysteria to left cerebral damage (Flor-Henry, 1983). In part this may be a function of the statistical permutations used in analyzing his data. However, this also may reflect the nature of the population studied (i.e., psychiatric rather than neurological) and, thus, the differential effect of long-standing and biochemical disturbances vs. gross anatomical lesions.

Facial–Emotional Recognition and Prosopagnosia

Possibly due in part to the visual–spatial complexity of the human face, the right hemisphere has been shown to be dominant in the perception and recognition of familiar and unfamiliar faces (Bradshaw, Taylor, Patterson, & Nettleton, 1980; DeRenzi, 1982; DeRenzi, Faglione, & Spinnler, 1968; DeRenzi & Spinnler, 1966; Geffen, Bradshaw, & Wallace, 1971; Hecaen & Angelergues, 1962; Levy, Trevarthen, & Sperry, 1972; Ley & Bryden, 1979; Rizzolatti, Umilta, & Berlucchi, 1971). There is some suggestion, however, that the left hemisphere is involved in the recognition of famous faces (Marzi & Berlucchi, 1977) and the differentiation of highly similar faces (presented in outline form) when analysis of fine detail is necessitated (Patterson & Bradshaw, 1975).

Whether the face of a friend or that of a stranger, right hemisphere superiority for facial recognition is augmented by the additional display of facial emotion (Ley & Bryden, 1979; Suberi & McKeever, 1977). Indeed, not only is it predominant in perceiving facial emotion, regardless of the emotion conveyed (Buchtel, Campari, DeRisio, & Rota, 1978; Dekosky, Heilman, Bowers, & Valenstein, 1980; Landis, Assal, & Perrot, 1979; Strauss & Moscovitch, 1981; Suberi & McKeever, 1977), but faces also are judged to be more intensely emotional when viewed exclusively by the right hemisphere (Heller & Levy, 1981). Thus, the right hemisphere is dominant for the perception of faces and facial emotion.

In addition, the left side of the face has been found to be more emotionally expressive (Campbell, 1978; Chaurasis & Goswami, 1975; Sackheim, Gur, & Saucy, 1978) and to be perceived as more intensely emotional as well (Borod & Caron, 1980; Sackheim & Gur, 1978). In response to emotional stimuli, the left half of the face becomes more activated, and a significant majority of patients respond with conjugate lateral eye movements to the left (Schwartz, Davidson, & Maer, 1975; Tucker, 1981).

Conversely, when the right hemisphere is damaged, particularly the occipital–temporal region, a severe disturbance in the ability to recognize the faces of friends, loved ones, or pets can result (DeRenzi, 1986; DeRenzi *et al.*, 1968; DeRenzi & Spinnler, 1966; Hecaen & Angelergues, 1962; Landis *et al.*, 1986; Levine, 1978; Whiteley & Warrington, 1977), a condition referred to as prosopagnosia. Some patients may be unable to recognize their own face in the mirror. For example, one patient could not identify his wife and, although tested for 7 hr by the same examiner, was unable to recognize him at the end of the session (De Renzi, 1986). Another patient was unable to recognize relatives or her pets or even discriminate between people on the basis of sex, but instead had to rely on the presence of details (such as lipstick, rouge, hair length, a mustache) to make discriminations (Levine, 1978).

In addition, lesions to the right cerebrum may result in difficulty recognizing, distinguishing, or differentiating facial emotion (DeKosky *et al.*, 1980). That is, patients are unable to recognize or determine what others are feeling as conveyed through their facial expression.

Electrical stimulation of the posterior portion of the right middle temporal gyrus also results in an inability to label the emotion shown in faces correctly, whereas posterior right temporal stimulation disrupts visual–spatial memory for faces in general (Fried *et al.*, 1982). Thus, the right hemisphere is clearly dominant for perceiving, recognizing, differentiating, expressing, and even recalling facial emotion.

In some instances, depending on the extent of damage, rather than a frank failure to recognize, patients may notice that friends, lovers, or their children, look different, strange, or unfamiliar—perceptions that may give rise to a host of abnormal emotional reactions and upheavals, including frank paranoia, for example, fear that one's wife may have been replaced by an imposter.

Delusional misperception of familiar and unfamiliar individuals, as well as disturbances such as Capgras syndrome (delusional doubles) or false identification, also can result from right hemisphere and/or (bilateral) frontal damage (Alexander, Stuss, & Benson, 1979; Benson, Gardner, & Meadows, 1976; Hecaen, 1964). For example, one patient who was looking into a dark tachistoscope suddenly said in an emotional voice, "I see my daughter—oh, she's gone" and was unable to recognize ward personel or relatives when present (Levine, 1978).

Disturbances of Emotion and Personality

Overview

The right cerebral hemisphere appears to be dominant in regard to most aspects of somesthesis, including the maintenance of the body image, visual–spatial–geometrical analysis, facial expression and perception, and musical and paralinguistic melodic–intonational processing. The right hemisphere also predominates in regard to most aspects of emotional functioning. However, it is important to note that some investigators believe that one half of the brain mediates so-called positive emotions, whereas the other is responsible for negative mediation (cf. Otto, Yeo, & Dougher, 1987; Silberman & Weingartner, 1986, for discussion.)

Nevertheless, when the right cerebrum is damaged there can result a myriad of peculiar disturbances that involve a number of modalities. Patients with body-image disturbances may seem emotionally abnormal and possibly hysterical, rather than neurologically impaired. Those with facial agnosia may become paranoid and convinced that friends or lovers have been replaced by imposters. Patients with intonational–melodic and emotional–linguistic deficiencies may fail to achieve adequate vocal expression of their feelings, fail to recognize or misinterpret the feelings conveyed by others, as well as "miss the point" or fail to recognize discrepancies in speech, such as when presented with implausible information. Conversely, their own speech patterns and behavior may become abnormal, tangential, disinhibited, and contaminated by implausible, confabulatory, and delusional ideation.

Thus, in all instances, regardless of where within the right hemisphere damage occurs, social-emotional abnormalities may result. Indeed, emotional disturbances may be the dominant or only manifestation of a patient's illness. Unfortunately, if not accompanied by gross neurological signs, the possibility of right hemisphere damage may be overlooked.

Mania and Emotional Incontinence

In December 1974, associate Supreme Court Justice William O. Douglas suffered a massive infarct in the right cerebral hemisphere that left him paralyzed and in pain for many years. As reviewed by Gardner et al. (1983):

For all public purposes, Douglas acted as if he were fine, as if he could soon assume full work on the Court. He insisted on checking himself out of the hospital where he was receiving rehabilitation and then refused to return. He responded to seriously phrased queries about his condition with off handed quips: Walking has very little to do with the work of the Court; If George Blanda can play, why not me? He insisted in a press release that his left arm had been injured in a fall, thereby baldly denying the neurological cause of his paralysis. Occasionally, he acted in a paranoid fashion, claiming, for example, that the Chief Justice's quarters were his and that he was the Chief Justice. During sessions of the Court, he asked irrelevant questions, and sometimes rambled on. Finally, after considerable pressure, Douglas did resign. But the Justice refused to accept that he was no longer a member of the Court. He came back, buzzed for his clerks and tried to inject himself into the flow of business. He took aggressive steps to assign cases to himself, asked to participate in, author, and even publish separately his own opinions, and he requested that a tenth seat be placed at the Justices' bench. (p. 170)

In short, this formerly highly impressive and dignified man acted for a long time period after his stroke in a highly unusual and bizzare manner.

Since the right hemisphere is dominant in the perception and expression of facial, somesthetic, and auditory emotionality, damage to this half of the brain can result in a variety of affective and social–emotional abnormalities, including indifference, lability, hysteria, florid manic excitement, pressured speech, ideas of reference, bizarre confabulatory responding, childishness, irritability, euphoria, impulsivity, promiscuity, and abnormal sexual behavior (Bear, 1977, 1983; Bear and Fedio, 1977; Clark & Davison, 1987; M. Cohen & Niska, 1980; Cummings and Mendez, 1984; Erickson, 1945; Forrest, 1982; Gardner et al., 1983; Gruzelier and Manchanda, 1982; Jamieson & Wells, 1979; Jampala & Abrams, 1983; Joseph, 1986a; Lishman, 1968; Offen, Davidoff, Troost, & Richey, 1976; Rosenbaum & Berry, 1975; Spencer, Spencer, Williamson, & Mattson, 1983; Spreen et al., 1965; Starkstein, Pearlson, Boston, & Robinson, 1987; Stern & Dancy, 1942).

For example, M. Cohen and Niska (1980) report on a patient with a subarachnoid hemorrhage and right temporal hematoma who developed an irritable mood; shortened sleep time; loud, grandiose, tangential speech; flight of ideas; and lability and who engaged in the buying of expensive commodities. Similarly, Oppler (1950) documented an individual with a good premorbid history who began to deteriorate over many years' time. Eventually, the patient developed flight of ideas, emotional elation, increased activity, hypomanic behavior, lability, extreme fearfulness, distractability, jocularity, and argumentativeness. The patient was also overly talkative and produced a great deal of tangential-circumstantial ideation with fears of persecution and delusions. Eventually a tumor was discovered (which weighed more than 74 g) and removed from the right frontal parietal area.

Similarly, Spreen et al. (1965) described a 65-year-old man who, following a right-sided stroke (with left hemiparesis), developed extremely unpredictable behavior and lability. Regardless of external circumstances he would begin crying at one moment and at the next demonstrate irritability, happiness, or extreme depression. Secondary mania also has been reported with right frontal encephalopathy accompanied by bioelectric epileptiform activity (Jack, Rivers-Bulkeley, & Rabin, 1983).

Over the course of the last several years, I have examined eight male patients who developed manic-like symptoms after suffering a right frontal stroke ($N=1$) or trauma ($N=7$) to the right hemisphere. All but one had good premorbid histories and had worked steadily at the same job for over 6 years. Upon recovering from their injuries, all developed delusions of grandeur, pressured speech, flight of ideas, decreased need for sleep, indiscriminant financial activity, extreme emotional lability, and increased libido. One patient, formerly very reserved, quiet, conservative, and dignified with more than 20 patents to his name, and who had been married to the same woman for more than 25 years, began patronizing up to four different prostitutes a day and continued this activity for months. He left his job, began thinking up and attempting to act out extravagant grandiose schemes, and camped out at Disneyland and attempted to convince personnel there to finance his ideas for developing an amusement park on top of a mountain. At night, he frequently had dreams in which either John or Robert Kennedy would appear and offer him advice—and he was a Republican!

CONSCIOUSNESS, AWARENESS, MEMORY, AND DREAMING

Right Hemisphere Mental Functioning

That the right brain is capable of conscious experience has now been well demonstrated in studies of patients who have undergone complete corpus callosotomies (i.e., split-brain operations) for the purposes of controlling intractable epilepsy. As described by Nobel Laureate Roger Sperry (1966),

> Everything we have seen indicates that the surgery has left these people with two separate minds, that is, two separate spheres of consciousness. What is experienced in the right hemisphere seems to lie entirely outside the realm of awareness of the left hemisphere. This mental division has been demonstrated in regard to perception, cognition, volition, learning and memory. (p. 299)

For example, when split-brain patients are tactually stimulated on the left side of the body, their left hemispheres demonstrate marked neglect when verbal responses are required, they are unable to name objects placed in the left hand, and they fail to report the presence of a moving or stationary stimulus in the left half of their visual fields (Bogen, 1979; Gazzaniga, 1970; Gazzaniga & LeDoux, 1978; Joseph, 1988b; Levy, 1983; Sperry, 1982). They (i.e., their left hemisphere) cannot verbally describe odors, pictures, or auditory stimuli tachistoscopically or dichotically presented to the right brain; they also have great difficulty explaining why the left half of their body responds or behaves in a particular purposeful manner (such as when the right brain is selectively given a command). In addition, they demonstrate marked difficulties in naming incomplete figures (and thus forming visual closure), as well as a reduced ability to name and identify nonlinguistic and environmental sounds (Joseph, 1988b)—capacities associated with the functional integrity of the right hemisphere.

However, by raising the left hand (which is controlled by the right half of the cerebrum) the disconnected right brain is able to indicate when the patient is tactually or visually stimulated on the left side. When tachistoscopically presented with words to the left of visual midline, although unable to name them the right hemisphere is usually able to point correctly with the left hand to the word viewed when offered multiple visual choices in full field (Figs. 15 and 16).

In this regard, when presented with words such as "toothbrush," such that the word "tooth" falls in the left visual field (and thus, is transmitted to the right brain) and the

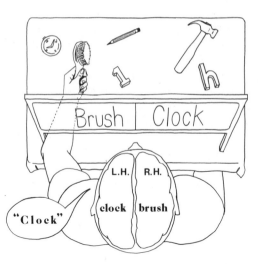

FIGURE 15. The split-brain patient is facing a screen upon which is flashed (via tachistoscope) the words "brush" and "clock." He is instructed to reach inside with his left hand to retrieve the object that corresponds to what he has seen. Because the word "brush" was viewed by the right brain, he retrieves the brush with his left hand. However, because the word "clock" was viewed by the left (speaking) brain, when asked what he saw he states, "clock."

word "brush" falls in the right field (and goes to the left hemisphere), when offered the opportunity to point to several words (e.g., hair, tooth, coat, brush), the left hand usually will point to the word viewed by the right brain (i.e., tooth) and the right hand to the word viewed by the left hemisphere (i.e., brush). When offered a verbal choice, the speaking (usually the left) hemisphere will respond "brush" and will deny seeing the word "tooth."

Overall, this indicates that the disconnected right and left cerebral hemispheres, although unable to communicate and directly share information, are nevertheless fully

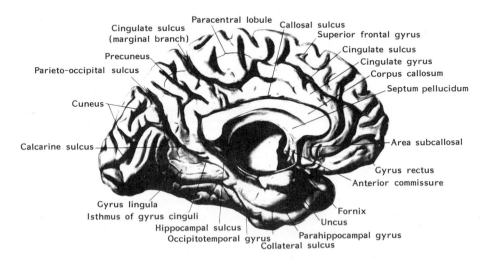

FIGURE 16. Gross anatomy of the brain. The medial surface of the left cerebral hemisphere. Diencephalic structures have been removed. Reproduced by permission from *Neuroanatomy* 2nd Ed., by F. A. Mettler, 1948, C. V. Mosby Company, St. Louis, MO.

capable of independently generating and supporting mental activity (Bogen, 1969, 1979; Gazzaniga, 1970; Gazzaniga & LeDoux, 1978; Joseph, 1988*b;* Levy, 1983, Sperry, 1982). Hence, in the right hemisphere we deal with a second form of awareness that accompanies in parallel what appears to be the "dominant" temporal–sequential, language-dependent stream of consciousness in the left cerebrum. Moreover, as has been demonstrated by Sperry, Bogen, Levy, Gazzaniga, and their colleagues, the isolated right cerebral hemisphere, like the left, is capable of self-awareness, can plan for the future, has goals and aspirations, has likes and dislikes, has social and political awareness, can purposefully initiate behavior, can guide responses choices and emotional reactions, as well as recall and act on certain desires, impulse situations, or environmental events—without the aid, knowledge or active (reflective) participation of the left half of the brain (Joseph, 1988*a,b*).

Right Brain Perversity

In that the brain of the normal as well as split-brain patient maintains the neuroanatomy to support the presence of two psychic realms, it is surprising that a considerable degree of conflict does not arise during the course of everyday activity. Frequently (such as in the case of the split-brain patient, L. B., described below), although isolated, the right half of the brain is fully willing to assist the left in a myriad of activities. Presumably such difficulties do not occur because both minds, having once been joined, share the same goals and interests. However, common experience seems to argue otherwise, for even in the intact individual, psychic functioning often is plagued by conflicts.

In its most subtle manifestations the disconnected right hemisphere may attempt to aid the left or provide it with clues when the left (speaking) brain is called upon to describe or guess what type of stimulus has been shown to the right (such as in a T-scope experiment). This may involve the right brain nodding the head, clearing the throat (so as to give clues or indicate to the left brain that it has guessed incorrectly) or by attempting to trace or write an answer on the back of the right hand (e.g., Sperry, Zaidel, & Zaidel, 1979). For example, after the right hemisphere was selectively shown a picture of Hitler, the patient signaled "thumbs down."

EX: That's another "thumbs-down"?

LB: Guess I'm antisocial.

EX: Who is it?

LB: GI came to mind, I mean. . . . Subject at this point was seen to be tracing letters with the first finger of the left hand on the back of his right hand.

EX: You're writing with your left hand; let's keep the cues out.

LB: Sorry about that.

Nevertheless, the behavior of the right hemisphere is not always cooperative, and sometimes it engages in behavior that the left brain finds objectionable, embarrassing, puzzling, mysterious, and/or quite frustrating. This is probably true for the normal as well as the "split-brain" person.

For example, Akelaitis (1945, p. 597) describes two patients with complete corpus callosotomies who experienced extreme difficulties in making the two halves of their bodies cooperate. "In tasks requiring bimanual activity the left hand would frequently perform oppositely to what she desired to do with the right hand. For example, she would be putting on clothes with her right and pulling them off with her left, opening a door or drawer with her right hand and simultaneously pushing it shut with the left. These uncontrollable acts made her increasingly irritated and depressed.''

Another patient experienced difficulty while shopping, the right hand would place something in the cart and the left hand would put it right back again. Both patients frequently experienced other difficulties as well. ''I want to walk forward but something makes me go backward.'' A recently divorced male patient noted that on several occasions while walking about town he found himself forced to go some distance in another direction. Later (although his left hemisphere was not conscious of it at the time), it was discovered (by Dr. Akelaitis) that this diverted course, if continued, would have led him to his former wife's new home.

Geschwind (1981) reports a callosal patient who complained that his left hand on several occasions suddenly struck his wife—much to the embarrassment of his left (speaking) hemisphere. In another case, a patient's left hand attempted to choke the patient himself and had to be wrestled away (Goldstein, cited by Geschwind, 1981).

Brion and Jedynak (cited by Geschwind, 1981) indicate that this type of independent left-sided (right hemisphere) activity was common in their split-brain patients and termed it the ''alien hand.'' (See Chapter 4 for further details.)

In addition, Bogen (1979, p. 333) indicates that almost all of his ''complete commissurotomy patients manifested some degree of intermanual conflict in the early postoperative period.'' One patient, Rocky, experienced situations in which his hands were uncooperative; the right would button up a shirt, and the left would follow right behind and undo the buttons. For years, he complained of difficulty getting his left leg to go in the direction he (or rather his left hemisphere) desired. Another patient often referred to the left half of her body as ''my little sister'' when she was complaining of its peculiar and independent actions.

A split-brain patient described by Dimond (1980, p. 434) reported that once when she had overslept, her ''left hand slapped me awake.'' This same patient, in fact, complained of several instances where her left hand had acted violently. Similarly, Sweet (1945) describes a female patient whose left hand sometimes behaved oppositionally and in a fashion which on occasion was quite embarrassing.

Similar difficulties plagued a split-brain patient on whom I reported recently (Joseph, 1988b). Indeed, after callosotomy, this patient (2-C) frequently was confronted with situations in which his left extremities not only acted independently, but engaged in purposeful and complex behaviors—some of which he (or rather, his left hemisphere) found objectionable and annoying.

For example, 2-C complained of instances in which his left hand would perform socially inappropriate actions (e.g., attempting to strike a relative) and would act in a manner completely opposite to what he expressively intended, such as turn off the TV or change channels, even though he (or rather his left hemisphere) was enjoying the program. Once, after he had retrieved something from the refrigerator with his right hand, his left took the food, put it back on the shelf, and retrieved a completely different item, ''even though that's not what I wanted to eat!'' On at least one occasion, his left leg refused to continue ''going for a walk'' and would only allow him to return home.

In the laboratory, he often became quite angry with his left hand, he struck it and expressed hate for it. Several times, his left and right hands were observed to engage in actual physical struggles. For example, on one task both hands were stimulated simultaneously (while out of view) with either the same or two different textured materials (e.g., sandpaper to the right, velvet to the left), and the patient was required to point (with the left and right hands simultaneously) to an array of fabrics that were hanging in view on the left and right of the testing apparatus. However, at no time was he informed that two different fabrics were being applied. After stimulation, the patient would pull his hands out from inside the apparatus and point with the left to the fabric felt by the left and with the right to the fabric felt by the right.

Surprisingly, although his left hand (controlled by the right hemisphere) responded correctly, his left hemisphere vocalized: "That's wrong!" Repeatedly, he reached over with his right hand and tried to force his left extremity to point to the fabric experienced by the right (the left hand responded correctly, but his left hemisphere didn't know this). His left hand refused to be moved and physically resisted being forced to point at anything different. In one instance, a physical struggle ensued, the right grappling with the left.

Moreover, while 2-C was performing this (and other tasks), his left hemisphere made statements such as; "I hate this hand" or "this is so frustrating," and would strike his left hand with his right or punch his left arm. In these instances, there could be little doubt that his right hemisphere was behaving with purposeful intent and understanding, whereas his left brain had absolutely no comprehension of why his left hand (right hemisphere) was behaving in this manner.

Lateralized Goals and Attitudes

Nevertheless, why the right and left cerebral hemispheres in some situations behave cooperatively and yet in others in an oppositional fashion is in part a function of lateralization. Each hemisphere is concerned with different types of information and, even when analyzing ostensibly the same stimulus, may interpret and process it differently and even reach different conclusions (Levy & Trevarthen, 1976). Moreover, even when the goals are the same, the two halves of the brain may produce and attempt to act on different strategies.

Functional lateralization may thus lead to the development of oppositional attitudes, goals, and interests. For example, Reuben Gur (personal communication, 1987) described one split-brain patient whose left hand would not allow the patient to smoke and would pluck lit cigarettes from his mouth or right hand and put them out. Apparently, although his left brain wanted to smoke, his right hemisphere did not approve. Even 2-C experienced conflicts when attempting to eat, watch TV, or go for walks, his right and left brain apparently enjoying different TV programs or types of food. Nevertheless, these difficulties are not limited to split-brain patients, for conflicts of a similar nature often plague the intact patient as well.

Lateralized Memory Functioning

Functional lateralization greatly determines what type of material can be memorized or even recognized by each half of the cerebrum. This is because the code or form in which a stimulus is represented in the brain and memory is determined by the manner in which it is processed and the transformations that take place. Because the right and left cerebral hemispheres differentially process information, the manner in which this information is represented will also be lateralized. Thus, some types of information can only be processed or stored by the right vs. the left cerebrum.

For example, it is well known that the left hemisphere is responsible for the encoding and recall of verbal memories, whereas the right cerebrum is dominant in regard to visual–spatial, nonverbal, and emotional memory functioning (Bogen, 1979; Fried *et al.*, 1982; Gazzaniga & LeDoux, 1978; Hecaen & Albert, 1978; Kimura, 1963; Levy, 1983; Luria, 1980; Milner, 1962, 1968; Sperry, 1974; Sperry *et al.*, 1979; Suberi & McKever, 1977; Wechsler, 1973; Whitehouse, 1981). If the left temporal lobe were destroyed, verbal memory functioning would be impaired, since the right brain does not readily store this type of information. Conversely, the left has great difficulty storing or remembering nonlinguistic information.

In the intact normal brain, some memory traces appear to be stored unilaterally rather than laid down in both hemispheres (Doty & Overman, 1977). Moreover, when one hemisphere learns, has certain experiences, and/or stores information in memory, this information is not always available to the opposing hemisphere, one hemisphere cannot always gain access to memories stored in the other half of the brain (Joseph, 1982; Risse & Gazzaniga, 1979).

To gain access to these lateralized memories, one hemisphere has to activate the memory banks of the other brain half via the corpus callosum (Doty & Overman, 1977). This has been demonstrated experimentally in primates. For example, after one hemisphere had been trained to perform a certain task, although either hemisphere could respond correctly once it was learned, when the commissures were subsequently cut, only the hemisphere that originally was trained was able to perform—i.e., could recall it. The untrained hemisphere, acted as though it never had been exposed to the task; its ability to retrieve the original memories was now abolished (Doty & Overman, 1977).

In a conceptually similar study, Risse and Gazzaniga (1979) injected sodium amytal into the left carotid arteries of intact patients in order to anesthetize the language dominant left cerebral hemisphere. After the left cerebrum was inactivated, the awake right hemisphere was still able to follow and behaviorally respond to commands, e.g., palpating an object with the left hand.

Once the left hemisphere had recovered from the drug, as determined by the return of speech and motor functioning, none of the eight patients studied was able to recall verbally what objects had been palpated with the left hand, "even after considerable probing." Although encouraged to guess, most patients refused to try and insisted that they did not remember anything. However, when offered multiple choices in full field, most patients immediately raised the left hand and pointed to the correct object!

According to Risse and Gazzaniga (1979), although the memory of touching and palpating the object was not accessible to the verbal (left hemisphere) memory system, it was encoded in a nonverbal form within the right hemisphere and was unavailable to the left hemisphere when normal function returned. The left (speaking) hemisphere was unable to gain access to information and memories stored within the right half of the brain. Nevertheless, the right brain not only remembered but was able to act on its memories.

This indicates that when exchange and transfer is not possible, is in some manner inhibited, or if for any reason the two halves of the brain become functionally disconnected and are unable to share information, the possibility of information transfer at a later time is precluded (Bures & Buresova, 1960; Risse & Gazzaniga, 1979)—even when the ability to transfer is acquired or restored. The information is lost to the opposite half of the cerebrum. Nevertheless, although lost, these memories and attached feelings can continue to influence whole-brain functioning in subtle as well as profound ways.

Lateralization of memory affects complex behavioral functioning in a number of ways, for one hemisphere may experience and store certain information in memory and at a later time in response to certain situations act on those memories, much to the surprise, perplexity, or chagrin of the other half of the brain (Joseph, 1980, 1982, 1988a); one hemisphere cannot always gain access to memories stored in the other half of the brain.

Dreaming

Complete functional deactivation is probably quite rare in the normal brain. However, there is some evidence to suggest that interhemispheric communication is reduced, for example, during sleep and possibly during dreaming (Banquet, 1983).

Most dreaming occurs during rapid eye movement (REM), which is possibly associated with right hemisphere activation and low-level left hemisphere arousal (Goldstein, Stoltzfus, & Gardocki, 1972; Hodoba, 1986; Meyer, Ishikawa, Hata, & Karacan, 1987). In this regard, it is interesting to note that it becomes progressively more difficult to recall one's dreams as one spends time in or awakens during non-REM (NREM) (Wolpert & Trosman, 1958), which is associated with high left hemisphere and low right brain activation (Goldstein et al., 1972). Thus, are dreams really forgotten, or are they locked away in a code that is not accessible to the speaking left hemisphere?

Dreaming and Hemispheric Oscillation

Although up to five stages of sleep have been identified in humans, for our purposes we will be concerned only with two distinct sleep states. These are the REM and NREM periods. NREM occurs during a stage referred to as slow-wave or synchronized sleep. By contrast, REM occurs during a sleep stage referred to as paradoxical sleep. It is called paradoxical, for electrophysiologically the brain seems quite active and alert, similar to its condition during waking. However, the body musculature is paralyzed, and the ability to perceive outside sensory events is greatly attenuated (for a recent detailed review, see Hobson et al., 1986).

Most people awakened during REM report dream activity approximately 80% of the time. When awakened during the NREM period, dreams are reported approximately 20% of the time (Foulkes, 1962; Goodenough, Shapiro, Holden, & Steinschriber, 1959; Monroe, Rechtschaffen, Foulkes, & Jensen, 1965). However, the type of dreaming that occurs during REM versus NREM is quite different. For example, NREM dreams (when they occur) are often quite similar to thinking and speech (i.e., linguistic thought), such that a kind of rambling verbal monologue is experienced in the absence of imagery (Foulkes, 1962; Monroe et al., 1965). It is also during NREM in which an individual is most likely to talk in his or her sleep (Kamiya, 1961). By contrast, REM dreams involve a considerable degree of visual imagery, emotion, and tend to be distorted and implausible to various degrees (Foulkes, 1962; Monroe et al., 1965).

REM is characterized by high levels of activity within the brainstem, occipital lobe, and other nuclei (see Hobson et al., 1986, for review). It also has been reported that electrophysiologically the right hemisphere becomes highly active during REM, whereas conversely the left brain becomes more active during NREM (Goldstein et al., 1972; Hodoba, 1986). Similarly, measurements of cerebral blood flow have shown an increase in the right temporal and parietal regions during REM sleep and in subjects who upon wakening report visual, hypnagogic, hallucinatory, and auditory dreaming (Meyer et al., 1987).

Interestingly, abnormal and enhanced activity in the right temporal and temporal–occipital area acts to increase dreaming and REM sleep for an atypically long time period. Similarly, REM sleep increases activity in this same region much more than in the left hemisphere (Hodoba, 1986), which indicates that there is a specific complementary relationship between REM sleep and right temporal–occipital electrophysiological activity. At least one group of investigators, however, have failed to find significant hemispheric electroencephalographic (EEG) differences between REM and NREM (Ehrlichman, Antrobus, & Wiener, 1985).

Daydreams, Night Dreams, and Hemispheric Oscillation

There is some evidence to suggest that during the course of the day and night the two cerebral hemispheres oscillate in activity every 90 to 100 minutes and are 180 degrees out of phase—a cycle that corresponds to changes in cognitive efficiency, the appearance of day dreams, REM (dream sleep), and, conversely, NREM sleep (Bertini, Violani, Zoccolotti, Antonelli, & DiStephano, 1983; Broughton, 1982; Gordon, Frooman, & Lavie, 1982, cited by Hodoba, 1986; Klein & Armitage, 1979; Kripke & Sonnenschein, 1973; Levie et al., 1983, cited by Hodoba, 1986). That is, like two pistons moving up and down, it appears that when the right brain is functionally at its peak of activity, the left brain is correspondingly at its nadir.

Similarly, shifts in cognitive abilities associated with the right and left hemisphere have been found during these cyclical changes during the day and after awakenings from REM and NREM sleep. That is, performance across a number of tasks associated with left hemisphere cognitive efficiency is maximal during NREM, whereas, conversely, right hemisphere performance (e.g., point localization, shape identification, orientation in space) is maximal after REM awakenings (Bertini et al., 1983; Gordon et al., 1982; Levie et al., 1983; cited by Hodoba, 1986). Moreover, Bertini et al., (1983) found that left hand motor dexterity (in right-handed subjects) was superior to the right when awakened during REM and that the opposite relationship was found during NREM, i.e., right hand superiority (Hodoba, 1986, for review.)

Conversely, there have been reports of patients with right cerebral damage who have ceased dreaming altogether or to dream only in words (Humphrey & Zangwill, 1951; Kerr & Foulkes, 1978, 1981). For example, defective dreaming, deficits that involve visual imagery, and loss of hypnagogic imagery have been found in patients with focal lesions or hypoplasia of the posterior right hemisphere and abnormalities in the corpus callosum

(Botez, Olivier, Vezina, Botez, & Kaufman, 1985; Kerr & Foulkes, 1981; Murri, Arena, Siciliano, Mazzotta, & Muratorio, 1984).

An absence or diminished amount of dreaming during sleep also has been reported after split-brain surgery; i.e., as reported by the disconnected left hemisphere (Bogen & Bogen, 1969; Hoppe & Bogen, 1977). Similarly, a paucity of REM episodes have been noted in other callosotomy patients, although these particular patients continued to report some dream activity (Greenwood, Wilson, & Gazzaniga, 1977).

On the other hand it has been reported that when the left hemisphere has been damaged, particularly the posterior portions (i.e., aphasic patients), the ability to verbally report and recall dreams also is greatly attenuated (Murri et al., 1984; Pena-Casanova & Roig-Rovira, 1985; Schanfald, Pearlman, & Greenberg, 1985). However, aphasics have difficulty describing much of anything, let alone their dreams. By contrast, in some respects, a parallel between these latter findings and those of Risse and Gazzaniga (1979) in their sodium amytal studies may be explanatory. That is, with left hemisphere damage or when the left brain is at a low level of arousal, the ability to verbally recall or report events experienced or generated by the right hemisphere appears to be reduced; i.e., the left (speaking) half of the brain cannot remember because it cannot gain access to right cerebral memory centers.

Thus, it appears that the right hemisphere provides the physiological foundation from which dreams in part derive their source and origin (Goldstein et al., 1972; Hodoba, 1986; Meyer et al., 1987). However, in some instances in which these dream centers are disconnected from the language-dominant left hemisphere as a result of posterior right or left hemisphere lesions or after callosotomy, the ability to recall, report, and/or produce vivid visual and hypnogogic dream imagery is attenuated. Frontal lobe damage and lobotomy also have been reported to abolish dreaming, however (Freeman & Watts, 1942, 1943).

It is important to note that some investigators believe the left hemisphere is responsible for dreaming (see Greenberg & Farah, 1986; Miller, 1988, for a detailed review). Nevertheless, although the left hemisphere no doubt makes a major contribution, it probably takes both hemispheres to dream.

Dream Patterns

Although dreams probably serve a number of purposes, and at times are highly improbable and bizarre, they often reflect something significant about the mental and emotional life of the dreamer, as well as other issues of concern to the right half of the brain. For example, when subjects are awakened repeatedly during REM over the course of several days, often an evolving thematic pattern, like an unfolding story, can be discerned. These patterns frequently reflect mental–emotional activity concerned with the solution of particular problems (Cartwright, Tipton, & Wicklund, 1980; Kramer, Whitman, Baldridge, & Lansky, 1964). For example, one subject, a student, noted that "after being woken many times and seeing three or four dreams a night, I could realize there was a certain problem being worked out, like coping with responsibilities that were thrust upon me, but that weren't necessarily my own but I took on anyway. It was working out the feelings of resentment of taking somebody else's responsibility, but I met them well in my dreams. A good thing about spending time in the sleep lab was you could relate a common bond to some of the'' dreams (Cartwright *et al.,* 1980, p. 277). Similar bonds and patterns were recognized by Freud (1900) and Jung (1945) many years ago.

Nevertheless, it might reasonably be asked: If dreams are of importance and not merely reflective of random and purely confabulatory ideation, why are they so difficult to recall? In part, as noted in the introduction to this section, this may be a function of lateralization, alterations in hemispheric arousal and activity, differential memory storage, and decreased interhemispheric communication during REM. Perhaps they only can be recalled by the right hemisphere. Nevertheless, in some instances, dreams are probably nothing more than mundane and confabulatory *noise.*

Long-Lost Childhood Memories

For most individuals it is extremely difficult, if not impossible, to recall events which occurred before the age of 4. There are several reasons for this. Information processed and experienced during infancy versus adulthood is stored by certain transformations and retrieval strategies that are quite different. As the brain matures and new information-processing strategies are learned and developed, the manner in which information is processed and stored is altered. Although these early memories are stored within the brain, the organism no longer has the means of retrieving them, i.e., the key no longer fits the lock.

That is, early experiences may be unrecallable because infants use a different system of codes to store memories, whereas adults use symbols and associations (such as language) that are not yet fully available to the child (Dollard & Miller, 1950; Joseph, 1982; Piaget, 1952, 1962, 1974). Much of what was experienced and committed to memory during early childhood took place before the development of linguistic labeling ability and was based on a pre- or nonlinguistic code (Dollard & Miller, 1950; Freud, 1900). Thus, the adult, who is relying on more sophisticated coding systems, cannot find the right set of neural programs to open the door to childhood memories. The key does not fit the lock because both the key and the lock have changed.

Emotional and Right Brain Functioning in Children

As we are now well aware, the developing organism is extremely vulnerable to environmental influences during infancy such that the nervous system and behavior may be altered dramatically as manifested in the adult (Casagrande & Joseph, 1978; 1980; Denenberg, 1981; Joseph & Casagrande, 1980; Joseph & Gallagher, 1980; Joseph, Hess, & Birecree, 1978; Langmeier & Matejcek, 1975). Interestingly, the right cerebral hemisphere seems to be more greatly affected (see Denenberg, 1981, for review). Moreover, during these same early years, our traumas, fears, and other emotional experiences, like those of an adult, are mediated not only by the limbic system, but also via the nonlinguistic, social–emotional right brain. And, just as they are in adulthood, these experiences are stored in the memory banks of the right cerebrum.

However, much of what was experienced and learned by the right brain during these early years was not always shared or available for left hemisphere scrutiny (and vice versa). That is, a child's two hemispheres are not only functionally lateralized but are limited in their ability to share and transfer information. In many ways, infants and young children have split brains (Finlayson, 1975; Galin, Diamond, & Herron, 1979; Galin, Johnstone, Nakell, & Herron, 1979; Joseph, 1982; Joseph & Gallagher, 1985; Joseph *et al.*, 1984; Kraft, Mitchell, Languis, & Wheatley, 1980; Molfese *et al.*, 1975; O'Leary, 1980; Salamy, 1978; Yakovlev & Lecours, 1967).

Indeed, because of the immaturity of the corpus callosum and lack of myelin (Yakoviev & Lecours, 1967), communication is so poor that children as old as age 4 have difficulty transferring tactile, auditory, or visual information between the hemispheres, e.g., accurately describing complex pictures shown to the right brain (Joseph *et al.*, 1984). Thus, the left hemisphere of a young child has at best incomplete knowledge of the contents and activity that are occurring within the right. This sets the stage for differential memory storage and a later inability to transfer information between the cerebral hemispheres. (For more information regarding pediatric neuropsychology, see Nkiokiktjien, 1988.)

Because of lateralization and limited exchange, the effects of early socializing experience can have potentially profound effects. As a good deal of this early experience is likely to have unpleasant, if not traumatic, moments, it is fascinating to consider the later ramifications of early emotional learning occurring in the right hemisphere unbeknownst to the left—learning and associated emotional responding that later may be completely inaccessible to the language centers of the left half of the brain. That is, although limited transfer in children confers advantages, it also provides for the eventual development of a number of very significant psychic conflicts—many of which do not become apparent until much later in life.

Moreover, because of the immaturity of the callosum, children frequently can encounter situations in which the right and left brain not only differentially perceive what is going on but are unable to link these experiences so as to understand fully what is occurring or to correct misperceptions (Galin, 1974; Joseph, 1982). Consider a young divorced mother with ambivalent feelings toward her young son (cf. Galin, 1974), who, although she does not express these feelings verbally, conveys them through her tone of voice, facial expression, and in the manner in which she touches her son. She knows that she should love him, and at some level she does. She wants to be a good mother and makes herself go through the motions. However, she also resents her son because she has lost her freedom, he is a financial burden, and he may hinder her in finding a desirable mate. She is confronted by two opposing attitudes, one of which is unacceptable to the image she has of a good mother. Like many of us, she must prevent these feelings from reaching linguistic consciousness. However, this does not prevent them from being expressed nonlinguistically via the right brain.

Her son also has a right brain that perceives her tension and ambivalance. His right brain notes the stiffness when his mother holds or touches him and is aware of the manner in which she sometimes looks at him. Worse, when she says, "I love you," his right brain senses the tension and tone of her voice and correctly perceives that what she means is, "I don't want you" or, "I hate you." His left brain hears, however, "I love you" and notes only that she is attentive. He is in a double-bind conflict, with no way for his two cerebral hemispheres to match impressions.

This little boy's right brain feels something painful when the words "I love you" are spoken. When his mother touches him, he becomes stiff and withdrawn because his right brain, through analysis of facial expression, emotional tone, and tactile sensation, is fully aware that she does not want him.

Later, as an adult, this same young man has one failed relationship after another. He feels that he cannot trust women and often feels rejected; when a girl or woman says "I love you," it makes him want to cringe, run away, or strike out. As an adult, his left brain hears "Love," and his right brain feels pain and rejection.

Because the two halves of his cerebrum were not in communication during early childhood, his ability to gain insight into the source of his problems is greatly restricted. His left brain cannot access these memories. It has "no idea" as to the cause of his conflicts.

In this regard, this curious asymmetrical arrangement of function and maturation may well predispose the developing child in later life to come upon situations in which it finds itself responding emotionally, nervously, anxiously, or neurotically, without linguistic knowledge, or without even the possibility of linguistic comprehension as to the cause, purpose, eliciting stimulus, or origin of its behavior (Joseph, 1982). As a child or an adult, it may find itself faced with behavior that is mysterious, embarrassing, etc. "I don't know what came over me."

Functional Commissurotomies and Limited Interhemispheric Transfer

The corpus callosum is the gateway through which information may travel from one brain half to the other. However, it also acts to limit information exchange, since almost 40% of the adult callosum lacks myelin (Selnes, 1974). Since myelin acts to insulate and thus preserve information transmission by minimizing leakage (Rogart & Ritchi, 1977), some information is lost and degraded even when transfer is possible (cf. Marzi, 1986).

Moreover, particularly when one is dealing with complex or emotional information, situations probably sometimes arise in which one brain half has little or no knowledge as to what is occurring in the other (Dimond, 1980; Dimond & Beaumont, 1974, Dimond, Gazzanniga, & Gibson, 1972; Geschwind, 1965; Joseph, 1980, 1982; Joseph et al., 1984; Marzi, 1986; Myers, 1959). In part, this is a consequence of lateralized specialization. Certain forms of information can only be processed and, thus, recognized by the right or left half of the brain. (See Merriam & Gardner, 1987 for a brief review of studies of interhemispheric transfer in normals and schizophrenics.) Even information that is transferred may be subject to interpretation and misinterpretation (Gazzangia & LeDoux, 1978; Joseph, 1980, 1982, 1986a,b, 1988a; Joseph et al., 1984).

In addition, one brain half can be prevented from knowing what is occurring in the opposite half because of inhibitory or suppressive actions initiated by, for example, the frontal lobes, such that certain forms of information are suppressed, censored, and interhemispheric (as well as intrahemispheric) information transmission prevented. Thus, there sometimes results a *functional commissurotomy* (Hoppe, 1977).

Therefore, these three conditions—lateralized specialization, frontal lobe inhibitory activity, and incomplete myelination of callosum axons—can reduce the ability of the two hemispheres to communicate among normal, intact individuals. Hence, in many ways the brain of even a normal adult is functionally split and disconnected, and for good reason. These conditions protect the brain and linguistic consciousness from becoming overwhelmed. As we have seen with frontal lobe damage, when communication is allowed to occur freely (due to disinhibition), the overall integrity of the brain to function normally is curtailed dramatically (Joseph, 1986a; Luria, 1973, 1980).

Nevertheless, a unique side effect of having two brains that are not always able to communicate completely and successfully is intrapsychic conflicts. That is, we sometimes find ourselves feeling happy, sad, depressed, angry, and so forth, without a clue as to the cause. In other instances, we actually may commit certain thoughtless, impulsive, overly emotional, or embarrassing actions and "have no idea" as to "what came over" us. To posit the notion that we have such experiences simply "because" is absurd. Nor, among "normals," are such experiences always attributable to biochemical fluctuations or the result of "unconscious" urges. Rather, unbeknownst to the left brain, sometimes the right perceives, remembers, or responds to some external or internal source of experience and/or to its own memories and, thus, reacts in an emotional manner. The left (speaking) hemisphere in turn only knows that it is feeling something but is unsure what or why, or conversely, it confabulates various denials, rationalizations, and explanations, which it accepts as fact (Joseph, 1980, 1982, 1986a).

CONCLUDING COMMENTS

Overall, based on numerous studies conducted on normal, brain-injured, and neurosurgical patients, the right cerebral hemisphere has been shown to dominate in the perception and identification of environmental and nonverbal sounds (e.g., wind, rain, thunder, birds singing); somesthesis; stereognosis; the maintenance of the body image; and the comprehension and expression of prosodic, melodic, and emotional features of speech, as well as the perception of most aspects of musical stimuli, i.e., chords, timbre, tone, pitch, loudness, melody, intensity. Moreover, the right predominates in the analysis of geometric and visual space, including depth perception, orientation, position, distance, figure ground, perspective, visual closure, and stereopsis.

It also appears to be more involved than the left in the production of certain forms of visual imagery (see Ehrlichman & Barrett, 1983, for contradictory evidence), dreams during REM sleep, as well as day dreams during waking. Conversely, the left brain appears to be associated with NREM sleep and the thinking type of mentation that sometimes occurs during this stage. However, the left hemisphere probably provides much of the dialogue and commentary that accompany dream activity.

A considerable body of evidence indicates that the right hemisphere is dominant in the comprehension and expression of prosodic, melodic, and emotional features of speech; the expression and perception of visual, facial, and verbal affect; and the ability to determine a person's mood, attitude, and intentions through the analysis of gesture, facial expression, vocal–melodic, and intonational qualities.

Because the right brain is dominant in regard to most, if not all, aspects of social–emotional functioning, when it is damaged a myriad of affective disturbances may result. These include mania, depression, hysteria, gross social–emotional disinhibition, euphoria, childishness, puerility, or, conversely, complete indifference and apathy. Patients may become delusional, engage in the production of bizarre confabulations, and experience a host of somatic disturbances ranging from pain and body-perceptual distortions to seizure-induced sexual activity and orgasm. They may fail to recognize the left half of their own bodies or, in other instances, fail to recognize the faces of friends, loved ones, or even their pets. In fact, patients with right-sided lesions show less recovery and are more likely to die than are patients with left-sided destruction (Denes, Semenza, Stoppa, & Lis, 1982; Hobhouse, 1936; Hurwitz & Adams, 1972; Knapp, 1959; Marquardsen, 1969).

By contrast, the range of emotional disturbances associated with left cerebral damage seems to be limited to apathy, depression, emotional blunting, and schizophrenia, although euphoria sometimes accompanies receptive aphasia and loss of comprehension (Gainotti, 1972; Gasparrini et al., 1978; Geschwind, 1981; Gruzelier & Manchanda, 1982; Hillbom, 1960; Robinson & Szetela, 1981; Robinson, Kubos, Starr, Rao, & Price, 1984; Sherwin, Peron-Magnan, & Bancaud, 1982; Sinyour et al., 1986).

Despite evidence of considerable functional overlap as well as interhemispheric cooperation on a number of tasks, it certainly appears that the mental system maintained by the right cerebral hemisphere is highly developed, social–emotional, bilateral, and in many ways dominant over the temporal–sequential, language-dependent half of the cerebrum. Indeed, the right cerebrum can independently recall and act on certain memories with purposeful intent; it is the dominant source of our dreams, psychic conflicts, and desires and is fully capable of motivating, initiating, as well as controlling behavioral expression—often without the aid or even active (reflective) participation of the left half of the brain.

REFERENCES

Akelaitis, A. J. (1945). Studies on the corpus callosum. IV. Diagnostic dyspraxia in epileptics following partial and complete section of the corpus callosum. *American Journal of Psychiatry, 101,* 594–599.

Alajoanine, T. (1948). Aphasia and artistic realization. *Brain, 71,* 229–241.

Albert, M. L. (1973). A simple test for visual neglect. *Neurology (New York), 23,* 658–664.

Albert, M. L., Sparks, R., & Helm, N. (1973). Melodic intonation therapy for aphasia. *Archives of Neurology, 29,* 334–339.

Albert, M. L., Sparks, R., von Strockert, T., & Sax, D. (1972). A case of auditory agnosia. Linguistic and nonlinguistic processing. *Cortex, 8,* 427–443.

Alexander, M. P., Stuss, D. T., & Benson, D. F. (1979). Capgras syndrome: A reduplicative phenomenon. *Neurology (New York), 29,* 130–131.

Arrigoni, G., & DeRenzi, E. (1964). Constructional apraxia and hemispheric locus of lesion. *Cortex, 1,* 170–197.

Axelrod, S., Noonan, M., & Atanacio, B. (1980). On the laterality of psychogenic somatic symptoms. *Journal of Nervous and Mental Disease, 168,* 517–525.

Banquet, J. P. (1983). Inter- and intrahemispheric relationships of the EEG activity during sleep in man. *Electroencephalography and Clinical Neurophysiology, 55,* 51–59.

Bear, D. (1977). The significance of behavioral change in temporal lobe epilepsy. *McLean Hospital Journal, 9,* 11–23.

Bear, D. M. (1983). Hemispheric specialization and the neurology of emotion. *Archives of Neurology, 40,* 195–202.

Bear, D. M., & Fedio, P. (1977). Quantitative analysis of interictal behavior in temporal lobe epilepsy. *Archives of Neurology, 34,* 454–467.

Beaumont, J. G. (1974). Handedness and hemisphere function. In S. J. Dimond & J. G. Beaumont (Eds.), *Hemispheric function in the human brain,* (pp. 89–120). New York: John Wiley & Sons.

Beck, E. C., Dustman, R. E., & Sakai, M. (1969). Electrophysiological correlates of selective attention. In C. R. Evans, & R. B. Mulholland (Eds.), *Attention in neurophysiology* (pp. 221–240). E. Norwalk, CT: Appleton & Lange.

Benson, D., & Barton, M. (1970). Disturbances in constructional ability. *Cortex, 6,* 19–46.

Benson, D. F., Gardner, H., & Meadows, J. C. (1976). Reduplicative paramnesia. *Neurology (New York),* 147–151.

Benton, A. (1979). Visuoperceptive, visuospatial and visuoconstructive disorders. In K. M. Heilman, & E. Valenstein (Eds.), *Clinical neuropsychology* (pp. 186–232). Oxford: Oxford University Press.

Bertini, M., Violani, C., Zoccolotti, P., Antonelli, A., & DiStephano, L. (1983). Performance on a unilateral tactile test during waking and upon awakenings from REM and NREM. In W. P. Koella (Ed.), *Sleep* (pp. 122–155). Basel: S. Karger.

Bhaskar, P. A. (1987). Scrotal pain with testicular jerking. An unusual manifestation of epilepsy. *Journal of Neurology, Neurosurgery and Psychiatry, 50,* 1233–1234.

Bisiach, E., Bulgarelli, C., Sterzi, R., & Vallar, G. (1983). Line bisection and cognitive plasticity of unilateral neglect of space. *Brain and Cognition, 2,* 32–38.

Bisiach, E., & Luzzatti, C. (1978). Unilateral neglect of representational space. *Cortex, 14,* 129–133.

Black, F. W., & Bernard, B. A. (1984). Constructional apraxia as a function of lesion locus and size in patients with focal brain damage. *Cortex, 20,* 111–120.

Black, F. W., & Strub, R. L. (1976). Constructional apraxia in patients with discrete missile wounds of the brain. *Cortex, 12,* 212–220.

Blumstein, S., & Cooper, W. E. (1974). Hemispheric processing of intonational contours. *Cortex, 10,* 146–158.

Blumstein, S., & Goodglass, H. (1972). Perception of stress as a semantic cue in aphasia. *Journal of Speech Hearing Research, 15,* 800–806.

Bogen, J. E. (1969). The other side of the brain. *Bulletin of the Los Angeles Neurological Societies, 34,* 135–162.

Bogen, J. E. (1979). The calosal syndrome. In K. M. Heilman & E. Valenstein (Eds.), *Clinical neuropsychology* (pp. 308–358). New York: Oxford University Press.

Bogen, J., & Bogen, C. (1969). The other side of the brain. III. The corpus callosum and creativity. *Bulletin of the Los Angeles Neurological Society, 34,* 191–220.

Boller, F., Cole, M. Vrtunski, P. B., Patterson, M., & Kim, Y. (1979). Paralinguistic aspects of auditory comprehension in aphasia. *Brain & Language, 9,* 164–174.

Boller, F., & Green, E. (1972). Comprehension in severe aphasics. *Cortex, 8,* 382–390.

Bornstein, R. A., & Matarasso, J. D. (1982). Wechsler VIQ versus PIQ differences in cerebral dysfunction: A review of the literature with emphasis on sex differences. *Journal of Clinical Neuropsychology, 4,* 319–334.

Borod, J. C., & Caron, H. S. (1980). Facedness and emotion related to lateral dominance, sex, and expression type. *Neuropsychologia, 18,* 237–241.

Botez, M. I., Olivier, M., Vezina, J.-L., Botez, T., & Kaufman, B. (1985). Defective revisualization: Dissociation between cognitive and imagistic thought case report and short review of the literature. *Cortex, 21,* 375–389.

Bowers, D., Coslett, B., Bauer, R. M., Speedie, L. J., & Heilman, K. (1987). Comprehension of emotional prosody following unilateral hemisphere lesions: Processing defect versus distraction defect. *Neuropsychologia, 25,* 317–328.

Bradshaw, J. L., Nettleton, N. C., & Spher, K. (1982). Braille reading and left and right hemispace. *Neuropsychologia, 20,* 493–500.

Bradshaw, J. L., Taylor, M. J., Patterson, K., & Nettleton, N. (1980). Upright and inverted faces, and housefronts, in the two visual fields: A right and a left hemisphere contribution. *Journal of Clinical Neuropsychology, 2,* 245–257.

Brain, R. (1941). Visual disorientation with special references to lesions of the right cerebral hemisphere. *Brain, 64,* 244–272.

Breasted, J. H. (1937). *A history of Egypt.* New York: Charles Scribner's.

Breitling, D., Guenther, W., & Rondot, P. (1987). Auditory perception of music measured by brain electrical activity mapping. *Neuropsychologia, 25,* 765–774.

Bronowski, J. (1973). *The ascent of man.* Boston: Little, Brown.

Broughton, R. (1982). Human consciousness and sleep/waking rhythms: A review and some neuropsychological considerations. *Journal of Clinical Neuropsychology, 4,* 193–218.

Brownell, H. H., Potter, H. H., & Bihrle, A. M. (1986). Inference deficits in right brain-damaged patients. *Brain and Language, 27,* 310–321.

Bryden, M. P., & Allard, F. (1976). Visual hemifield differences depend on typeface. *Brain and Language, 3,* 191–200.

Bryden, M. P., Ley, R. G., & Sugarman, J. H. (1982). A left-ear advantage for identifying the emotional quality of tonal sequences. *Neuropsychologia, 20,* 83–87.

Buchtel, H., Campari, F., De Risio, C., & Rota, R. (1978). Hemispheric differences in the discrimination reaction times to facial expression. *Italian Journal of Psychology, 5,* 159–169.

Bures, J., & Buresova, O. (1960). The use of Leao's spreading depression in the study of interhemispheric transfer of memory traces. *Journal of Comparative and Physiological Psychology, 59,* 211–214.

Butters, N., & Barton, M. (1970). Effect of parietal lobe damage on the performance of reversible operations in space. *Neuropsychologia, 8,* 205–214.

Calvanio, R., Petrone, P. N., & Levine, D. N. (1987). Left visual spatial neglect is both environment-centered and body-centered. *Neurology (New York), 37,* 1179–1183.

Campbell R. (1978). Asymmetries in interpreting and expressing a posed facial expression. *Cortex, 15,* 327–342.

Caramazza, A., Gordon, J., Zurif, E. B., & DeLuca, D. (1976). Right-hemispheric damage and verbal problem solving behavior. *Brain and Language, 3,* 41–46.

Carmazza, A., & Zurif, E. B. (1976). Dissociation of algorithmic and heuristic process in language comprehension: Evidence from aphasia. *Brain and Language, 3,* 572–582.

Carmon, A., & Bechtoldt, H. P. (1969). Dominance of the right cerebral hemisphere for stereopsis. *Neuropsychologia, 7,* 29–39.

Carmon, A., & Benton, A. L. (1969). Tactile perception of direction and number in patients with unilateral cerebral disease. *Neurology (New York), 19,* 525–532.

Carmon, A., & Nachshon, I. (1971). Effect of unilateral brain damage on perception of temporal order. *Cortex, 7,* 410–418.

Carmon, A., & Nachshon, I. (1973). Ear asymmetry in perception of emotional non-verbal stimuli. *Acta Psychologica, 37,* 351–357.

Cartwright, R. D., Tipton, L. W., & Wicklund, J. (1980). Focusing on dreams. *Archives of General Psychiatry, 37,* 275–288.

Casagrande, V. A., & Joseph, R. (1978). Effects of monocular deprivation on geniculostriate connections in prosimian primates. *Anatomical Record, 190,* 359.

Casagrande, V. A., & Joseph, R. (1980). Morphological effects of monocular deprivation and recovery on the dorsal lateral geniculate nucleus in galago. *Journal of Comparative Neurology, 194,* 413–426.

Catchpole, C. K. (1979). *Vocal communication in birds.* Baltimore: University Park Press.

Chase, R. A. (1967). Discussion. In F. L. Darley (Ed.), *Brain mechanisms underlying speech and language* (pp. 136–139). Orlando, FL: Grune & Stratton.

Chaurasis, B. D., & Goswami, H. K. (1975). Functional asymmetry in the face. *Acta Anatomica, 91,* 154–160.

Cicone, M., Wapner, W., & Gardner, H. (1980). Sensitivity to emotional expressions and situations in organic patients. *Cortex, 16,* 145–158.

Clark, A. F., & Davison, K. (1987). Mania following head injury. *British Journal of Psychiatry, 150,* 841–844.

Cohen, H. D., Rosen, R. C., & Goldstein, I. (1976). Electroencephalographic laterality changes during human sexual orgasm. *Archives of Sexual Behavior, 5,* 189–200.

Cohen, M. R., & Niska, R. W. (1980). Localized right cerebral hemisphere dysfunction and recurrent mania. *American Journal of Psychiatry, 137,* 847–848.

Corkin, S., Milner, B., & Rasmussen, T. (1970). Somotosensory thresholds: Contrasting effects of post-central gyrus and posterior parietal-lobe excisions. *Archives of Neurology, 23,* 41–58.

Critchley, M. (1953). *The parietal lobes.* New York: Hafner.

Cubelli, R., Caselli, M., & Neri, I. (1984). Pain endurance in unilateral cerebral lesions. *Cortex, 20,* 369–375.

Cummings, J. L., & Mendez, M. F. (1984). Secondary mania with focal cerebrovascular lesions. *American Journal of Psychiatry, 41,* 1084–1087.

Curry, F. K. W. (1967). A comparison of left-handed and right-handed subjects on verbal and non-verbal dichotic listening tasks. *Cortex, 3,* 343–352.

Davidson, C., & Schick, W. (1935). Spontaneous pain and other subjective sensory disturbances. *Archives of Neurology and Psychiatry, 34,* 1204–1237.

Day, J. (1977). Right hemisphere language processing in normal right-handers. *Journal of Experimental Psychology: Human Perception and Performance, 3,* 518–528.

Day, R., Cutting, J. E., & Copeland, P. (1971). Perception of linguistic and non-linguistic dimensions of dichotic stimuli. *Status Report of Haskins Laboratories, 27,* 1–6.

DeKosky, S. T., Heilman, K. M., Bowers, D., & Valenstein, E. (1980). Recognition and discrimination of emotional faces and pictures. *Brain and Language, 9,* 206–214.

Delis, D. C., Robertson, L. C., & Efron, R. (1986). Hemispheric specialization of memory for visual hierarchical stimuli. *Neuropsychologia, 24,* 410–433.

Deloche, G., Serion, X., Scius, G., & Segui, J. (1987). Right hemisphere language processing: Lateral difference with imageable and nonimageable ambiguous words. *Brain and Language, 30,* 197–205.

Denenberg, V. H. (1981). Hemispheric laterality in animals and the effects of early experience. *Behavioral Brain Sciences, 4,* 1–49.

Denes, G. Semenza, C., Stoppa, E., & Lis, A. (1982). Unilateral spatial neglect and recovery form hemiplegia. *Brain, 105,* 543–552.

Denny-Brown, D., Meyer, J. S., & Horenstein, S. (1952). The significance of perceptual rivalry resulting from parietal lobe lesion. *Brain, 75,* 433–471.

DeRenzi, E. (1982). *Disorder of space exploration and cognition.* New York: John Wiley & Sons.

DeRenzi, E. (1986). Prosopagnosia in two patients with CT-scan evidence of damage confined to the right hemisphere. *Neuropsychologia, 24,* 385–389.

DeRenzi, E., & Faglioni, P. (1965). The comparative efficiency of intelligence and vigilance tests in detecting hemisphere cerebral damage. *Cortex, 1,* 410–433.

DeRenzi, E., Faglioni, P., & Spinnler, H. (1968). The performance of patients with unilateral brain damage on face recognition tasks. *Cortex, 4,* 17–34.

DeRenzi, E., & Scotti, G., (1969). The influence of spatial disorders in impairing tactual discrimination of shapes. *Cortex, 5,* 53–62.

DeRenzi, E., Scotti, G., & Spinnler, H. (1969). Perceptual and associative disorders of visual recognition: Relationship to the side of the cerebral lesion. *Neurology (New York), 19,* 634–642.

DeRenzi, E., & Spinnler, H. (1966). Facial recognition in brain-damaged patients. An experimental approach. *Neurology (New York), 16,* 145–152.

DeRenzi, E., Zambolini, A., & Crisi, G. (1987). The pattern of neuropsychological impairment associated with left posterior cerebral artery infarcts. *Brain, 110,* 1099–1116.

Desmedt, J. E. (1977). Active touch exploration of extrapersonal space elicits specific electrogenesis in the right cerebral hemisphere of intact right-handed man. *Proceedings of the National Academy of Sciences (U.S.A.), 74,* 4037–4040.

DeUrso, V., Denes, G., Testa, S., & Semenza, C. (1986). The role of the right hemisphere in processing negative sentences in context. *Neuropsychologia, 24,* 289–292.

Dimond, S. J. (1980). *Neuropsychology.* London: Butterworths.

Dimond, S. J., & Beaumont, J. G. (1974). Experimental studies of hemisphere function in the human brain. In S. J. Dimond & J. G. Beaumont (Eds.), *Hemisphere function in the human brain* (pp. 77–110). New York: John Wiley & Sons.

Dimond, S. J., Gazzaniga, M. S., & Gibson, A. R. (1972). Cross field and within field integration of visual information. *Neuropsychologia, 10,* 379–381.

Dodds, A. G. (1978). Hemispheric differences in tactuo-spatial processing. *Neuropsychologia, 16,* 247–254.

Dollard, J., & Miller, N. E. (1950). *Personality and psychotherapy.* New York: McGraw-Hill.

Doty, R. W., & Overman, W. H. (1977). Mnemonic role of forebrain commissures in macaques. In S. Harnad, R. W. Doty, L. Goldstein, J. Jaynes, & G. Krauthamer, (Eds.), *Lateralization in the nervous system* (pp. 75–88). Orlando, FL: Academic Press.

Durant, W. (1939). *The life of Greece.* New York: Simon & Schuster.

Dwyer, J. W., & Rinn, W. E. (1981). The role of the right hemisphere in contextual inference. *Neuropsychologia, 19,* 479–482.

Efron, R. (1963). The effect of handedness on the perception of simultaneity and temporal order. *Brain, 86,* 261–284.

Ehrlichman, H. M., Antrobus, J. S., & Wiener, M. (1985). EEG assymetry and sleep mentation during REM and NREM. *Brain and Cognition, 4,* 477–485.

Ehrlichman, H., & Barrett, J. (1983). Right hemisphere specialization for mental imagery. A review of the evidence. *Brain and Cognition, 2,* 55–76.

Ellis, H. D., & Shepherd, J. W. (1975). Recognition of upright and inverted faces presented in the left and right visual fields. *Cortex, 11,* 3–7.

Erickson, T. (1945). Erotomania (nymphomania) as an expression of cortical epileptiform discharge. *Archives of Neurology and Psychiatry, 53,* 226–231.

Ettlinger, G. (1960). The description and interpretation of pictures in cases of brain lesion. *Journal of Mental Science, 106,* 1337–1346.

Ferro, J. M., Kertesz, A., & Black, S. E. (1987). Subcortical neglect. *Neurology (New York), 37,* 1487–1492.

Finlayson, M. A. J. (1975). A behavioral manifestation of the development of interhemispheric transfer of learning in children. *Cortex, 12,* 290–295.

Flor-Henry, P. (1983). *Cerebral basis of psychopathology.* Boston: John Wright.

Foldi, N. S., Cicone, M., & Gardner, H. (1983). Pragmatic aspects of communication in brain-damaged patients. In S. S. Segalowitz (Ed.), *Language functions and brain organization* (pp. 230–250). Orlando, FL: Academic Press.

Fontenot, D. J. (1973). Visual field differences in the recognition of verbal and nonverbal stimuli in man. *Journal of Comparative and Physiological Psychology, 85,* 564–569.

Fontenot, D. J., & Benton, A. L. (1971). Tactile perception of direction in relation to hemispheric locus of lesion. *Neuropsychologia, 9,* 83–88.

Forrest, D. V. (1982). Bipolar illness after right hemispherectomy. *Archives of General Psychiatry, 39* 817–819.

Foulkes, W. D. (1962). Dream reports from different stages of sleep. *Journal of Abnormal and Social Psychology, 65,* 14–25.

Franco, L., & Sperry, R. W. (1977). Hemispheric lateralization for cognitive processing of geometry. *Neuropsychologia, 15,* 107–111.

Freeman, W., & Watts, J. W. (1942). *Psychosurgery.* Springfield, IL: Charles C Thomas.

Freeman W., & Watts, J. W. (1943). Prefrontal lobotomy. *American Journal of Psychiatry, 99,* 798–806.

Freeman, W., & Williams, J. M. (1953). Hallucinations in Braille. *Archives of Neurology and Psychiatry, 70,* 630–634.

Freud, S. (1900). *The interpretation of dreams,* standard edition (Vol. 5). London: Hogarth Press.

Fried, I., Mateer, C., Ojemann, G., Wohns, R., & Fedio, P. (1982). Organization of visuospatial functions in human cortex. *Brain, 105,* 349–371.

Gainotti, G. (1972). Emotional behavior and hemispheric side of lesion. *Cortex, 8,* 41–55.

Gainotti, G., D'Erme, P., Monteleone, D., & Silveri, M. C. (1986). Mechanisms of unilateral spatial neglect in relation to laterality of cerebral lesions. *Brain, 109,* 599–612.

Gainotti, G., Messerlie, P., & Tissot, R. (1972). Qualitative analysis of unilateral neglect in relation to laterality of cerebral lesion. *Journal of Neurology, Neurosurgery and Psychiatry, 35,* 545–550.

Galin, D. (1974). Implications for psychiatry of left and right cerebral specialization. *Archives of General Psychiatry, 31,* 572–583.

Galin, D., Diamond, D. R., & Braff, D. (1977). Lateralization of conversion symptoms: More frequent on the left. *American Journal of Psychiatry, 134,* 578–580.

Galin, D., Diamond, R., & Herron, J. (1979). Development of crossed and uncrossed tactile localization on the fingers. *Brain and Language, 4,* 588–590.

Galin, D., Johnstone, J., Nakell, L., & Herron, J. (1979). Development of the capacity for tactile information transfer between hemispheres in normal children. *Science, 204,* 1330–1332.

Gardner, H. (1975). *The shattered mind.* New York: Vintage Books.

Gardner, H., Brownell, H. H., Wapner, W., & Michelow, D. (1983). Missing the point: The role of the right hemisphere in the processing of complex linguistic materials. In E. Perceman (Ed.), *Cognitive processing in the right hemisphere* (pp. 201–244). Orlando, FL: Academic Press.

Gardner, H., Ling, P. K., Flamm, L., & Silverman, J. (1975). Comprehension and appreciation of humorus material following brain damage. *Brain, 98,* 399–412.

Gasparrini, W. G., Satz, P., Heilman, K. M., & Coolidge, F. L. (1978). Hemispheric asymmetry of affective processing as determined by the MMPI. *Journal of Neurology Neurosurgery and Psychiatry, 41,* 470–473.

Gates, A., & Bradshaw, J. L. (1977). The role of the cerebral hemispheres in music. *Brain and language, 3,* 451–460.

Gazzaniga, M. S. (1970). *The bisected brain.* E. Norwalk, CT: Appleton & Lange.

Gazzaniga, M. S., & LeDoux, J. E. (1978). *The integrated mind.* New York: Plenum Press.

Geffen, G., Bradshaw, J. L., & Wallace, G. (1971). Interhemispheric effects on reaction time to verbal and nonverbal visual stimuli. *Journal of Experimental Psychology 87,* 415–422.

Geschwind, N. (1965). Disconnexion syndromes in animals and man. *Brain, 88,* 585–644.

Geschwind, N. (1981). The perverseness of the right hemisphere. *Behavioral and Brain Sciences, 4,* 106–107.

Goldstein, K. (1942). *After effects of brain injuries in war.* Orlando, FL: Grune & Stratton.

Goldstein, L., Stoltzfus, N. W., & Gardocki, J. F. (1972). Changes in interhemispheric amplitude relationships in the EEG during sleep. *Physiology and Behavior, 8,* 811–815.

Goodenough, D. R., Shapiro, A., Holden, M., & Steinschriber, R. (1959). Comparison of "dreamers" and "non-dreamers." *Journal of Nervous and Mental Disease, 59,* 295–302.

Goodglass, H., & Berko, J. (1960). Agrammatism and inflectional morphology in English. *Journal of Speech and Hearing Research, 3,* 257–267.

Goodglass, H., & Kaplan, E. (1972). *Boston diagnostic aphasia examination.* Philadelphia: Lea & Febiger.

Gordon, H. W. (1970). Hemispheric asymmetries in the perception of musical chords. *Cortex, 6,* 387–398.

Gordon, H. W., & Bogen, J. E. (1974). Hemispheric lateralization of singing after intracarotid sodium amylobarbitone. *Journal of Neurology, Neurosurgery and Psychiatry, 37,* 727–737.

Gordon, H. W., Frooman, B., & Lavie, P. (1982). Shift in cognitive asymmetries between wakings from REM and NREM sleep. *Neuropsychologia, 20,* 99–103.

Gorelick, P. B., & Ross, E. D. (1987). *Journal of Neurology, Neurosurgery and Psychiatry, 37,* 727–737.

Greenberg, M. S., & Farah, M. J. (1986). The laterality of dreaming. *Brain and Cognition, 5,* 307–321.

Greenwood, P., Wilson, D. H., & Gazzaniga, M. S. (1977). Dream report following commissurotomy. *Cortex, 13,* 311–316.

Gruzelier, J., & Manchanda, R. (1982). The syndrome of schizophrenia: Relations between elecrodermal response, lateral asymmetries and clinical rating. *British Journal of Psychiatry, 141,* 488–495.

Halperin, Y., Nachshon, I., & Carmon, A. (1973). Shift of ear superiority in dichotic listening to temporally patterned nonverbal stimuli. *Journal of Experimental Psychology, 101,* 46–54.

Hannay, H. J., Falgout, J. C., Leli, D. A., Katholi, C. R., Halsey, J. H., & Wills, E. L. (1987). Focal right temporo-occipital blood flow changes associated with judgment of line orientation. *Neuropsychologia, 25,* 755–763.

Hartshorne, C. (1973). *Born to sing. An interpretation and world survey of bird songs.* London: Indiana University Press.

Haslam, D. R. (1970). Lateral dominance in the perception of size and pain. *Quarterly Journal of Experimental Psychology, 22,* 503–507.

Hatta, T. (1978) The functional asymmetry of tactile pattern learning in normal subjects. *Psychologia, 21,* 83–89.

Head, H., & Holmes, G. (1911). Sensory disturbances from cerebral lesions. *Brain, 34,* 102–254.

Hecaen, H. (1962). Clinical symtamology in right and left hemispheric lesions. In V. B. Mountcastle (Ed.), *Interhemispheric relations and cerebral dominance* (pp. 122–140). Baltimore: Johns Hopkins Press.

Hecaen, H. (1964). Mental changes associated with tumors of the frontal lobes. In J. M. Warren & K. Akert (Eds.), *The frontal granular cortex and behavior* (pp. 335–352). New York: McGraw-Hill.

Hecaen, H., & Albert, M. L. (1978). *Human neuropsychology,* New York: John Wiley & Sons.

Hecaen, H., & Angelergues, R. (1962). Agnosia for faces (prospagnosia). *Archives of Neurology, 7,* 92–100.

Hecaen, H., & Assal, G. (1970). A comparison of construction deficits following right and left hemisphere lesions. *Neuropsychologia, 8,* 289–304.

Heilman, K. M. (1979). Neglect and related disorders. In K. M. Heilman & E. Valenstein (Eds.), *Clinical neuropsychology* (pp. 300–320). New York: Oxford University Press.

Heilman, K. M., Bowers, D., Speedie, L., & Coslett, H. B. (1984). Comprehension of affective and nonaffective prosody. *Neurology (New York), 34,* 917–921.

Heilman, K. M., Rothi, L., & Kertesz, A. (1983). Localization of apraxia-producing lesions. In A. Kertesz (Ed.), *Localization in neuropsychology* (pp. 180–200). Orlando, FL, Academic Press.

Heilman, K., & Scholes, R. J. (1976). The nature of comprehension errors in Broca's conduction, and Wernicke's aphasia. *Cortex, 12,* 258–265.

Heilman, K., Scholes, R., & Watson, R. T. (1975). Auditory affective agnosia. *Journal of Neurology, Neurosurgery and Psychiatry, 38,* 69–72.

Heilman, K. M., Schwartz, H. D., & Watson, R. T. (1978). Hypoarousal in patients with a neglect syndrome and emotional indifference. *Neurology (New York), 28,* 229–232.

Heilman, K. M., & Van Den Abell, T. (1979). Right hemispheric dominance for mediating cerebral activation. *Neuropsychologia, 17,* 315–322.

Heilman, K. M., Watson, R. T., Valenstein, E., & Damasio, A. R. (1983). Localization of lesions in neglect. In A. Kertesz (Ed.), *Localization in neuropsychology* (pp. 150–180). Orlando, FL: Academic Press.

Heller, W., & Levy, J. (1981). Perception and expression of emotion in right-handers and left-handers. *Neuropsychologia, 19,* 263–272.

Hellige, J. B., & Webster, R. (1979). Right hemisphere superiority for initial stages of letter processing. *Neuropsychologia, 17,* 653–660.

Helm-Estabrooks, N. (1983). Exploiting the right hemisphere for language rehabilitation: Melodic intonation therapy. In E. Perecman (Ed.), *Cognitive processing in the right hemisphere* (pp. 165–190). Orlando, FL: Academic Press.

Hermelin, B., & O'Connor, N. (1971). Functional asymmetry in reading of Braille. *Neuropsychologia, 9,* 431–435.

Hernandez-Peon, R., Chavez-Iberra, G., & Aguilar-Figuerua, E. (1963). Somatic evoked potentials in one case of hysterical anesthesia. *Electroencephalography and Clinical Neurophysiology, 15,* 889–896.

Hier, D. B., Mondlock, J., & Caplan, L. R. (1983). Behavioral abnormalities after right hemisphere stroke. *Neurology (New York), 33,* 337–344.

Hillbom, E. (1960). After-effects of brain injuries. *Acta Psychiatrica Scandinavica, 142* (suppl.).

Hines, D. (1976). Recognition of verbs, abstract nouns and concrete nouns from the left and right visual half-fields. *Neuropsychologia, 14,* 211–216.

Hobhouse, N., (1936). Prognosis in hemiplegia in middle life. *Lancet, 1,* 327–328.

Hobson, J. A., Lydic, R., & Baghdoyan, H. A. (1986). Evolving concepts of sleep cycle generation: From brain centers to neuronal populations. *Behavioral and Brain Sciences, 9,* 371–448.

Hodoba, D. (1986). Paradoxic sleep facilitation by interictal epileptic activity of right temporal origin. *Biological Psychiatry, 21,* 1267–1278.

Hom, J., & Reitan, R. (1982). Effects of lateralized cerebral damage on contalster and ipsilateral sensorimotor performance. *Journal of Clinical Neuropsychology, 3,* 47–53.

Hoppe, K. D. (1977). Split brains and psychoanalysis. *Psychoanalytic Quarterly, 46,* 220–244.

Hoppe, K. D., & Bogen, J. E. (1977). Alexithymia in twelve commissurotomized patients. *Psychotherapy and Psychosomatics, 28,* 148–155.

Howes, D., & Boller, F. (1975). Simple reaction times: Evidence for focal impairment from lesions of the right hemisphere. *Brain, 98,* 317–322.

Humphrey, M. E., & Zangwill, O. L. (1951). Cessation of dreaming after brain injury. *Journal of Neurology, Neurosurgery and Psychiatry, 14,* 322–325.

Hurwitz, L. J., & Adams, G. F. (1972). Rehabilitation of hemiplegia: Indices of assessment and prognosis. *British Medical Journal, 1,* 94–98.

Jack, R. A., Rivers-Bulkeley, N. T., & Rabin, P. L. (1983). Secondary mania as a presentation of progressive dialysis encephalopathy. *Journal of Nervous and Mental Disease, 171,* 193–195.

Jamieson, R. C., & Wells, C. E. (1979). Manic psychosis in a patient with multiple metastic brain tumours. *Journal of Clinical Psychiatry, 40,* 280–282.

Jampala, V. C., & Abrams, R. (1983). Mania secondary to right and left hemisphere damage. *American Journal of Psychiatry, 140,* 1197–1199.

Jeannerod, M. (1987). *Neurophysiological and neuropsychological aspects of spatial neglect.* New York: North-Holland.

Joseph, R. (1980). Awareness, the origin of thought and the role of conscious self-deception in resistance and repression. *Psychological Reports, 46,* 767–781.

Joseph, R. (1982). The neuropsychology of development: Hemispheric laterality, limbic language and the origin of thought. *Journal of Clinical Psychology, 38,* 4–33.

Joseph, R. (1986a). Confabulation and elusional denial: Frontal lobe and lateralized influences. *Journal of Clinical Psychology, 42,* 507–518.

Joseph, R. (1986b). Reversal of cerebral dominance for language and emotion in a corpus callosotomy patient. *Journal of Neurology, Neurosurgery and Psychiatry, 49,* 628–634.

Joseph, R. (1988a). The right cerebral hemisphere. *Journal of Clinical Psychology, 44,* 630–673.

Joseph, R. (1988b). Dual mental functioning in a split-brain patient. *Journal of Clinical Psychology, 44,* 770–779.

Joseph, R., & Casangrande, V. A. (1980). Visual deficits and recovery following monocular lid closure in a prosimian primate. *Behavioral Brain Research, 1,* 165–186.

Joseph, R., & Gallagher, R. E. (1980). Gender and early environmental influences on activity, overresponsiveness, and exploration. *Developmental Psychobiology, 13,* 527–544.

Joseph, R., & Gallagher, R. E. (1985). Interhemispheric transfer and the completion of reversible operations in non-conserving children. *Journal of Clinical Psychology, 41,* 796–800.

Joseph, R., Gallagher, R. E., Holloway, W., & Kahn, J. (1984). Two brains—one child. Interhemispheric transfer deficits and confabulation in children aged 3,7,10. *Cortex, 20,* 317–331.

Joseph, R., Hess, S., & Birecree, E. (1978). Effects of sex hormone manipulations and exploration on sex differences in learning. *Behavioral Biology, 24,* 364–377.

Jung, C. G. (1945). On the nature of dreams (translated by R. F. C. Hull.), *The collected works of C. G. Jung* (pp. 473–507). Princeton, NJ: Princeton University Press.

Jung, C. G. (1964). *Man and his symbols.* New York: Dell.

Kamiya, J. (1961). Behavioral, subjective and physiological aspects of drowsiness and sleep. In D. W. Fiske, & S. R. Maddi (Eds.), *Function of varied experience* (pp. 145–174). Homewood, IL: Dorsey Press.

Kerr, N. H., & Foulkes, D. (1978). Reported absence of visual dream imagery in a normally sighted subject with Turner's syndrome. *Journal of Mental Imagery, 2,* 247–264.

Kerr, N. H., & Foulkes, D. (1981). Right hemisphere mediation of dream visualization: A case study. *Cortex, 17,* 603–611.

Kertesz, A. (1983a). Localization of lesions in Wernicke's aphasia. In A. Kertesz (Ed.), *Localization in neuropsychology* (pp. 150–170). Orlando, FL: Academic Press.

Kertesz, A. (1983b). Right-hemisphere lesions in constructional apraxia and visuospatial deficit. In A. Kertesz (Ed.), *Localization in neuropsychology* (pp. 301–313). Orlando, FL: Academic Press.

Kim, Y., Morrow, L., Passafiume, D., & Boller, F. (1984). Visuoperceptual and visuomotor abilities and locus of lesion. *Neuropsychologia, 2,* 177–185.

Kimura, D. (1961). Cerebral dominance and the perception of verbal stimuli. *Canadian Journal of Psychology, 15,* 156–171.

Kimura, D. (1963). Right temporal lobe damage: perception of unfamiliar stimuli after damage. *Archives of Neurology, 18,* 264–271.

Kimura, D. (1964). Left–right differences in the perception of melodies. *Quarterly Journal of Psychology, 16,* 355–358.

Kimura, D. (1966). Dual functional asymmetry of the brain in visual perception. *Neuropsychologia, 4,* 275–285.

Kimura, D. (1969). Spatial localization in left and right visual fields. *Canadian Journal of Psychology, 23,* 445–448.

Kimura, D. (1977). Acquisition of motor skill after left-hemisphere damage. *Brain, 100,* 527–542.

King, F. L., & Kimura, D. (1972). Left ear superiority in dichtoic perception of vocal nonverbal sounds. *Canadian Journal of Psychology, 26,* 111–116.

Klein, R., & Armitage, R. (1979). Rhythms in human performance: 1-1/2 hour oscillations in cognitive style. *Science, 204,* 1326–1328.

Knapp, M. E. (1959). Problems in rehabilitation of the hemiplegic patient. *Journal of the American Medical Association, 169,* 224–229.

Knox, C., & Kimura, D. (1970). Cerebral processing of nonverbal sounds in boys and girls. *Neuropsychologia, 8,* 227–237.

Kraft, R. H., Mitchell, O. R., Languis, M. L., & Wheatley, G. H. (1980). Hemispheric asymmetries during six-to-eight year-olds' performance on Piagetian conservation and reading tasks. *Neuropsychologia, 18,* 637–644.

Kramer, M., Whitman, R. M., Baldridge, B. J., & Lansky, L. M. (1964). Patterns of dreaming: The interrelationship of the dreams of a night. *Journal of Nervous and Mental Disease, 139,* 426–439.

Kripke, D. F., & Sonnenschein, D. (1973). A 90 minute daydream cycle. *Sleep Research, 2,* 187–188.

Lackner, J. L., & Teuber, H.-L. (1973). Alterations in auditory fusion thresholds after cerebral injury in man. *Neuropsychologia, 11,* 409–415.

Landis, T., Assal, G., & Perrot, E. (1979). Opposite cerebral hemisphere superiorities for visual associative processing of emotional facial expressions and objects. *Nature (London)*, *278*, 739–740.

Landis, T., Cummings, J. L., Christen, L., Bogen, J. E., & Imhof, H.-G. (1986). Are unilateral right posterior cerebral lesions sufficient to cause prospagnosia? Clinical and radiological findings in six additional patients. *Cortex*, *22*, 243–252.

Landis, T., Graves, R., & Goodglass, H. (1982). Aphasic reading and writing: possible evidence for right hemisphere participation. *Cortex*, *18*, 105–112.

Langmeier, J., & Matejcek, Z. (1975). *Psychological deprivation in childhood*. New York: John Wiley & Sons.

Lansdell, H. (1968). Extent of temporal lobe ablations on two lateralized deficits. *Physiology and Behavior*, *3*, 271–273.

Lansdell, H. (1970). Relation of extent of temporal removal to closure and visuomotor factors. *Perceptual and Motor Skills*, *31*, 491–498.

Lebrun, Y. (1987). Anosognosia in aphasics. *Cortex*, *23*, 251–263.

Leicester, J., Sidman, M., Stoddard, L. T., & Mohr, J. P. (1969). Some determinants of visual neglect. *Journal of Neurology, Neurosurgery and Psychiatry*, *32*, 580–587.

Lenneberg, E. (1967). *Biological foundations of language*. New York: John Wiley & Sons.

Levine, D. N. (1978). Prosopagnosia and visual object agnosia: A behavioral study. *Brain and Language*, *5*, 341–365.

Levine, D. N., & Sweet, E. (1983). Localization of lesions in Broca's motor aphasia. In A. Kertesz (Ed.), *Localization in neuropsychology* (pp. 185–207). Orlando, FL: Academic Press.

Levy, J. (1974). Psychological implications of bilateral asymmetry. In S. Dimond & J. G. Beaumont (Eds.), *Hemisphere function in the human brain* (pp. 121–183). London: Paul Elek.

Levy, J. (1983). Language, cognition and the right hemisphere. *American Psychologist*, *38*, 538–541.

Levy, J., & Trevarthen, C. (1976). Metacontrol of hemispheric function in human split-brain patients. *Journal of Experimental Psychology: Human perception and Performance*, *2*, 299–312.

Levy, J., Trevarthen, C., & Sperry, R. W. (1972). Perception of bilateral chimeric figures following hemispheric deconnection. *Brain*, *95*, 61–78.

Ley, R. G. (1980). An archival examination of an asymmetry of hysterical conversion symptoms. *Journal of Clinical Neuropsychology*, *2*, 1–9.

Ley, R. G., & Bryden, M. P. (1979). Hemispheric differences in processing emotions and faces. *Brain and Language*, *7*, 127–138.

Lishman, W. A. (1968), Brain damage in relation to psychiatry disability after head injury. *British Journal of Psychiatry*, *114*, 373–410.

Luria, A. (1973). *The working brain*. New York: Basic Books.

Luria, A. (1980). *Higher cortical functions in man*. New York: Basic Books.

Mahoney, A. M., & Sainsbury, R. S. (1987). Hemispheric asymmetry in the perception of emotional sounds. *Brain and Cognition*, *6*, 216–233.

Mannhaupt, H. R. (1983). Processing of abstract and concrete nouns in lateralized memory-search tasks. *Psychological Research*, *45*, 91–105.

Marquardsen, J. (1969). The natural history of acute cerebrovascular disease. *Acta Neurologica Scandinavica* *45* (suppl.), 1–133.

Marzi, C. A. (1986). Transfer of visual information after unilateral input to the brain. *Brain and Cognition*, *5*, 163–173.

Marzi, I. A., & Berlucchi, G. (1977). Right visual field superiority for accuracy of recognition of famous faces in normals. *Neuropsychologia*, *15*, 751–756.

Mateer, C. A. (1983). Motor and perceptual functions of the left hemisphere and their interaction. In S. J. Segalowitz (Ed). *Language functions and brain organization* (pp. 80–110). Orlando, FL: Academic Press.

McClain, E. G. (1978). *The Pythagorian Plato*. Denver, CO: Great Eastern Books.

McFarland, H. R., & Fortin, D. (1982). Amusia due to right temporal-parietal infarct. *Archives of Neurology*, *39*, 725–727.

McFie, J., & Zangwill, O. L. (1960). Visual-constructive disabilities associated with lesions of the left cerebral hemisphere. *Brain*, *83*, 243–260.

Meador, K. J., Loring, D. W., Bowers, D., & Heilman, K. M. (1987). Remote memory and neglect syndrome. *Neurology (New York)*, *37*, 522–526.

Mehta, Z., Newcombe, F., & Damasio, H. (1987). A left hemisphere contribution to visiospatial processing. *Cortex*, *23*, 447–461.

Merriam, A. E., & Gardner, E. B. (1987). Corpus callosum function in schizophrenia: A neuropsychological assessment of interhemispheric information processing. *Neuropsychologia, 25,* 185–193.

Meyer, J. S., Ishikawa, Y., Hata, T., & Karacan, I. (1987). Cerebral blood flow in normal and abnormal sleep and dreaming. *Brain and Cognition, 6,* 266–294.

Miller, L. (1984). Neuropsychological conceptus of somatoform disorders. *International Journal of Psychiatry in Medicine, 14,* 31–46.

Miller, L. (in press). On the neuropsychology of dreams. *Psychoanalytic Review.*

Mills, L., & Rollman, G. B. (1980). Hemispheric asymmetry for auditory perception of temporal order. *Neuropsychologia, 18,* 41–47.

Milner, B. (1962). Laterality effect in audition. In V. Mountcastle, (Ed.), *Interhemispheric relations and cerebral dominance* (pp. 173–201). Baltimore: John Hopkins University Press.

Milner, B. (1964). Some effects of frontal lobectomy in man. In J. M. Warren & K. Akert (Eds.), *The frontal granular cortext and behavior* (pp. 313–334). New York: McGraw-Hill.

Milner, B. (1968). Visual recognition and recall after right temporal lobe excision in man. *Neuropsychologia, 6,* 191–209.

Milner, B. (1970). Memory and the medial temporal regions of the brain. In K. Pribram & D. E. Broadbent (Eds.) *Biology of memory.* New York: Academic Press.

Molfese, D., Freeman, R. B., & Palermo, D. S. (1975). The ontogeny of brain lateralization for speech and nonspeech stimuli. *Brain and Language, 2,* 356–368.

Monrad-Krohn, G. (1963). Prosody and its disorders. In L. Halpern (Ed.), *Problems of dynamic neurology* (pp. 237–291). Jerusalem: Jerusalem Post Press.

Monroe, B., Rechtschaffen, A., Foulkes, D., & Jensen, J. (1965). Discriminability of REM and NREM reports. *Personality and Social Psychology, 2,* 456–460.

Motomura, N., Yamadori, A., Mori, E., Ogura, J., Sakai, T., & Sawada, T. (1986). Unilateral spatial neglect due to hemorrhage in the thalamic region. *Acta Neurologica Scandinavica, 74,* 190–194.

Murray, F. S., & Hagan, B. C. (1973). Pain threshold and tolerance of hands and feet. *Journal of Comparative and Physiological Psychology, 84,* 639–643.

Murri, L., Arena, R., Siciliano, G., Mazzotta, R., & Muratorio, A. (1984). Dream recall in patients with focal cerebral lesions. *Archives of Neurology, 41,* 183–185.

Myers, R. E. (1959). Interhemispheric communication through the corpus callosum: Limitations under conditions of conflict. *Journal of Comparative and Physiological Psychology, 52,* 6–9.

Nathanson, M., Bergman, P. S., & Gordon, G. G. (1952). Denial of illness. *Archives of Neurology and Psychiatry, 68,* 380–387.

Nebes, R. B. (1971). Handedness and the perception of whole-part relationship. *Cortex, 7,* 350–356.

Nielsen, J. M. (1937). Unilateral cerebral dominance as related to mind blindness: Minimal lesions capable of causing visual agnosia for objects. *Archives of Neurology and Psychiatry, 38,* 108–135.

Neilsen, J. M. (1946). *Agnosia, apraxia, aphasia. Their value in cerebral localization.* New York: Hoeber.

Njiokiktjien, C. (1988). *Pediatric behavioural neurology.* Amsterdam: Suyi.

Offen, M. L., Davidoff, R. A., Troost, B. T., & Richey, E. T. (1976). Dacrystic epilepsy. *Journal of Neurology, Neurosurgery and Psychiatry, 39,* 829–834.

O'Leary, D. S. (1980). A developmental study of interhemispheric transfer in children aged 5 to 10. *Child Development, 51,* 743–750.

Oppler, W. (1950). Manic psychosis in a case of parasagittal meningioma. *Archives of Neurology and Psychiatry, 47,* 417–430.

Otto, M. W., Yeo, R. A., & Dougher, M. J. (1987). Right hemisphere involvement in depression: Toward a neuropsychological theory of negative affective experiences. *Biological Psychiatry, 22,* 1201–1215.

Patterson, K., & Bradshaw, J. L. (1975). Differential hemispheric mediation of nonverbal visual stimuli. *Journal of Experimental Psychology: Human Perception and Performance, 1,* 246–252.

Pena-Casanova, J., & Roig-Rovira, T. (1985). Optic aphasia, optic apraxia, and loss of dreaming. *Brain and Language, 26,* 63–71.

Penfield, W., & Perot, P. (1963). The brain's record of auditory and visual experience. *Brain, 86,* 595–696.

Piaget, J. (1952). *The origins of intelligence in children.* New York: Norton.

Piaget, J. (1962). *Play, dreams and imitation in childhood.* New York: Norton.

Piaget, J. (1974). *The child and reality.* New York: Viking Press.

Piazza, D. M. (1980). The influence of sex and handedness in the hemispheric specialization of verbal and nonverbal tasks. *Neuropsychologia, 18,* 163–176.

Piercy, M., Hecaen, H., & Ajuriaguerra, J. (1960). Constructional apraxia associated with unilateral cerebral lesions—left and right sided cases compared. *Brain, 83,* 225–242.

Poeck, K., Kerschensteiner, M., Hartje, W., & Orgass, B. (1973). Impairment in visual recognition of geometric figures in patients with circumscribed retrorolandic brain lesions. *Neuropsychologia, 11,* 311–319.

Redlich, F. C., & Dorsey, J. E. (1945). Denial of blindness by patients with cerebral disease. *Archives of Neurology and Psychiatry, 53,* 407–417.

Reese, H. H. (1948). The relation of music to diseases of the brain. *Occupational Therapy and Rehabilitation, 27,* 12–18.

Risse, G. L., & Gazzaniga, M. S. (1979). Well-kept secrets of the right hemisphere: A carotid amytal study of restricted memory transfer. *Neurology (New York), 28,* 950–953.

Rizzolatti, G., Umilta, C., & Berlucchi, G. (1971). Opposite superiorities of the right and left cerebral hemispheres in discriminative reaction time to physiognomical and alphabetical material. *Brain, 94,* 431–442.

Robinson, R. G., & Benson, D. F. (1981). Depression in aphasic patients: Frequency, severity, and clinical–pathological correlations. *Brain and Language, 14,* 282–291.

Robinson, R. G., Kubos, K. L., Starr, L. B., Rao, K., & Price, T. R. (1984). Mood disorders in stroke patients. *Brain, 107,* 81–93.

Robinson, R. G., & Szetela, B. (1981). Mood change following left hemisphere brain injury. *Annals of Neurology, 9,* 447–453.

Rogart, R. B., & Ritchie, J. M. (1977). Pathophysiology of conduction in demyelinated nerve fibers. In P. Morell (Ed.), *Myelin* (pp. 144–288). New York: Plenum Press.

Roland, P. E., Skinhoj, E., & Lassen, N. A. (1981). Focal activation of human cerebral cortex during auditory discrimination. *Journal of Neurophysiology, 45,* 1139–1150.

Rosenbaum, A. H., & Berry, M. J. (1975). Positive therapeutic response to lithium in hypomania secondary to organic brain syndrome. *American Journal of Psychiatry, 132,* 1072–1073.

Ross, E. (1981). The aprosodias: Functional-anatomic organization of the affective components of language in the right hemisphere. *Archives of Neurology, 38,* 561–589.

Roth, M. (1949). Disorders of the body image caused by lesions of the right parietal lobe. *Brain, 72,* 89–111.

Roth, N. (1944). Unusual types of anosognosia and their relation to the body-image. *Journal of Nervous and Mental Disease, 100,* 35–43.

Ruff, R. L. (1980). Orgasmic epilepsy. *Neurology (New York), 30,* 1252–1253.

Sackheim, H. A., & Gur, R. C. (1978). Lateral asymmetry in intensity of emotional expression. *Neuropsychologia, 16,* 473–481.

Sackheim, H. A., Gur, R. C., & Saucy, M. C. (1978). Emotions are expressed more intensely on the left side of the face. *Science, 202,* 424–435.

Safer, M., & Leventhal, H. (1977). Ear differences in evaluating emotional tones and verbal content. *Journal of Experimental Psychology, Human Perception and Performance, 3,* 75–82.

Salamy, A. (1978). Commissural transmission: Maturational changes in humans. *Science, 200,* 1409–1411.

Sandifer, P. H. (1946). Anosognosia and disorders of body scheme. *Brain, 69,* 122–137.

Schanfald, D., Pearlman, C., & Greenberg, R. (1985). The capacity of stroke patients to report dreams. *Cortex, 21,* 237–247.

Schwartz, G. E., Davidson, R. J., & Maer, F. (1975). Right hemisphere lateralization for emotion in the human brain: Interaction with cognition. *Science, 190,* 286–288.

Segalowitz, S. J., & Plantery, P. (1985). Music draws attention to the left and speech draws attention to the right. *Brain and Cognition, 4,* 1–6.

Selnes, O. A. (1974). The corpus callosum: Some anatomical and functional considerations with special reference to language. *Brain and Language, 1,* 111–139.

Semmes, J., Weinstein, S., Ghent, L., & Teuber, H. L. (1960). *Somatosensory changes after penetrating head wounds in man.* Cambridge, MA: Harvard University Press.

Shankweiler, D., & Studdert-Kennedy, M. (1966). Lateral differences in perception of dichotically presented synthetic consonant–vowel syllables and steady-state vowels. *Journal of the Acoustic Society of America, 39,* 1256A.

Shankweiler, D., & Studdert-Kennedy, M. (1967). Identification of consonants and vowels presented to left and right ears. *Quarterly Journal of Experimental Psychology, 19,* 59–63.

Shapiro, B. E., Alexander, M. P., Gardner, H., & Mercer, B. (1981). Mechanisms of confabulation. *Neurology (New York)*, *31*, 1070–1076.

Shapiro, B. E., & Danly, M. (1985). The role of the right hemisphere in the control of speech prosody in propositional and affective contexts. *Brain and Language*, *1*, 111–139.

Sherwin, I., Peron-Magnan, P., & Bancaud, J. (1982). Prevalence of psychosis in epilepsy as a function of the laterality of the epileptogenic lesion. *Archives of Neurology*, *39*, 621–625.

Silberman, E. K., & Weingartner, H. (1986). Hemispheric lateralization of functions related to emotion. *Brain and Cognition*, *5*, 322–353.

Silverberg R., Bentin, S., Gaziel, T., Obler, L. K., & Albert, M. L. (1979). Shift of visual field preference for English words in native Hebrew speakers. *Brain and Language*, *8*, 184–190.

Sinyour, D., Jacques, P., Kaloupek, D. G., Becker, R., Goldenberg, M., & Coopersmith, H. (1986). Poststroke depression and lesion location. *Brain*, *109*, 537–546.

Smith, A. (1966). Speech and other functions after left (dominant) hemispherectomy. *Journal of Neurology, Neurosurgery and Psychiatry*, *29*, 467–471.

Smith, A., & Burklund, C. W. (1966). Dominant hemispherectomy. *Science*, *153*, 1280–1282.

Spellacy, F. (1970). Lateral preference in the identification of patterned stimuli. *Journal of the Acoustical Society of America*, *47*, 574–578.

Spencer, S. S., Spencer, D. D., Williamson, P. D., & Mattson, R. H. (1983). Sexual automatisms in complex partial seizures. *Neurology (New York)*, *33*, 527–533.

Sperry, R. (1966). Brain bisection and the neurology of consciousness. In J. C. Eccles (Ed). *Brain and conscious experience* (pp. 298–313). New York: Springer-Verlag.

Sperry, R. (1974). Lateral specialization in the surgically separated hemispheres. In F. O. Schmitt & F. G. Worlden (Eds.), *The neurosciences: Third study program* (pp. 1–12). Cambridge, MA: MIT Press.

Sperry, R. (1982). Some effects of disconnecting the cerebral hemispheres. *Science*, *217*, 1223–1226.

Sperry, R. W., Zaidel, E., & Zaidel, D. (1979). Self recognition and social awareness in the deconnected minor hemisphere. *Neuropsychologia*, *17*, 153–166.

Spreen, O., Benton, A. L., & Fincham, R. W. (1965). Auditory agnosia without aphasia. *Archives of Neurology*, *13*, 84–92.

Starkstein, S. E., Pearlson, G. E., Boston, J., & Robinson, R. G. (1987). Mania after brain injury. *Archives of Neurology*, *44*, 1069–1073.

Stern, D. B. (1977). Handedness and the lateral distribution of conversion reactions. *Journal of Nervous and Mental Disease*, *164*, 122–130.

Stern, K., & Dancy, T. (1942). Glioma of the diencephalon in a manic patient. *American Journal of Psychiatry*, *98*, 716.

Strauss, E., & Moscovitch, M. (1981). Perception of facial expressions. *Brain and Language*, *13*, 308–332.

Studdert-Kennedy, M., & Shankweiler, D. (1970). Hemispheric specialization for speech perception. *Journal of the Acoustical Society of America*, *48*, 579–594.

Stuss, D. T., Alexander, M. P., Lieberman, A., & Levine, H. (1978). An extraordinary form of confabulation. *Neurology (New York)*, *28*, 1166–1172.

Suberi, M., & McKeever, W. F. (1977). Differential right hemispheric memory storage of emotional and non-emotional faces. *Neuropsychologia*, *5*, 757–768.

Sweet, W. H. (1945). Intracranial aneurysm simulating neoplasm. Syndrome of the corpus callosum. *Archives of Neurology and Psychiatry*, *45*, 86–103.

Swisher, L. P., Dudley, J. G., & Doehring, D. G. (1969). Influence of contralateral noise on auditory intensity discrimination. *Journal of Acoustical Society of America*, *45*, 1532–1536.

Teuber, H.-L., & Weinstein, S. (1956). Ability to discover hidden-figures after cerebral lesions. *Archives of Neurology and Psychiatry*, *76*, 369–379.

Tucker, D. (1981). Lateral brain function, emotion, and conceptualization *Psychological Bulletin*, *89*, 19–46.

Tucker, D., Watson, R. T., & Heilman, K. M. (1977). Affective discrimination and evocation of affectively toned speech in patients with right parietal disease. *Neurology (New York)*, *27*, 947–950.

Tsunoda, T. (1975). Functional differences between right- and left-cerebral hemispheres detected by the key-tapping method. *Brain and Language*, *2*, 152–170.

Vignolo, L. A. (1983). Modality-specific disorders of written language. In A. Kertesz (Ed.), *Localization in neuropsychology* (pp. 357–370). Orlando, FL: Academic Press.

Wapner, W., Hamby, S., & Gardner, H. (1981). The role of the right hemisphere in the apprehension of complex linguistic materials. *Brain and Language, 14,* 15–33.

Warrington, E. K., James, M., & Maciejewski, C. (1986). The WAIS as a lateralizing and localizing instrument: A case study of 656 patients with unilateral cerebral lesions. *Neuropsychologia, 24,* 223–239.

Watson, R. T., Valenstein, E., & Heilman, K. M. (1981). Thalamic neglect: The possible role of the medial thalamus and nucleus reticularis in behavior. *Archives of Neurology, 38,* 501–506.

Wechsler, A. F. (1973). The effect of organic brain disease on recall of emotionally charged versus neutral narrative texts. *Neurology (New York), 23,* 130–135.

Weinstein, E. A., & Sersen, E. A. (1961). Tactual sensitivity as a function of handedness and laterality. *Journal of Comparative and Physiological Psychology, 54,* 665–669.

Weinstein, E. A., & Kahn, R. L. (1950). The syndrome of anosognosia. *Archives of Neurology and Psychiatry, 64,* 772–791.

Weinstein, E. A., & Kahn, R. L. (1952). Non-aphasic misnaming (paraphasia) in organic brain disease. *Archives of Neurology and Psychiatry, 67,* 72–78.

Weinstein, S. (1978). Functional cerebral hemispheric asymmetry. In M. Kinsbourne (Ed.), *Asymmetrical function of the brain* (pp. 17–48). New York: Cambridge University Press.

Weintraub, S., Mesulam, M.-M., & Kramer, L. (1981). Disturbances in prosody: A right hemisphere contribution to language. *Archives of Neurology, 38,* 742–744.

Wertheim, N. (1969). The amusias. In P. J. Vinkin & G. W. Bruyn (Eds.), *Handbook of clinical neurology* (Vol. 4, pp. 195–206). Amsterdam: North-Holland.

Whitehouse, P. J. (1981). Imagery and verbal encoding in left and right hemisphere damage patients. *Brain and Language, 14,* 315–332.

Whiteley, A. M., & Warrington, E. K. (1977). Prosopagnosia: A clinical, psychological and anatomical study of three patients. *Journal of Neurology, Neurosurgery and Psychiatry, 40,* 395–403.

Wilkinson, H. A. (1973). Epileptic pain. *Neurology (New York), 23,* 518–520.

Wolpert, E. A., & Trosman, H. (1958). Studies in psychophysiology of dreams. I. Experimental evocation of sequential dream episodes. *Archives of Neurology, 79,* 603–606.

Worner, K. H. (1973). *History of music.* New York: Free Press.

Yakovlev, P. I., & Lecours, A. (1967). The myelogenetic cycles of regional maturation of the brain. In A. Minkowski (Ed.), *Regional development of the brain in early life* (pp. 404–491). London: Blackwell.

Yamadori, A., Osumi, U., Mashuara, S., & Okuto, M. (1977). Preservation of singing in Broca's aphasia. *Journal of Neurology, Neurosurgery and Psychiatry, 40,* 221–224.

York, G. K., Gabor, A. J., & Dreyfus, P. M. (1979). Paroxysmal genital pain: An unusual manifestation of epilepsy. *Neurology (New York), 29,* 516–519.

Zaidel, E. (1983). Language in the right hemisphere, convergent perspectives. *American Psychologist, 38,* 542–546.

Zurif, E. B. (1974). Auditory lateralization: Prosodic and syntactic factors. *Brain and Language, 1,* 391–404.

Zurif, E. B., & Carson, G. (1970). Dyslexia in relation to cerebral dominance and temporal analysis. *Neuropsychologia, 8,* 239–244.

The Left Cerebral Hemisphere
Aphasia, Alexia, Agraphia, Agnosia, Apraxia, Language, and Thought

OVERVIEW

It is now well known that among more than 80% of the right-handed population and among 50% of those who are left-handed, the left cerebral hemisphere provides the neural foundation for the verbal perception, comprehension, differentiation, identification, and linguistic labeling of visual, auditory, and somesthetic information. The left hemisphere dominates in the perception and processing of real words, word lists, rhymes, numbers, backwards speech, Morse code, consonants, consonant vowel syllables, nonsense syllables, the transitional elements of speech, and single phonemes (Blumstein & Cooper, 1974; Cutting, 1974; Kimura, 1961; Kimura & Folb, 1968; Levy, 1974, Mills & Rollman, 1979; Papcun, Krashen, Terbeek, *et al.,* 1974; Shankweiler & Studdert-Kennedy, 1966, 1967; Studdert-Kennedy & Shankweiler, 1970). It is also dominant for recognizing phonetic, conceptual, and verbal (but not physical) similarities, e.g., determining whether two letters (g and p versus g and q) have the same vowel ending (Levy, 1974; Moscovitch, 1973).

The left half of the cerebrum mediates most aspects of expressive and receptive linguistic functioning, such as reading, writing, speaking, spelling, naming, and the comprehension of the grammatical, syntactical, and descriptive components of language, including time sense, rhythm, verbal concept formation, analytical reasoning, and verbal memory (Albert, Sparks, von Strockert, & Sax, 1972; Carmazza & Zurif, 1976; DeRenzi, Zambolini, & Crisi, 1987; Efron, 1963; Goodglass & Kaplan, 1972; Hecaen & Albert, 1978; Heilman & Scholes, 1976; Kertesz, 1983*a,b*; Levine & Sweet, 1983; Luria, 1980; B. Milner, 1970; Vignolo, 1983; Zurif & Carson, 1970).

The perception, organization, and categorization of information into discrete temporal units or within a linear and sequential time frame are also left hemisphere-mediated activities, including the sequential control of finger, hand, arm, and articulatory movements (Beaumont, 1974; Efron, 1963; Heilman *et al.,* 1983; Kimura, 1977; Lenneberg,

1967; Luria, 1980; Mateer, 1983). Indeed, the left half of the brain is sensitive to rapidly changing acoustics cues, be they verbal or nonverbal, and is specialized for sorting, separating, and extracting in a segmented fashion, the phonetic and temporal–sequential or articulatory features of incoming auditory information so as to identify speech units (Shankweiler & Studdert-Kennedy, 1967; Studdert-Kennedy & Shankweiler, 1970). However, its superiority regarding temporal sequencing includes the visual domain, for the left half of the brain is superior to the right in visual sequential memory and in detecting nonverbal sequences (Halperin; Nachson, & Carmon, 1973; Zaidel, 1977).

EGOCENTRIC AND LINQUISTIC THOUGHT

A multitude of neuronal structures and fibers pathways are involved in the formulation, expression, and comprehension of speech, language, and thought. Nevertheless, within the left cerebrum, specific regions are known to govern particular functions. For example, an area in the left frontal convexity (i.e., Broca's area) mediates expressive speech, whereas the superior temporal lobule (Wernicke's area), the left inferior parietal lobe (the angular and supramarginal gyrus), and various thalamic nuclei (e.g., the pulvinar) are involved in linguistic comprehension. These regions and the multiple interaction that link them comprise the language axis of the left hemisphere (Joseph, 1982).

Limbic language. Language, in part, is a fusion of motor and sensory–limbic activities and consists of denotative, syntactical–grammatical (left hemisphere), as well as prosodic–emotional (right hemispheric and limbic) components (Joseph, 1982, 1988*a*) Language springs forth from roots buried within the ancient limbic lobe (Joseph, 1988*b*) (see Chapter 3, The Limbic System). Limbic speech, however, is not bound up with thinking, the expression of thought, or conscious reflection. Although communicative, limbic speech occurs essentially independent of thought, as it is predominantly emotional and is concerned with the immediacy of the "here and now."

Right hemisphere speech. Right cerebral language is social, melodic, emotional, contextual, inferential, and highly communicative of meaning and intent. In part, limbic speech is hierarchically rerepresented, refined, and elaborated by right hemisphere language structures.

Left hemisphere speech. Denotative syntactical–grammatical language is concerned with nominal functions, descriptive statements of fact, and temporal–sequential relations (i.e., first and last) and serves explanatory as well as communicative functions, indeed, language (as manifested through linguistic thought) often serves as a means of explaining as well as organizing impulses originating in the nonlinguistic regions of the cerebrum so that the temporal–sequential and language-dependent regions of the brain may achieve understanding (Joseph, 1982, 1986).

Thought

Thinking is clearly a form of communication and, as such, is a form of language, an organized hierarchy of associations, symbols, and labels that appear before an observer— within the mind's "eye." In the process of thinking, one often acts to organize information that is "not thought out" and that is not clearly understood, so that it may become thought out and thereby comprehended (Ach, 1951; James, 1961; Joseph, 1980, 1982; Schilder, 1951).

Thought (i.e., directed thinking) can be a means of deduction, clarification, plan and goal formation, and reality manipulation (Craik, 1943; Freud, 1900; Miller, Galanter, & Pribram, 1960; Piaget, 1962). However, it is also a progression, an associative advance that leads from an inner or outer perception to linguistic–motor expression (Freud, 1900), and an elaboration that some have argued appears with an initial or leading idea that is followed by a series of related ideations or as originating developmentally from the nonaccessible regions of the mind (Freud, 1900; James, 1961; Jung, 1954; Piaget, 1962).

By contrast, sometimes the "train of thought" emerges spontaneously and reflexively, as if related ideas simply become strung together with no specific goal or purpose in mind. Moreover, in these instances, sometimes these thoughts rapidly alternate in content and fluctuate between seemingly unrelated ideas, as if triggered by some agent external to the left half of the brain (such as the right hemisphere) or via the production of random neural activity. Indeed, sometimes it is exactly that—random and reflexive.

The Purpose of Thought

Directed or spontaneous, the substance that is thought always unfolds before an observer. It is a series of transactions that are witnessed and experienced, a sometimes purposeful means of explanation through which ideas, impulses, desires, or thing-in-the-world may be understood, comprehended, and possibly acted on. Paradoxically, it is often a process by which one explains things to oneself. Indeed, as a means of deduction or explanation, and as a form of internal language, it is almost as if one is talking to oneself inside one's head. Nevertheless, the fact that one acts as both the explainee and the explainer raises a curious question: "Who is explaining what to whom?" A functional duality is thus implied in the production and reception of thought.

Assuming that the subject of thought originates in me, the thinker, and given that the organization of this often linear arrangement is also a product of self-generated activity, it should be expected in some instances that "I" should already know not only what "I" am about to think prior to thinking it but that I should also know the conclusion before it is communicated. In fact, often we do know before we think (and while we think), and often we do not think simply because the question–answer–implications are simultaneously understood without the aid of thought. Thus, some redundancy is built into the thinking process.

Because thinking is often a form of communication, it seems that one aspect of the self, or rather, the brain, sometimes does not have access to the information (or at least an understanding of the material) to be explained, until after it is presented and organized in a linear sequence of language-related ideas and images. In this regard, thinking is sometimes a form of communication through which one part of the brain gains access and understanding regarding information or knowledge possessed in yet other regions of the brain.

Indeed, thinking often serves in part as a means of organizing, interpreting, and explaining impulses that arise in the nonlinguistic portions of the nervous system so that the language-dependent regions may achieve understanding (Joseph, 1980, 1982). In fact, although thought may take various nonlinguistic forms (e.g., musical thought, visual imagery), one need only listen to one's own thoughts in order to realize that thinking often consists of an internal linguistic monologue, a series of words heard within one's own head.

THE DEVELOPMENT OF LANGUAGE AND THOUGHT

Three Linguistic Stages

As pertaining to the development of thought and language, we will be concerned with three maturational stages of linguistic expression. Initially, linguistic expression in the infant is reflexive and/or indicative of generalized and diffuse feeling states. It is largely emotional–prosodic in quality and is mediated by limbic and brainstem nuclei (Joseph, 1982; 1989). (See also Chapter 3, The Limbic System.)

At approximately 3–4 months of age, the infant's utterances begin to assume meaningful as well as imitative qualities, are indicative of specific feelings states, and begin to become influenced by both the right and left cerebral hemisphere. It is during this period that a second babbling stage develops and the child's prosodic utterances begin to assume temporal–sequential characteristics. That is, the left hemisphere begins to provide rhythm and specification to the melody and associated feelings states expressed by the right hemisphere and limbic system. From this point on, true language begins to develop. However, it is not until a third stage of linguistic functioning makes it appearance that the child begins not to only speak words but to think them. This final stage coincides with the development of egocentric speech.

Limbic and Brainstem Cognitions

For some time after birth, due to immaturity of the neocortex and its subcortical and thalamic interconnections, most behavior is initially mediated by limbic, brainstem, and spinal nuclei (see Joseph, 1982, 1989, for review). Indeed, at this stage of neocortical immaturity, the psychic functioning of the newborn is probably no more than a vague, undifferentiated awareness, consisting of a multitude of excitatory and inhibitory neuronal interactions and a series of transient feeling states and emotional upheavals that lack psychological referants or distinctive features (Joseph, 1982). The neonate is essentially internally oriented, its psychic attentional functions almost entirely directed toward stimuli impinging on the body surface and sensations transmitted by the mouth (E. Milner, 1967).

Cognition consists largely of generalized and diffuse feeling states aimed at the alleviation of displeasure or painful affect and with the reactivation of experiences associated with pleasurable sensations. In fact, from birth to 1 month of age, the infant displays only two attitudes—accepting and rejecting—and a very limited range of vocalization—crying and cooing (Milner, 1967; Spitz & Wolf, 1946). These feeling states and vocalizations are largely mediated and expressed by the limbic system.

Limbic Speech

Indeed, the original impetus to speak springs forth from roots buried within the depths of the ancient limbic lobe and is bound with, and tied to, mood, impulse, feeling, desire, pleasure, pain, and fear (Joseph, 1982, 1989; Robinson, 1967). The infant cries, coos, and produces various prosodic inflectional variations that are without temporal–

sequential organization that serve no true communicative purpose. It is only over the course of the first few months that these prosodic–melodic utterances become associated with specific moods and emotions (Piaget, 1952) and babbling makes its appearance (Brain & Walton, 1969).

Early and Late Babbling and Probable Speech

However, although the diffuse prosodic–melodic utterances of the infant are limbic, much of early babbling is a product of random and reflexive motor activity, motor overflow, and self-stimulation. Early babbling is also representative of the neocortical maturational changes that occur within the language axis and the initial exercise and activation of these developing pathways.

By approximately 3–4 months of age, the neocortex of the right cerebral hemisphere has greatly increased its hierarchical acquisition of, and synaptic control over, various limbic nuclei (Joseph, 1982). Prosodic output begins to assume an imitative quality, which in turn is context specific (Piaget, 1952); the infant's largely intonational–melodic vocal repertoire becomes more elaborate and increasingly tied to certain feeling states and begins to acquire probable meanings (Hoff-Ginsberg & Shatz, 1982; Piaget, 1952). For example, the infant may purposefully cry or call "mama," whereas initially "mama" signified nothing beyond the random universal babbling produced by all infants.

As cries, babbles, or, for example, the word "mama" first assume probable meanings, they initially signify a variety of diffuse feelings and needs. Hence, "mama" might mean "mama come here," "mama give me," "mama I hurt," "I am hungry" (Piaget, 1952; Vygotsky, 1962). Moreover, "mama" at times may continue to signify nothing more than reflexive (early) babbling for several months.

Late Babbling and Temporal Sequential Speech

By the time the infant has reached 3–4 months of age, a second babbling stage develops, i.e., late babbling. Whereas the first babbling stage reflects motor self-stimulation, late babbling heralds the first real shift from emotional–prosodic–melodic speech to temporal–sequential language (Leopold, 1947), i.e., left hemisphere speech. Indeed, these developmental changes coincide with the maturation of the arcuate fasciculus, the major pathways by which auditory–linguistic input is transmitted from Wernicke's area to Broca's area for motoric sequencing and expression. Its appearance also corresponds to the completion of the myelogenetic cycle within Heschyl's gyrus and the primary and association auditory receiving areas (Lecours, 1975). Moreover, during this later period, infants begin to respond behaviorally to specific speech sounds and their phonemic characteristics. This is because Wernicke's area is now functionally capable of beginning to process these signals appropriately.

As the infant's left cerebral hemisphere begins to mature and respond to and influence auditory–linguistic stimuli, it begins to stamp and impose temporal sequences onto the stress, pitch, and melodic intonational contours, which up to that time have characterized speech output. This is part of what the late babbling stage heralds: the ability to sequence. That is, syllabication is imposed on the intonational contours of the child's speech by the left hemisphere, such that the melodic features of generalized vocal expression come to be punctuated, sequenced, and segmented, and vowel and consonantal elements begin to be produced. (cf. De Boysson-Bardies, Bacri, Sagart, & Poizet, 1980). Left hemisphere speech comes to be superimposed over right hemisphere melodic language output.

Thus, as the left hemisphere matures and wrests control of the peripheral and cranial musculature from subcortical influences, a second form of language emerges, one that arises through interactions and nominal associations with external stimulatory activities and through the production of sequences, i.e., left hemisphere speech. Left hemisphere speech is thus grammatical, temporal–sequential, denotative, and social and is closely bound with the eventual expression and development of thought. Thinking, however, does not appear until much later in development, an unfolding event that corresponds to the appearance of a third form of language: egocentric speech.

EGOCENTRIC SPEECH

Egocentric speech is self-directed speech consisting of an explanatory monologue in which children comment on their play and other actions, usually after the action has occurred. According to Vygotsky (1962), egocentric speech makes its first appearance at approximately 3 years of age. According to Piaget (1952, 1962, 1974), at its peak, egocentric speech comprises almost 40–50% of the preoperational child's language, the remainder consisting of social speech (denotative, interactional, and emotional). Social speech is produced in order to communicate with others. Egocentric speech is produced in order to communicate with no one other than the child who produces it.

Before the development of egocentric speech, communication is directed strictly toward outside sources. There is no attempt to communicate with the self, for there is no internal dialogue as thought has not yet developed. At around age 3, egocentric speech—the peculiar linguistic structure from which thought will arise—appears within the context of social–denotative vocalizations (Vygotsky, 1962). That is, part of the time the child engages in social speech, whereas the remainder of speech activities are egocentric. Egocentric speech is essentially a self-directed form of communication that heralds the first attempts at self-explanation. It is essentially speech for oneself (Joseph, 1982; Piaget, 1962; Vygotsky, 1962).

While the child is engaging in egocentric speech, he does not appear concerned with the listening needs of his audience simply because to all appearances his words are meant for his ears alone (Piaget, 1952, 1962, 1974; Vygotsky, 1962). The child is essentially thinking out loud in an explanatory fashion (Joseph, 1982; Vygotsky, 1962).

When engaged in an egocentric monologue, there is no interest in influencing or explaining to others what in fact is being explained. In fact, the child will keep up a running verbal accompaniment to his actions, commenting on his behavior, while or after it occurs, in an explanatory fashion, even while alone. Moreover, while engaged in this self-directed external monologue, the child appears oblivious to the responses of others to his statements (Piaget, 1952, 1962, 1974; Vygotsky, 1956). It is as if the child has no awareness that others hear him.

Egocentric speech is explanatory, and initially it is produced only after an action has been completed. The child observes what he has done and then comments on and/or explains what has taken place. At this stage, egocentric speech is completely external. There are no (or few) internally generated linguistic thoughts. It is only as the child grows older that the child's comments and explanations occur earlier in the sequence of expression, until finally the child begins to explain his actions before they are performed instead of after they have occurred.

Egocentric speech presents us with a curious anomaly, for we must accept that the child knows what he has done without commenting on or explaining his actions; moreover, he must know why he has performed certain behaviors without the need to explain them to himself. Nevertheless, the fact that he explains and comments on his behaviors after they occur argues otherwise. Paradoxically, the child acts as both actor and witness, explainer and the one explained to. Clearly, the child explains his actions to himself (Vygotsky, 1962).

According to Vygotsky (1962), after its initial appearance and elaboration, egocentric speech also begins to occur internally and in fact becomes progressively more covert as the child grows older. Egocentric speech occurs internally as linguistic thought (Joseph, 1982). At its overt maximum, when it appears to be fully developed (comprising by age 4 years almost 50% of the child's speech), its traits and structures are simultaneously being internalized and strengthened and comprise a greater portion of the child's cognitive activities than may be witnessed (like an iceberg). That is, egocentric speech never disappears but becomes completely internalized in the form of inner speech, i.e., thought. The child has now learned to think words as well as to speak them and to think them in a temporal and organized sequence that retains its original and primary function—self-communication.

Self-Explanation

The essential feature of the external components of egocentric speech is that it is based on stimuli and actions that occur outside the child's immediate sphere of understanding and experience, for initially it is evoked while the child is observing his behavior or after he has completed his action. This suggests that the child (or at least the speaking half of his brain) has access to the impulses to behave only on an external basis. He does not know why he has performed a particular action, so he must interpret and explain them after they occur. In this regard, when they "misbehave," children are probably sometimes telling the truth when they say they "don't know why" they did such and such. That is, the left hemisphere does not know why.

As the child ages, the egocentric commentary occurs progressively earlier during the course of a particular behavior. For example, the 3-year-old will first comment or explain a picture that she has drawn after it is finished, whereas at a later age she will state what a picture is while she is drawing it, until finally the child will announce what she will draw and then draws it (Vygotsky, 1962). Essentially, as the child matures, she appears to receive advanced warning of her intentions and actions, until finally this information is available before rather than after she acts (Joseph, 1982). At this later stage, however, egocentric speech has been greatly internalized as thought.

Although egocentric speech is a self-directed monologue, it is nevertheless a product of the left cerebral hemisphere. That egocentric speech appears initially only after an action has occurred indicates that the left hemisphere of the young child is responding to impulses and actions initiated outside its immediate realm of experiences and comprehension. It seems that the left hemisphere in the production of egocentric speech is not only "thinking out loud" but is attempting to interpret what it observes and experiences externally, creating a meaningful explanatory sequence, which it then linguistically communicates to itself.

Interhemispheric Communication

The appearance and eventual internalization of egocentric speech occurs in response to several maturational changes in the central nervous system and parallels the development of the corpus callosum and an increased ability for the cerebral hemispheres to communicate (Joseph, 1982). As has been demonstrated by a number of independent researchers, communication between the right and left half of the brain is exceedingly poor before age 3 and remains limited until approximately age 5 (Galin, Diamond, & Braff, 1977; Galin, Diamond, & Herron, 1979a; Gallagher & Joseph, 1982; Joseph *et al.*, 1984; O'Leary, 1980; Salamy, 1978). Presumably this is a function of the immaturity of the corpus callosal fiber connections between the hemispheres (Yakovlev & Lecours, 1967). In this regard, it appears that the left hemisphere of the young child's brain has at best incomplete knowledge of the contents and activity occurring in the right, hence the development of egocentric speech.

Essentially, egocentric speech is a function of the left hemisphere's attempt to organize, interpret, and make sense of behavior initiated by the right hemisphere and limbic system. Because interhemispheric communication is at best grossly incomplete, the left brain uses language to explain to itself the behavior that it observes itself to be engaged in. As the commissures mature and information flow within and between the hemispheres increases, the left brain gains increased access to these impulses as they are formulated in the nonlinguistic portions of the brain; it begins internally to organize linguistically what it experiences internally (rather than externally). Essentially, increased commissural transmission allows the left hemisphere access to right hemisphere impulses to action before the action occurs, rather than forcing it to make sense of the behavior after its completion. Even in the adult, commissural transmission is not complete, however. (See Chapter 1, The Right Cerebral Hemisphere.) As such, the adult left hemisphere sometimes finds itself witnessing and participating in behaviors that it not only did not initiate, but that it does not understand.

DISORDERS OF LANGUAGE

Broca's Aphasia

Within the left frontal convexity is a large region that is responsible for the expression of speech. This is known as Broca's area, named after Paul Broca, who more than 100 years ago delineated the symptoms associated with damage to this area. Immediately adjacent to Broca's area is the portion of the primary motor area that subserves control over the oral–facial musculature and the right hand.

Various forms of linguistic information are transferred from Wernicke's area and the inferior parietal lobule and converge on Broca's area, where they receive their final sequential (syntactical, grammatical) imprint so as to become organized and expressed as temporally ordered motoric linguistic articulations, i.e., speech. From Broca's area these impulses are then transferred to the motor areas, which in turn control the oral musculature. Thus, verbal communication and the expression of thought in linguistic form are made possible.

Expressive Aphasia

As a result of massive damage to the left frontal convexity, a person's ability to speak would be dramatically curtailed. Often immediately following a stroke in this region, patients are almost completely mute and suffer a paralysis of the right upper extremity. This disorder is called Broca's (or expressive) aphasia (Goodglass & Kaplan, 1972; Levine & Sweet, 1983).

Although symptoms differ depending on the severity of the lesion, in general, individuals with Broca's aphasia are very limited in their ability to speak. In severe cases, speech may be restricted to a few stereotyped phrases and expressions, such as "Jesus Christ" or to single words such as "fine," "yes," "no," which are produced with much effort. Even if capable of making longer statements, much of what these people say is either poorly articulated or mumbled, or both, such that only a word or two is intelligible. They are able to make one-word answers in response to questions. Speech beyond one-word statements is almost always agrammatical (i.e., the production of some correct words but in the wrong order) and contaminated by verbal paraphasias (i.e., "orrible" for "auto") and/or the substitution of semantically related words (e.g., mother for father and characterized by the omission of relational words such as those that tie language together (i.e., the prepositions, modifiers, articles, and conjunctions). Similarly, they have difficulty comprehending these same grammatical features (Samuels & Benson, 1979; Zurif, Caramazza, & Myerson, 1972), as well as related verbal material such as demonstrated on the Token test (DeRenzi & Vignolo, 1962). The ability of these patients to repeat what is said to them, although grossly deficient, is usually not as severely reduced as conversational speech.

The ability to write is always affected. Similarly, their capacity to write to dictation is severely limited. However, the ability to copy is much better preserved. In addition, reading comprehension is usually intact, although these persons are unable to read aloud.

Patients with moderate and severe expressive abnormalities also have difficulty performing three-step commands, although two-step requests may be performed without difficulty. However, they are better able to comprehend as well as verbalize semantically significant words. Even in moderate and mild cases, a consistent defect in the syntactical structure of speech is noted, including reductions in vocabulary and word fluency in both speech and writing (Goodglass & Berko, 1960; Levine & Sweet, 1983; Milner, 1964).

Persons with expressive aphasia, although greatly limited in their ability to speak, are nevertheless capable of making emotional statements or even singing (Gardner, 1975; Goldstein, 1942; Joseph, 1982; Smith, 1966; Smith & Burklund, 1966; Yamadori, Osumi, Mashuara, & Okuto, 1977). In fact, they may be able to sing words they are unable to say.

Except for emotional speech, however, language production is largely monotonic (Goodglass & Kaplan, 1972) or characterized by prosodic distortions such that in some cases they sound as if they are speaking with a foreign accent (Graff-Radford, Cooper, Colsher, & Damasio, 1986). This is often due to shifts in the enunciation of vowels, i.e., increased duration of the utterance and the pauses between words as they struggle to speak. However, in some instances, this is secondary to deep lesions involving perhaps the anterior cingulate and other nuclei. (See Chapter 4, The Frontal Lobes.)

Depression and Broca's Aphasia

Patients with left frontal damage and Broca's aphasia often become frustrated, sad, tearful, and depressed (Robinson & Szetela, 1981). Presumably this is because individuals with Broca's aphasia are fairly (but not completely) able to comprehend, hence are aware of their deficit and appropriately depressed. Indeed, those with the smallest lesions become the most depressed (Robinson & Benson, 1981)—the depression as well as the ability to sing presumably mediated by the intact right cerebral hemisphere (Joseph, 1982, 1988a). Nevertheless, it has also been reported that psychiatric patients classified as depressed (who presumably have no signs of neurological impairment) often demonstrate, electrophysiologically, insufficient activation of the left frontal lobe (d'Elia & Perris, 1974; Perris, 1974). With recovery from depression, left hemisphere activation returns to normal levels.

Apathetic States

Depression and depressive-like features also occur with left frontal and medial lesions that spare Broca's area (Robinson & Szetela, 1981). However, rather than depression per se, such patients (particularly when the frontal pole is damaged) frequently appear severely apathetic and hypoactive with reduced motor functioning and are poorly motivated. When questioned, rather than being worried or truly concerned about their condition, the overall picture is one of bland confusion and lack of interest. Patients also frequently seem motorically and emotionally blunted.

These depressive-like and apathetic states are sometimes attributable to disconnection from the limbic system and/or right cerebral hemisphere. Unfortunately, with frontal pole injury, tumor, or degeneration, the underlying neurological precursors to their condition are not very apparent until late in the disease, making misdiagnosis likely. (We will return to these issues in Chapter 4, The Frontal Lobe.)

Anomia or Word-Finding Difficulty

Everyone with aphasia has some degree of word-finding difficulty, i.e., dysnomia (or, if severe, anomia). Dysnomia is very common and can occur with fluent output, good comprehension, and ability to repeat, in the absence of paraphasias or other aphasic abnormalities. Although many normal individuals who have trouble finding a word sometimes experience it as being on the "tip of the tongue," anomia is a much more pervasive abnormality and may involve naming objects, describing pictures, and so forth, even when hints are provided.

In general, anomic difficulties suggest left hemisphere functional impairment and are sometimes secondary to disconnection or to a deficit in activating the correct phonological sound–word patterns (Kay & Ellis, 1987). Frequently, if dysnomia is the only predominant problem, the patient may erroneously ascribe it to deficient memory; i.e., complain of memory problems when in fact it is a word-finding difficulty. However, this is not due to mnemonic deficits. For example, providing hints or even the initial letter results in little improvement (Goodglass *et al.*, 1976). Moreover, once the word is supplied, the patient may again experience the same problem almost immediately. In general, the ability to generate nouns is more affected than the ability to produce verbs.

In severe cases, while conversing the patient may be so plagued with word-finding difficulty that speech becomes "empty" and characterized by many pauses as the patient searches for words. This condition is sometimes referred to as *anomic aphasia* (Hecaen & Albert, 1978). These same patients may erroneously substitute phrases or words for the ones that cannot be found, for example, calling a "spoon" the "stirrer," a "pencil" a "writer," or various objects "the whatchmacallit." This can lead to circumlocution, as these patients tend to talk around the word they are after: "Get me the uh, the uh thing over on the uh, on the top over there."

If accompanied by problems with reading and writing, the lesion is most likely situated in the posterior portion of the left hemisphere near the angular gyrus. However, lesions anywhere within the left hemisphere can result in anomic difficulties.

Wernicke's (Receptive) Aphasia

Wernicke's area is located within the left superior temporal lobe extending from the border zones of the primary auditory reception area toward the inferior parietal lobule. Auditory information is recived in the adjacent primary auditory area and is transferred to Wernicke's area. Wernicke's area acts to decode and encode auditory–linguistic information (be it externally or internally generated), so as to extract or impart temporal–sequential order and related linguistic features. In this manner, denotative meaning may be discerned or applied (Efron, 1963; Lackner & Teuber, 1973; Lenneberg, 1967). That is, this area acts to label information verbally that is transmitted from external sources as well as from other brain regions. For example, it may act to provide the auditory equivalent of a visually perceived written word. In this manner, we know what the words we read sound like.

If Wernicke's area is damaged, the patient has great difficulty comprehending spoken or written language (Goodglass & Kaplan, 1972; Kertesz, 1983a; Hecaen & Albert, 1978). Naming, reading, writing, and the ability to repeat are severely affected. This is referred to as Wernicke's (receptive) aphasia. However, if reading ability proves to be intact, the patient is probably suffering from *pure word deafness* rather than receptive aphasia (to be explained).

Frequently, disturbances involving linguistic comprehension are caused by an impaired capacity to discern the individual units of speech and their temporal order. Sounds must be separated into discrete interrelated linear units or they will be perceived as a blur, or even as a foreign language (Efron, 1963; Lackner & Teuber, 1973). Thus, a patient with Wernicke's aphasia may perceive a spoken sentence such as the "big black dog" as "the klabgigdod." However, comprehension is improved, if the spoken words are separated by long intervals.

Many receptive aphasics can comprehend frequently used words but have difficulty with those that are less frequently heard. Thus, loss of comprehension is not an all-or-none phenomenon. They will usually have greatest difficulty understanding relational or syntactical structures, including the use of verb tense, possessives, and prepositions. However, by speaking slowly and by emphasizing the pauses between each individual word, comprehension can be modestly improved.

Nevertheless, patients with damage to Wernicke's area are still capable of talking, due to preservation of Broca's area. However, because Wernicke's area also acts to code linguistic stimuli for expression (prior to its transmission to Broca's area), expressive speech is severely abnormal, lacking in content, containing neologistic distortions (e.g., "the razgabin"), and/or characterized by nonsequiturs, literal (sound substitution) and verbal paraphasic (word substitution) errors, a paucity of nouns and verbs, and the omission of pauses and sentence endings (Goodglass & Kaplan, 1972; Kertesz, 1983a; Hecaen & Albert, 1978). Patients may speak in a rush (e.g., press of speech), and what is said often conveys very little actual information. For this reason, this aspect of their language problem is referred to as *fluent aphasia*. These patients may also have difficulty establishing the boundaries of phonetic (confusing "love" for "glove") and semantic (e.g., cigarette for ashtray) auditory information (Fig. 17).

The speech of these patients may also be characterized by long, seemingly complex (albeit unintelligible) grammatically correct sentences, such that speech is often hyper-fluent and produced at an excessive rate. Thus, they have difficulty bringing sentences to a close such that many words are unintelligibly strung together. They also suffer severe word-finding difficulty, which adds a circumlocutory aspect to their speech. When severe, it deteriorates into jargon aphasia, preventing meaningful communication (Kertesz, 1983a; Marcie & Hecaen, 1979). For example, one patient with severe receptive aphasia responded in the following manner:

> Oh hear but that was a long time ago that was when that when before I even knew that much about this place although I am a little suspicious about what the hell is the part there is one part scares, uh estate spares, Ok that has a bunch of drives in it and a bunch of good googin, nothing real big but that was in the same time I coached them I said hey stay out of the spear struggle stay out of trouble so dont get and my kidds, uh except for the body the boys are pretty good although lately they have become winded or something . . . what the hell . . . kind of a platz goasted klack. . . .

Presumably because the coding mechanisms involved in organizing what these patients are planning to say are the same mechanisms that decode what they hear, expressive as well as receptive speech becomes equally disrupted. In fact, one gauge of comprehension can be based on the amount of normalcy in their language use. That is, if they can repeat only a few words normally, it is likely that they can only comprehend a few words as well. Nevertheless, in testing for comprehension, it is important to establish that the patient's major difficulty is not apraxia rather than aphasia.

In addition, like speech, the ability to write may be preserved, although what is written is usually completely unintelligible, consisting of jargon and neologistic distortions. Copying written material is possible, although it is also often contaminated by errors.

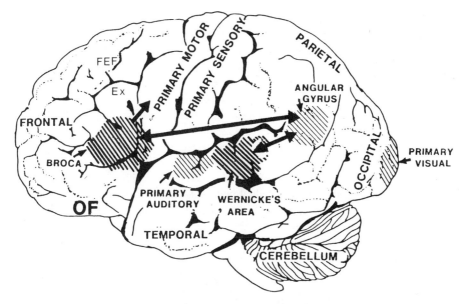

FIGURE 17. The lateral surface of the left cerebral hemisphere depicting the language axis (the angular gyrus, Broca's and Wernicke's areas), Exner's writing area (Ex), the frontal eye fields (FEF), and the orbital frontal lobes (OF).

Anosognosia

Nevertheless, although their speech is bizarre patients with damage to Wernicke's area usually do not realize that what they say is meaningless. Moreover, they may fail to comprehend that what they hear is meaningless as well (Lebrun, 1987). Nor can they be told that this is so, since they are unable to comprehend. This is because when Wernicke's area is damaged, there is no other region left to analyze the linguistic components of speech and language. The brain cannot be alerted to the patient's disability. They don't know that they don't know, that they don't understand. However, they may be somewhat more capable of recognizing that their writing is abnormal (Marcie & Hecaen, 1979).

"Schizophrenia"

Presumably, as a consequence of loss of comprehension, patients with Wernicke's aphasia may display euphoria or, in other cases, paranoia, as there remains a nonlinguistic or emotional awareness that something is not right. Emotional functioning and affective comprehension remain somewhat intact, although sometimes disrupted due to erroneously processed verbal input (Boller & Green, 1972; Boller Cole, Vrtunski, Patterson, & Kim, 1979). That is, the patient's right hemisphere continues to respond to signals generated by the left, even though these signals are abnormal. Similarly, the ability to read and write emotional words (as compared with nonemotional or abstract words) is also somewhat preserved among Wernicke's aphasics (Landis, Graves, & Goodglass, 1982). This is because the right hemisphere is intact.

Since these paralinguistic and emotional features of language are analyzed by the intact right cerebral hemisphere, the aphasic patient is able to grasp in general the meaning or intent of a speaker, although verbal comprehension is reduced. This in turn enables them to react in a somewhat appropriate fashion when spoken to. Unfortunately, this also makes them appear to comprehend much more than they are capable of. Similarly, Wernicke's aphasics retain the melodic, prosodic, and intonation contours of speech. In fact, at times their speech can become hypermelodic as well as characterized by inappropriate abnormal fluctuations in melodic contour. In addition, these patients often show normal gestural and facial expressions (Marcie & Hecaen, 1979).

Because these patients display unusual speech, loss of comprehension, a failure to comprehend that they no longer comprehend or "make sense" when speaking, as well as paranoia and/or euphoria, they are at risk of being misdiagnosed as psychotic or suffering from a formal thought disorder, i.e., "schizophrenia." Indeed, patients with abnormal left temporal lobe functioning sometime behave and speak in a "schizophrenic-like" manner (see Chapter 7, The Temporal Lobes).

According to Benson (1979), "those with Wernicke's aphasia often have no apparent physical or elementary neurological disability. Not infrequently, the individual who suddenly fails to comprehend spoken language and whose output is contaminated with jargon is diagnosed as psychotic. Patients with Wernicke's aphasia certainly inhabited some of the old lunatic asylums and probably are still being misplaced" (p. 42). Conversely, it has frequently been reported that schizophrenics often display significant abnormalities involving speech processing, such that the semantic, temporal–sequential, and lexical aspects of speech organization and comprehension are disturbed and deviantly constructed (Chaika, 1982; Flor-Henry, 1983; Hoffman, 1986; Hoffman, Stopek, & Andreasen, 1986; Rutter, 1979). Indeed, significant similarities between schizophrenic discourse and aphasic abnormalities have been reported (Faber, Abrams, Taylor, Kasprisin, Morris, & Weisz, 1983). In this regard, it is often difficult to determine what a schizophrenic person may be talking about. Indeed, these same people have sometimes been known to complain that what they say often differs from what they intended to say (Chapman, 1966). Temporal–sequential (i.e., syntactical) abnormalities have also been noted in their ability to reason, the classic example being: "I am a virgin. The Virgin Mary was a virgin. Therefore, I am the Virgin Mary." Thus, there is some possibility that a significant relationship exists between abnormal left hemisphere and left temporal lobe functioning and schizophrenic language, thought, and behavior. (We will return to this issue in Chapter 7, The Temporal Lobes.)

Pure Word Deafness

Located within the superior temporal lobe of both hemispheres are the primary auditory receiving areas. If these areas are destroyed bilaterally, the individual becomes cortically deaf. Although able to hear, these patients cannot perceive or comprehend nonverbal sounds or understand spoken language. When the primary auditory area is destroyed, the auditory association areas (Wernicke's area in the left hemisphere) are disconnected from all sources of auditory input, and cannot extract meaning from the auditory environment. When a patient is unable to perceive and identify linguistic and nonlinguistic sounds, the deficit is described as a *global* or *generalized auditory agnosia*. Cerebrovascular disease is the most common cause of this abnormality.

These patients are not deaf, however, as this can be ruled out by testing pure-tone thresholds. In fact, even with complete bilateral destruction of the primary auditory cortex, there is no permanent loss of acoustic sensitivity (Rubens, 1979). This is because sounds continue to be received in thalamic and subcortical centers. Hence, patients can still detect sounds. They just don't know what the sounds are. Moreover, deficits in loudness discrimination and sound localization are apparent.

In some instances, damage may be unilateral and involve predominantly the primary auditory receiving area of the left hemisphere as well as the underlying white matter such that Wernicke's region becomes disconnected from all sources of auditory input. Although the patient can hear and identify nonlinguistic sounds, they are unable to comprehend spoken language. These patients do not have Wernicke's aphasia, however, and are very aware of their deficits. Their own verbal output is normal (albeit sometimes loud and dysprosodic); frequently, they describe the sounds they hear as being "muffled," or they may complain that voices sound like "echos" or "noise" (Tanaka, Yamadori, and Mori, 1987).

Although they cannot repeat what is said to them, patients can read and write in a normal manner, and there is little or no evidence of aphasic symptoms. Nor do they demonstrate difficulty understanding nonverbal or pantomime actions. Nevertheless, some patients, as they recover from Wernicke's aphasia move to the stage of pure word deafness. However, in these instances, there are remnants of aphasic abnormalities.

Many such patients, like those who suffer some forms of deafness, may experience auditory hallucinations and/or exhibit paranoid ideation (Rubens, 1979). The hallucinations are likely a consequence of the attribution or erroneous extraction of meaning from randomly produced neural "noise." The paranoia is largely a normal reaction arising secondarily from the confusion associated with reduced environmental contact. That is, patients become fearful and mistrustful, as they are not sure what is "going on."

In part, pure word deafness is sometimes due to disturbances in processing rhythm and temporal sequences (Tanaka *et al.*, 1987; Albert & Bear, 1974) or making phonemic discriminations (Denes & Semenza, 1975). Indeed, slowing the rate of sound presentation or rate of speech can improve comprehension.

The Inferior Parietal Lobule

The primary sensory receiving areas for vision, audition, and somesthesis are located in the occipital, temporal, and parietal lobe, respectively. Adjacent to each primary zone is a secondary-association region, where higher-level information processing occurs. Wernicke's region is one such zone.

The inferior parietal lobule (including the angular and supramarginal gyri) is located at the junction where the three secondary association areas meet and overlap. In this regard, the inferior parietal region receives converging higher-order information from each sensory modality and is in fact involved in the multimodal assimilation of this input. (See Chapter 5, The Parietal Lobes.) Because of this, one can feel an object while blindfolded and know what it would look like and be able to name it as well.

Through its involvement in the construction of cross-modal associations, this region acts so as to increase the capacity for abstraction, categorization, differentiation, and the linguistic as well as visual labeling of sensorimotor experience. One is thus able to multiply classify a single stimulus or event.

When the inferior parietal region of the left hemisphere is damaged, a host of language-related disturbances may arise. This includes conduction aphasia, anomia, dyslexia, and agnosia. In addition, disturbances involving temporal–sequential programming, reasoning, and comprehension may occur. This includes apraxia and abnormalities involving the ability to perform calculations.

The Language Axis

When listening to someone speak, the information is first received in the primary auditory cortex and then transferred to Wernicke's area, where the temporal–sequential, semantic, and related linguistic features are stabilized, extracted, analyzed, and labeled. If it is a question that has been asked, the message is transferred from Wernicke's area to the inferior parietal lobule, where various ideational associations are aroused and organized via its vast interconnections with other cortical regions. Presumably a series of interactions continue to occur between Wernicke's area and the inferior parietal lobe until a reply is formulated and properly organized for possible expression (See Joseph, 1982, for greater detail). Lastly, the semantically correct and suitably chosen reply is transferred from Wernicke's region and the inferior parietal lobe, via a large fiber bundle (the arcuate fasciculus) to Broca's area, which then programs the speech musculature and neocortical motor areas so that the reply can be expressed.

Conduction Aphasia

Damage involving either the arcuate fasciculus or the supramarginal gyrus of the left hemisphere, or both, can result in a condition referred to as conduction aphasia (Benson, Sheremata, Bouchard, Segarram, Price, & Geschwind, 1973). However, in some cases, the lesion may extend to the insular and auditory cortex and underlying white matter of the left temporal lobe. Patients with this disorder have great difficulty communicating because a lesion in this vicinity disconnects Broca's area from the posterior language zones. Although a patient knows what he wants to say, he is unable to say it. Nor is he able to repeat simple statements, read out loud, or write to dictation, although the ability to comprehend speech and written language does remain intact.

Nevertheless, these patients are still able to talk. Unfortunately, most of what they say is contaminated by fluent paraphasic errors, phonetic word substitutions, and the telescoping of words caused by impaired sequencing. Patients also tend to confuse words that are phonetically similar. Because they can comprehend, they are aware of their disturbances and will try to come up with the correct words by generating successive approximations (Marcie & Hecaen, 1979). Hence, speech may be circumlocutous, seemingly tangential, as well as contaminated by paraphasic distortions; sentences are usually short and often unrelated (Marcie & Hecaen, 1979).

When writing, grapheme formation is usually normal. However, because these patients produce the wrong words and/or misspell what they produce, they may frequently cross out words and perform overwriting (i.e., writing over various letters with additional strokes). Patients are frequently very frustrated, irritable, and upset regarding their condition.

Global Aphasia

Global aphasia is essentially a total aphasia caused by massive left hemisphere damage involving the entire language axis, i.e., the frontal, parietal, and temporal convexity. Comprehension is severely reduced, as is the ability to speak, read, write, or repeat. Patients are usually, but not always paralyzed on the right side (Legatt, Rubin, Kaplan, Healton, & Brust, 1987) as a result of damage extending into the motor areas of the frontal lobe. Frequently this disturbance is secondary to cerebrovascular disease involving the middle cerebral artery. However, tumors and head injuries can also create this condition.

Isolation of the Speech Area (Transcortical Aphasia)

Isolation of the speech area is a condition in which the cortical border zones surrounding the language axis have been destroyed due to occlusion of the tiny tertiary blood vessels that supply these regions. That is, the language axis of the left hemisphere becomes completely disconnected from surrounding cortical tissue but remains (presumably) an intact functional unit. This is in contrast to global aphasia, in which the three major zones of language have been destroyed.

Nevertheless, like global aphasia, the rest of the cerebrum is unable to communicate with the language zones. As such, patients are unable to describe verbally what they see, feel, touch, or desire. Moreover, because the language axis cannot communicate with the rest of the brain, linguistic comprehension is largely abolished. That is, although communication among Wernicke's area, Broca's area, and the inferior parietal lobule is maintained, associations from other brain regions cannot reach the speech center. Although able to talk, these patients have nothing to say. Moreover, although able to see and hear, these patients are unable to understand linguistically what they perceive. However, they are capable of generating automatic-like responses to well-known phrases, prayers, or songs.

In an interesting case described by Geschwind, Quadfasel, and Segarra (1968), a 22-year-old woman with massive destruction of cortical tissue due to gas asphyxiation was found to have a preserved language axis. These investigators noted (pp. 343–346), once the patient regained "consciousness," that

> . . . she sang songs and repeated statements made by the physicians. However, she would follow no commands, resisted passive movements of her extremities, and would become markedly agitated and sometimes injured hospital personnel. In all other regards, however, she was completely without comprehension or the ability to communicate. The patient's spontaneous speech was limited to a few stereotyped phrases, such as "Hi daddy," "So can daddy," "mother," or "Dirty bastard." She never uttered a sentence of propositional speech over the nine years of observation. She never asked for anything and she never replied to questions and showed no evidence of having comprehended anything said to her. Occasionally, however, when the examiner said, "ask me no questions," she would reply "I'll tell you no lies," or when told, "close

your eyes'' she might say ''go to sleep.'' When asked, ''Is this a rose?'' she might say, ''roses are red, violets are blue, sugar is sweet and so are you.'' to the word ''Coffee'' she sometimes said, ''I love coffee, I love tea, I love the girls and the girls love me.'' An even more striking phenomenon was observed early in the patients illness. She would sing along with songs or musical commercials sung over the radio or would recite prayers along with the priest during religious broadcasts. If a record of a familiar song was played the patient would sing along with it. If the record was stopped she would continue singing correctly both words and music for another few lines and then stop. If the examiner kept humming the tune, the patient would continue singing the words to the end. New songs were played to her and it was found she could learn these as evidenced by her ability to sing a few lines correctly after the record had been stopped. Furthermore, she could sing two different sets of words to the same melody. For example, she could sing ''Let me call you sweetheart'' with the conventional words, but also learned the parody beginning with ''Let me call you rummy.'' Her articulation of the sounds and her production of melody were correct although she might sometimes substitute the words ''dirty bastard'' for some of the syllables.

Nevertheless, although such patients are able to sing, curse, and even pray, it is not clear whether these expressions are the product of right hemisphere activity or reflexive activation of the intact language zones, or both. I favor the former rather than the later explanations. In some cases, the isolation is only partial, involving either than anterior or posterior regions. In these instances, the disorder is referred to as *transcortical motor* or *transcortical sensory* aphasia, respectively (see Hecaen & Albert, 1978, for greater detail). Individuals with a partial transcortical aphasia have been reported to be able to read out loud, to write to dictation, and to repeat simple verbal statements. However, although repetition is somewhat preserved, spontaneous speech is severely limited. In sensory transcortical disturbances, comprehension is largely lost, whereas with motor transcortical aphasia, there is a greater preservation of comprehension.

ALEXIA AND AGRAPHIA

Alexia: Reading Abnormalities

A variety of theories purport to explain the mechanisms involved in reading and the comprehension of written language. These will not be discussed here. From a neurodynamic perspective, the process of reading involves the reception of visual impulses in the primary visual receiving areas, where various forms of perceptual analyses are initiated. This information is next transferred to the visual association cortex, where higher-level information processing is carried out and visual associations formed. These visual associations are next transmitted to a variety of areas (see Chapter 6, The Occipital Lobe), including the inferior and middle temporal lobe, inferior parietal lobule, and Wernicke's area. It is in these latter cortical regions that multimodal and linguistic assimilation take place so that the auditory equivalent of the visual stimulus may be retrieved. That is, through these interactions, visual grapheme clusters become translated into phonological sound images (Barron, 1980; Ellis, 1982; Friderici, Schoenle, & Goodglass, 1981). Thus, we know what a written word looks and sounds like. It is also possible, however, to bypass this phonological transcoding phase so that word meanings can be directly accessed (i.e., lexical reading).

Although it is likely that most individuals use both lexical and phonological strategies when reading, in either case the lingual, fusiform, and in particular the angular gyrus is involved (Gloning *et al.,* 1968; Greenblatt, 1973). With lesions involving the angular gyrus, or when damage occurs between the fiber pathways linking the left inferior parietal lobule with the visual cortex (i.e., disconnection), a condition referred to as *pure word blindness* sometimes occurs. Patients can see without difficulty but are unable to recognize written language. Written words evoke no meaning.

There are, however, several subtypes of reading disturbances that may occur with left cerebral damage. These include literal, verbal, and global alexia, and alexia for sentences. In addition, alexia can sometimes result from right hemisphere lesions, a condition referred to as *spatial alexia.* All these disorders, however, are acquired and should be distinguished from developmental dyslexia, which is present since childhood (Njiokiktjien, 1988).

Pure Word Blindness

The condition of pure word blindness is also referred to as pure alexia or alexia without agraphia (due to the preservation of the ability to write). Patients are totally unable to read written words or even recognize single letters. However, if words are spelled out loud, these patients have no difficulty with comprehension (because of the intact pathways from Wernicke's area to the angular gyrus). Moreover, they are able to speak, spell, as well as write without difficulty, but despite their ability to write, they are unable to read what they have written.

In general, the lesion appears to be between the left angular gyrus and the occipital lobe (in the arterial distribution of the left posterior cerebral artery), extending to within the splenium of the corpus callosum (Benson, 1979; Vignolo, 1983) and preventing right hemisphere visual input from being transferred to the inferior parietal lobe of the left half of the brain. In some cases, this condition is caused by a tumor or follows a head injury accompanied by a hematoma involving the white matter underlying the inferior parietal lobule (Greenblatt, 1973). In these instances, the left angular gyrus is unable to receive visual input from the left and right visual cortex, and visual input cannot be linguistically translated. The patient cannot gain access to the auditory equivalent of a written word.

Although unable to read written language, this syndrome is not always accompanied by a visual-field defect (hemianopsia). Moreover, objects may be named correctly (Hecaen & Kremin, 1976). However, patients may suffer from *color agnosia* (Benson & Geschwind, 1969), the inability to name colors correctly. These patients often (but not always) are unable to copy written material (because of disconnection from the visual areas), and many have difficulty performing math problems. In some cases, the patient suffers not only pure word blindness but blindness for numbers as well. This condition has been described as *global alexia* by some workers. However, global alexia is a more pervasive disorder, in which the ability to write (agraphia) and name objects is also compromised.

Alexia for Sentences

In general, patients are able to read letters and single words but are unable to comprehend sentences. However, patients may have difficulty with unfamiliar or particularly long words, whereas more familiar material is easily understood. Lesions are usually localized within the dominant occipital lobe but may extend into the inferior parietal area.

Verbal Alexia

In verbal alexia, the patient is able to read and recognize letters but is unable to comprehend or recognize whole words. However, if presented with short words, his ability improves. Thus, the longer the word, the greater the difficulty reading (Hecaen & Albert, 1978). Verbal alexia usually results from a lesion involving the dominant medial occipital lobe (Hecaen & Albert, 1978; Hecaen & Kremin, 1976).

Literal Alexia

Literal alexia is a condition in which the patient is unable to recognize or read letters and has been referred to as *pure letter blindness*. Moreover, the patient is usually unable to read by spelling a word out loud, and the ability to read numbers and even musical notation is often disturbed. Some investigators have attributed literal alexia to left inferior occipital lesions (Hecaen & Kremin, 1976). This disorder has also been referred to as *frontal alexia*. This is because patients with Broca's aphasia or lesions involving the left frontal convexity have difficulty reading aloud and have the most difficulty with single letters rather than whole words (Benson, 1977).

Spatial Alexia

Spatial alexia is associated predominantly with right hemisphere lesions. In part this disorder is due to visual–spatial abnormalities including neglect and inattention. With right cerebral lesions the patient may fail to read the left half of words or sentences and may in fact fail to perceive or respond to the entire left half of a written page.

Right posterior injuries may also give rise to spatial disorientation such that the patient is unable to visually track and keep place properly, their eyes darting haphazardly across the page. For example, they may skip to the wrong line. Spatial alexia may also result from left cerebral injuries, in which case it is the right half of letters, words, and sentences that is ignored (Marshall & Newcombe, 1966).

Agraphia: Writing Abnormalities

Just as one theory of reading proposes that visual graphemes are converted into phonological units (visual images into sound), it has been proposed that in writing one transcodes speech sounds into grapheme clusters—a phoneme-to-grapheme conversion (Barron, 1980; Ellis, 1982; Friderici *et al.,* 1981). In the lexical route, there is no phonological step. Instead, the entire word is merely retrieved.

Regardless of which theory one adheres to, it appears that the angular gyrus plays an important role in writing. Presumably, the angular gyrus provides the word images (probably through interaction with Wernicke's area), which are to be converted to graphemes. These representations are then transmitted to the left frontal convexity (i.e.,

Broca's and Exner's area) for grapheme conversion and motoric expression, However, it is possible that the initial graphemic representations are formed in the inferior parietal lobule (Roeltgen, Sevush, & Heilman, 1983).

Nevertheless, it appears that at least two stages are involved in the act of writing: a linguistic stage and a motor–expressive–praxic stage. The linguistic stage involves the encoding of information into syntactical–lexical units (Goldstein, 1948); this stage is mediated through the angular gyrus, which provides the linguistic rules that subserve writing. The motor stage is the final step in which the expression of graphemes is subserved; this stage is mediated presumably by Exner's writing area (located in the left frontal convexity) in conjunction with the inferior parietal lobule.

Disturbances involving the ability to write can occur due to disruptions at various levels of processing and expression and may arise secondary to lesions involving the left frontal or inferior parietal cortices. As with alexia, several subtypes of agraphia may become manifest, depending on which level and anatomical region is compromised. These include frontal agraphia, pure agraphia, alexic agraphia, apraxic agraphia, and spatial agraphia.

Disturbances of Exner's Writing Area

Within a small area along the lateral convexity of the left frontal region lies Exner's writing area (Hecaen & Albert, 1978). Exner's area appears to be the final common pathway whereby linguistic impulses receive a final motoric stamp for the purposes of writing. Exner's area, however, also seems to be very dependent on Broca's area, with which it maintains extensive interconnections; i.e., Broca's area acts to organize impulses received from the posterior language zones and relays them to Exner's area for the purpose of written expression.

Lesions localized to this vicinity have been reported to result in disturbances in the elementary motoric aspects of writing, i.e., frontal agraphia (Penfield & Roberts, 1959), sometimes referred to as pure agraphia. However, pure agraphia has also been attributed to left parietal lesions (Basso, Taborelli, & Vignolo, 1978; Strub & Geschwind, 1983). In general, with frontal agraphia, grapheme formation becomes labored and incoordinated and takes on a sloppy appearance. Cursive handwriting is usually more disturbed than printing. The ability to spell per se may or may not be affected, whereas with parietal lesions spelling is often abnormal. Rather, there are disturbances in grapheme selection; the patient may either seem to have forgotten how to form certain letters or may abnormally sequence or even add unnecessary letters when writing, or both (Hecaen & Albert, 1978).

With severe damage, the left hand is more affected than the right (because of disconnection from the left hemisphere language axis). However, with either hand, patients may not be able to write or spell correctly, even if given block letters.

Frontal agraphia can also result from lesions involving Broca's area. These patients are unable to write spontaneously or to dictation; when they do write, their samples may be contaminated by perseverations or the addition of extra strokes to letters (e.g., when writing an "m"). Often such patients are able to write their name or other well-learned (automatic) items without difficulty; therefore, when tested, these patients should be required to write spontaneously as well as to dictation.

Pure Agraphia

In pure agraphia, patients have difficulty in the motor control of grapheme selection and production, frequently misspell words, and may insert the wrong letters or place them in the wrong order or sequence when attempting to write (Marcie & Hecaen, 1979). By contrast, reading, oral speech, and the ability to name objects or letters are usually unimpaired.

Most commonly, pure agraphia is associated with lesions involving the superior and midparietal regions of the left hemisphere, areas 5 and 7 (Basso *et al.,* 1978; Vignolo, 1983), and/or the inferior parietal region (Strub & Geschwind, 1983). Patients are unable to write because the area involved in organizing visual-letter organization (i.e., the inferior parietal lobe) is cut off from the region controlling hand movements in the frontal lobe (Strub & Geschwind, 1983). However, according to Vignolo (1983), the posterior superior left parietal lobule (area 7) is crucial for the sensorimotor linguistic integration needed for writing.

Alexic Agraphia

Alexic agraphia is a disturbance involving the ability to read and to write. It is a disruption of both the ability to decode and to encode written language. However, reading and writing may not be equally affected. Usually recognition of letters is better than words, and the longer the word, the greater the difficulty with recognition.

These patients have severe difficulty forming graphemes and spelling, even when block letters are employed (Marcie & Hecaen, 1979). Although words are misspelled, syntactical sequencing is preserved such that what is written remains grammatically correct. Nevertheless, patients often display some degree of anomia and apraxia (due to inferior parietal involvement). Verbal–auditory comprehension is generally intact, as is expressive speech.

Often alexia with agraphia is caused by a lesion involving the left inferior parietal lobule and angular gyrus (Benson & Geschwind, 1969; Hecaen & Kremin, 1976) and for this reason has also been called parietal alexia. Because the angular gyrus is destroyed, a massive disconnection results such that the auditory areas cannot completely communicate with the visual areas. Nor can the frontal areas interact with the inferior parietal lobe. There are thus two separate disconnections. Patients are unable to perceive visual–linguistic symbols correctly and are unable to reproduce them; i.e., they cannot read or write.

Apraxic Agraphia

It has been argued that the sensorimotor engrams necessary for the production and perception of written language are stored within the inferior parietal lobule of the left hemisphere (Strub & Geschwind, 1983). When this region is damaged, patients sometimes have difficulty forming letters owing to an inability to access these engrams (Strub & Geschwind, 1983). Writing samples are characterized by misspellings, letter omissions, distortions, temporal–sequential misplacements, and inversions (Kinsbourne &

Warrington, 1964). This type of agraphia is often seen in conjunction with Gerstmann's syndrome (see under Finger Agnosia).

Because the patient is also apraxic, the ability to make gestures or complex patterned movements such as those involved in writing is also deficient. That is, the ability to temporally sequence hand movements correctly, independent of writing, is affected (see under Apraxia). The patient no longer knows how to hold or manipulate a pen correctly or how to move the hand when writing.

Spatial Agraphia

Right cerebral injuries can secondarily disrupt writing skills due to generalized spatial and constructional deficiencies. Thus, words and letters will not be properly formed and aligned, even when copying. There may be difficulty keeping lines straight, and letters may be slanted at abnormal angles. In some cases, the writing may be reduced to an illegible scrawl. In addition, patients may write only on the right half of the paper, with the left-hand margin becoming progressively larger and the right side smaller. If allowed to continue, patients may end up writing only along the edge of the right-hand margin of the paper.

Patients with right hemisphere lesions may tend to segment the letters in words abnormally when writing cursively (i.e., *cu siv e ly*). This is caused by a failure to perform closure as well as a release over the left hemisphere (i.e., left hemisphere release). That is, the left acting unopposed begins to temporally sequence abnormally and thus produce segments unnecessarily. It is also important to note that the insertion of gaps between letters within words can also occur following left hemisphere lesions.

Aphasia and Agraphia

Although every patient with agraphia does not necessarily suffer from aphasic abnormalities, all those who have aphasia do have some degree of agraphia. In some instances, the aphasia may be mild and the agraphic disturbance may be severe or conversely quite subtle and only demonstrated through special testing. In general, it is best to require the patient to write cursively rather than to print. Moreover, the more complex the writing task, the more likely it is that an agraphic disturbance will be demonstrated. In testing, one should not be satisfied with the writing of simple words or sentences if agraphia is truly to be ruled out.

Verbal Memory

It has long been established that the left cerebral hemisphere is "dominant" in regard to linguistic memory. Patients with left temporal lobe damage, removal, or posterior cerebral strokes have significant difficulty recalling short prose or verbal narrative passages. They also do poorly on paired associate learning, the repetition of digits, and perform more deficiently than those with right cerebral dysfunction when recalling consonant trigrams or recognizing recurring verbal material (DeRenzi *et al.*, 1987; Hecaen & Albert, 1978; Kimura, 1963; B. Milner, 1967; B. Milner & Teuber, 1968; E. Milner,

1970). Similarly, verbal memory, and the recollection of verbally labeled material is more seriously and significantly disrupted after sodium amytal injection to the left but not right hemisphere (personal observation).

LANGUAGE AND TEMPORAL–SEQUENTIAL MOTOR CONTROL

The left cerebral hemisphere is specialized in regard to motor control and the mediation of temporal–sequential information processing and expression (Corballis & Morgan, 1978; Joseph, 1982; Kimura, 1982). Indeed, both language and thought are related to, and in part an outgrowth of, motor activity (Faaborg-Anderson, 1957; Jacobsen, 1932; Joseph, 1982; McGuigan, 1978). Thus, we find that when the left hemisphere is damaged, performance on problems involving not only language but temporal order is selectively impaired (Efron, 1963; Lackner & Teuber, 1973), as is nonverbal manual or oral performance (Mateer & Kimura, 1976; Heilman, Scholes, & Watson, 1975), the copying of meaningless movements (Kimura & Archibald, 1974) rapidity of limb and pursuit–motor movements (Heilman et al., 1975; Wyke, 1968), and the analysis of temporal speech sequences (Lenneberg, 1967).

Temporal sequencing is a fundamental property of language, as demonstrated by the use of syntax and grammar. That is, syntax is a system of rules that govern the positioning of various lexical items and their interrelations. This allows us to do more than merely name but to describe and analyze how various parts and segments of speech interrelate. We can determine what comes first or last (e.g., "point to the door after you point to the window"), and what is the subject and object. When the left hemisphere is damaged, particularly the anterior portions, expressive and receptive aspects of synactical information processing suffer.

By contrast, the right brain has great difficulty using syntactical or temporal–sequential rules. For example, if the isolated right brain is given a command, such as "pick up the yellow triangle and then the blue star," it may pick up the yellow star and the blue triangle (Zaidel, 1977). It responds to the first object in the sentence, regardless of grammatical relationship.

Thus, we find that the ability to extract denotative meaning from language is dependent on the ability to organize and coordinate speech into temporal and interrelated units—an ability in which the left hemisphere excels and that is at least in part an outgrowth or a function of motoric processing (Kimura, 1976, 1977, 1979, 1982).

Handedness and Language

There is some suggestion that language, in particular its grammatical and syntactical components, is directly related to handedness. Among most of the population the right hand is dominant for grasping, manipulating, exploring, writing, creating, destroying, and communicating. That is, although the left hand assists, it is usually the right that is more frequently used for orienting, pointing, gesturing, expressing, and gathering information concerning the environment. We use the right hand predominantly for waving goodbye, throwing a kiss, delivering a vulgar gesture, greeting, and so forth. The right hand appears to serve as a kind of motoric extension of language and thought in that it acts at the behest of linguistic impulses (Joseph, 1982).

Moreover, while talking, most people display right hand/arm gestural activity, which appears to accompany and even emphasize certain aspects of speech (Kimura, 1977). When speaking, the neural centers controlling right hand use become activated. In part this is attributed to the spread of neural excitation from the speech area to the immediately adjacent cortical regions controlling hand movement. Indeed, both speech and hand-control neurons occupy to some degree the same space and rely on similar neural centers in regard to programming. Hence, because they are so intimately linked, speaking can trigger hand movement.

Because they partially occupy the same neuronal space, sometimes dual and simultaneous activation of these two modalities results in competitive interference. For example, while speaking, the ability to simultaneously track, manually sequence, position, or maintain stabilization of the arms and hands is concurrently disrupted (Hicks, 1975; Lomas & Kimura, 1976; Kimura & Archibald, 1974; Kinsbourne & Cook, 1971); as the phonetic difficulty of the verbalizations increases (Hicks, 1975), motor control decreases—a function presumably of simultaneous activation of (and therefore competition for) the same neurons.

Naming, Knowing, Counting, Finger Recognition, and Hand Control

A variety of theories have been proposed so as to explain the evolution of handedness and language (Bradshaw & Nettleton, 1982; MacNeilage, Studdert-Kennedy, & Lindblom, 1987). Nevertheless, from an evolutionary, pyhlogenetic, and ontogenetic perspective, handedness and temporal–sequential motor control probably preceded the development of language-specialized neurons. Indeed, it is through the hand that one first comes to know the world, so that it may be named and identified. Hence, the infant first uses the hand to grasp various objects so they may be placed in the mouth and orally explored. As the child develops, rather than mouthing, more reliance is placed solely on the hand (as well as on the visual system), so that information may be gathered through touch and manipulation.

As the child and its brain matures, instead of predominantly touching, grasping, and holding, the fingers of the hand are used for pointing and then naming the object indicated. The fingers are later used for counting and the development of temporal–sequential reasoning; i.e., the child learns to count on his or her fingers, then to count (or name) by pointing at objects in space. In this regard, counting, naming, object identification, finger utilization, and hand control are ontogenetically linked. In fact, these capacities seem to rely on the same neural substrates for their expression, i.e., the left inferior parietal lobule. Thus, when the more posterior portions of the left hemisphere are damaged, naming (anomia), object identification (agnosia), arithmetical abilities (acalculia), finger recognition (finger agnosia), and temporal–sequential control over the hands and extremities (apraxia) are frequently compromised. It is relationships such as these that lend considerable credence to the argument that over the course of evolution the predominant usage of the right hand enabled the left brain to develop neurons specialized for counting, naming, and subserving the development of the temporal–sequential properties necessary for the mediation of grammatical–syntactical speech and language.

Agnosia, Apraxia, Acalculia, and Orientation in Space

Disturbances involving spatial–perceptual motor functioning can occur with lesions to either hemisphere. (See Chapter 1, The Right Cerebral Hemisphere.) However, the nature of the disturbance (as well as the severity) differ depending on which half of the brain has been compromised. For example, right cerebral injuries generally have a more pronounced effect on visual–spatial and related perceptual abilities and more greatly disrupt the overall perception and expression of configurational relationships (e.g., disruption of the overall gestalt), as demonstrated on drawing or constructional tasks. Patients with left-sided damage tend to preserve spatial relations but show a reduction in the number of parts represented. Moreover, left hemisphere lesions tend to affect motoric aspects of spatial–perceptual functioning more severely. As such, left hemisphere-injured patients tend to recognize their errors. Nevertheless, it sometimes occurs that patients not only fail to recognize their errors but fail even to recognize whatever object they are attempting to examine or reproduce. This condition is referred to as agnosia, a term presumably coined by Sigmund Freud during his studies in neurology.

Visual Agnosia

Visual agnosia is a condition in which the patient loses the capacity to recognize objects visually, although visual sensory functioning is largely normal. That is, objects are detected, but the ability to evoke or assign meaning is lost, and the object cannot be identified (Critchley, 1964*b*; Teuber, 1968). The percept becomes stripped of its meaning. For example, if shown a comb, the patient might have no idea as to what it is or what it might be used for. However, the patient may be capable of giving a rough estimate of its size and proportions and other features. In general, this disturbance is associated with damage involving the medial and deep mesial portion of the left occipital lobe. However, the lesion may extend into the left posterior temporal lobe.

Nevertheless, this is not a naming disorder. Patients with anomia have difficulty naming an object if it is presented by touch, sound, visual inspection, or auditory description. Patients with agnosia may have difficulty only through a single modality. If shown a comb, they may be unable to name or describe its use. However, if placed in their hand and encouraged to palpate and tactually explore it, they may be able to identify it without difficulty. (Conversely, patients who can recognize an item by sight but not by touch suffer from stereognostic abnormalities due to parietal lesions.) Hence, anomia occurs across modalities, whereas agnosia is usually (but not always) limited to a single modality.

Simultanagnosia

Simultanagnosia is the inability to see more than one thing or one aspect of an object at a time, although individual details are correctly perceived. However, the patient is unable to relate the different details in order to discern what is being viewed. For example, if shown a picture of a man holding an umbrella and a suitcase, they may see the suitcase and the man and the umbrella but be unable to relate these items into a meaningful whole. In fact, by surrounding the object with other objects, perceptual recognition may deteriorate even further. With severe damage, the patient may be unable even to recognize individual objects. Indeed, one patient I examined with bilateral posterior parietal–occipital damage (following stroke) could only identify parts of objects, but not the object itself.

As described by Luria (1980), this is due to a breakdown in the ability to perform serial feature-by-feature visual analysis and is sometimes accompanied by abnormal eye movements. Nevertheless, when compromised, a variety of anatomical regions can give rise to this abnormality. For example, simultanagnosia has been noted to occur with left, right, and bilateral superior occipital lobe lesions or with injuries involving the frontal eye fields (Kinsbourne & Warrington, 1962; Luria, 1980; Rizzo & Hurtig, 1987). Moreover, I have frequently observed patients with diffuse degenerative disturbances who demonstrate simultanagnosic deficiencies.

Right–Left Disorientation

Right–left disorientation is usually associated with left hemisphere and left parietal–occipital damage. It occurs only rarely among patients with right cerebral injuries (Gerstmann, 1930; McFie & Zangwill, 1960; Sauguet, Benton, & Hecaen, 1971).

In general, these patients have difficulty differentiating between the right and left halves of their body or of the bodies of others. This may be demonstrated in a number of ways: by asking the patient to touch or point to the side named by the examiner (e.g., "touch your left cheek," or "point to my right ear"), to point on their own body to the body part the examiner has pointed to on his/her body, or in performing crossed commands ("touch your left ear with your right hand"). In mild cases, patients have difficulty only with the crossed commands (Strub & Geschwind, 1983).

In part, it seems somewhat odd that right–left spatial disorientation is more associated with left than with right cerebral injuries, given the tremendous involvement the right half of the brain has in spatial synthesis and geometrical analysis. However, orientation to the left or right transcends geometrical space, as it relies on language. That is, left and right are designated by words and defined linguistically. In this regard, left and right become subordinated to language usage and organization (Luria, 1980). Thus left–right confusion is strongly related to problems in integrating spatial coordinates within a linguistic framework. It is perhaps for this reason that patients with aphasic disorders generally perform the most poorly of all brain-damaged groups on left–right orientation tasks (Sauguet *et al.*, 1971).

Finger Agnosia

Finger agnosia is not a form of finger-blindness, as the name suggests, nor is it an inability to recognize a finger as a finger. Rather, the difficulty involves naming and differentiating among the fingers of either hand as well as the hands of others (Gerstmann, 1930). This includes pointing to fingers named by the examiner or moving or indicating a particular finger on one hand when the same finger is stimulated on the opposite hand. In addition, if the examiner touches the patient's finger while his eyes are closed and asks him to touch the same finger, the patient may have difficulty. Often patients who have difficulty identifying fingers by name or simply differentiating between them nonverbally also suffer from receptive language abnormalities (Sauguet *et al.,* 1971). However, disturbances differentiating between the different fingers can occur independent of language abnormalities or with right parietal injuries (in which case the problem is seen only with the patient's left hand).

Usually, however, finger agnosia is associated with left parietal lesions, in which case the agnosia is demonstrable in both hands. It is also part of the constellation of symptoms often referred to as Gerstmann's syndrome, i.e., agraphia, acalculia, left–right disorientation, finger agnosia. Gerstmann's symptom complex is most often associated with lesions in the area of the supramarginal gyrus and superior parietal lobule (Hrbek, 1977; Strub & Geschwind, 1983).

Acalculia

When a patient has difficulty working with numbers or performing arithmetical operations secondary to a brain injury, the manner and level at which the problem is expressed will differ depending on which part of the cerebrum has been compromised. For example, a patient with a parietal–occipital lesion may suffer an alexia/agnosia for numbers, in which case he is unable to read or recognize different numerals. A patient with a posterior right cerebral injury may have difficulties with spatial–perceptual functioning and therefore misalign numbers when adding or subtracting (referred to as spatial acalculia).

Thus, in many instances, a patient may appear to have difficulty performing math problems when in fact the basic ability to calculate per se is intact. That is, the difficulty is attributable to spatial, linguistic, agnosic, or alexic abnormalities. By contrast, with left posterior lesions localized to the vicinity of the inferior parietal lobe, patients may have severe difficulty performing even simple arithmetic calculations, such as carrying, stepwise computation, borrowing (Boller & Grafman, 1983; Hecaen & Albert, 1978). When this occurs in the absence of alexia, aphasia, or visual–spatial abnormalities and is accompanied by finger agnosia, agraphia, and right–left orientation, it is considered part of Gerstmann's syndrome (Gerstmann, 1930). This deficit is the purest form of acalculia. It is caused by an impairment in the ability to maintain order, to plan correctly in sequence, and to manipulate numbers appropriately. (Calculation disturbances are discussed in greater detail in Chapter 5, The Parietal Lobes.)

Apraxia

The left cerebral hemisphere has been shown to be superior to the right in the control of certain types of complex sequenced motor acts (Kimura, 1980). If the left hemisphere is damaged, the patient's ability to acquire or perform tasks involving sequential changes in the hand or upper musculature or those requiring skilled movement may be impaired (Kimura, 1979, 1982). Indeed, the deficit may extend to well-learned and even stereotyped motor tasks, such as lighting a cigarette or using a key. This condition is referred to as apraxia.

Apraxia is a disorder of skilled movement in the absence of impaired motor functioning or paralysis (Heilman, 1979). Apraxic patients usually show the correct intent but perform the movement in a clumsy fashion. As with many other types of deficiencies following brain damage, patients and their families may not notice or complain of apraxic abnormalities. This is particularly true for those who are aphasic or paralyzed on the right side. That is, clumsiness with either extremity may not seem significant. Hence, direct examination is necessary to rule out the presence of this problem, even in the absence of complaints.

Apraxia is usually mildest when objects are used. Performance deteriorates most obviously when required to imitate or pantomime the correct action. For example, the patient may be asked to show the examiner, "how you would use a key to open a door" or "hammer a nail into a piece of wood." In many cases, the patient may erroneously use a body part (e.g., a finger) as an object (e.g., a key). That is, the patient may pretend that her finger is the key (inserting it into a "key hole" and turning it) rather than the finger and thumb holding an imaginary key. Although performance usually improves when these patients use actual objects (Goodglass & Kaplan, 1972), a rare few may show the disturbance when using the real object as well (Heilman, 1979).

In addition, patients with apraxia may demonstrate difficulty in properly sequencing their actions. For example, if the examiner were to pretend to place a cigarette and matches in front of the patient and ask him to demonstrate by pantomime how he would light it and take a drag, he might pretend to hold up the match, blow it out, strike it, and then pretend to suck on the cigarette. These patients incorrectly sequence a series of acts, but individual acts may be performed accurately.

Broadly speaking, there are several forms of apraxia, which like many of the disturbances already discussed may be attributable to a number of causes or anatomical lesions. These include ideational apraxia, ideomotor apraxia, buccal–facial apraxia, and dressing apraxia. With the exception of dressing apraxia (which is caused by a right cerebral injury), apraxic abnormalities are usually secondary to left hemisphere damage, in particular, injuries involving the left frontal and inferior parietal lobes.

The inferior parietal lobule appears to be the central region of concern in regard to the performance of skilled temporal–sequential motor acts. This is because the motor engrams for performing these actions appear to be stored in the left angular and supramarginal gyri (Heilman, 1979). These engrams assist in the programming of the motor frontal cortex, where the actions are actually executed.

If the inferior parietal region is destroyed, the patient loses the ability to appreciate when he has performed an action incorrectly. If the motor region is destroyed, although the act is still performed inaccurately (because of disconnection from the inferior parietal lobule), the patient is able to recognize the difference (Heilman, 1979). Thus, apraxic abnormalities secondary to left cerebral lesions tend to involve either destruction of the inferior parietal lobule or lesions resulting in disconnection of the frontal motor areas (or the right cerebral hemisphere) from this more posterior region of the brain. (Apraxia is discussed in more detail in Chapter 5, The Parietal Lobes.)

Pantomime Recognition

Patients with left inferior parietal or occipital lobe lesions have difficulty not only performing motor acts but comprehending, recognizing, and discriminating between different types of motor acts performed and pantomimed by others (Heilman, Rothi, & Valenstein, 1982; Rothi, Mack, Heilman, 1986). In the extreme, if asked to pantomime pouring water into a glass versus lighting and smoking a cigarette, these patients would have difficulty describing what was viewed or in choosing which was which.

SUMMARY

The left cerebral hemisphere maintains the neural substrates that mediate linguistic expression and comprehension, reading and writing, the performance of verbal abstract associations, verbal concept formation, the assigning of verbal labels to experience, the distinction of sound and sign by specific articulatory and linguistic features, mathematical and analytical reasoning, and temporal–sequential and gestural communication. In part, there is considerable evidence that left hemisphere superiority in regard to linguistic processing is related to, and an outgrowth of, handedness and temporal–sequential motor control. It has also been argued in detail elsewhere (Joseph, 1982) that linguistic thought and language often serve as an internalized means of organizing and labeling impulses that arise in the nonlinguistic portions of the nervous system so that the temporal–sequential– linguistic dependent regions of the brain may achieve understanding.

When damaged, a host of temporal–sequential, motoric, and language-related abnor- malities may result. These include expressive and receptive aphasia, alexia, agraphia, agnosia, apraxia, and acalculia. In addition, disorders of thought formation, including schizophrenic-like, depressive, and apathetic states are associated with left cerebral abnormalities.

REFERENCES

Abrams, R., & Taylor, M. A. (1980). Psychopathology and the electroencephalogram. *Biological Psychiatry, 15*, 871–878.

Ach, N. (1951). Determining tendencies. In D. Rapaport (Ed.), *Organization and pathology of thought* (pp. 37– 53). New York: Columbia University Press.

Albert, M. L., & Bear, D. (1974). Time to understand. A case study of word deafness with reference to the role of time in auditory comprehension. *Brain, 97*, 383–394.

Albert, M. L., Sparks, R., von Strockert, T., & Sax, D. (1972). A case of auditory agnosia Linguistic and nonlinguistic processing. *Cortex, 8*, 427–443.

Barron, R. W. (1980). Visual and phonological strategies in reading and spelling. In U. Frith (Ed.), *Cognitive processes in spelling* (pp. 201–230). London: Academic Press.

Basso, A., Taborelli, A., & Vignolo, A. (1978). Dissociated disorders of speaking and writing in aphasia. *Journal of Neurology, Neurosurgery and Psychiatry, 41*, 556–563.

Beaumont, J. G. (1974). Handedness and hemisphere function. In S. J. Dimond & J. G. Beaumont (Eds.), *Hemispheric function in the human brain* (pp. 89–120). New York: John Wiley & Sons.

Benson, D. F. (1977). The third alexia. *Archives of Neurology, 34*, 327–331.

Benson, D. F. (1979). *Aphasia, alexia, agraphia.* New York: Churchill-Livingstone.

Benson, D. F., & Geschwind, N. (1969). The alexias. In P. J. Vinken & G. W. Bruyn (Eds.), *Handbook of clinical neurology,* (Vol. 4) (pp. 427–473). Amsterdam: North-Holland.

Benson, D. F., Sheremata, W. A., Bouchard, R., Segarram, J., Price, D., & Geschwind, N. (1973). Conduc- tion aphasia. *Archives of Neurology, 28*, 339–346.

Blumstein, S., & Cooper, W. E. (1974). Hemispheric processing of intonational contours, *Cortex, 10*, 146– 158.

Boller, F., Cole, M., Vrtunski, P. B., Patterson, M., & Kim, Y. (1979). Paralinguistic aspects of auditory comprehension in aphasia *Brain & Language, 9*, 164–174.

Boller, F., & Grafman, J. (1983). Acalculia: Historical development and current significance. *Brain and Cognition, 2*, 205–223.

Boller, F., & Green, E. (1972). Comprehension in severe aphasics. *Cortex, 8*, 382–390.

Bradshaw, J. L., & Nettleton, N. C. (1982). Language lateralization to the dominant hemisphere: Tool use, gesture and language in hominid evolution. *Current Psychological Reviews, 2*, 171–192.

Brain, R., & Walton, J. N. (1969). *Brain's diseases of the nervous system.* New York: Oxford University Press.

Carmazza A., & Zurif, E. B. (1976). Dissociation of algorithmic and heuristic process in language comprehension: Evidence from aphasia. *Brain and Language, 3*, 572–582.

Chaika, E. (1982). A unified explanation for the diverse structural deviations reported for adult schizophrenics with disrupted speech. *Journal of Communication Disorders, 15*, 167–189.

Chapman, J. (1966). The early symptoms of schizophrenia. *British Journal of Psychiatry, 12*, 225–251.

Corballis, M. C., & Morgan, M. J. (1978). On the biological bais of lateality. I. *Behavioral and Brain Sciences, 1*, 261–269.

Craik, K. J. W. (1943). *The nature of explanation.* Cambridge: Cambridge University Press.

Critchely, M. (1964a). The neurology of psychotic speech. *British Journal of Psychiatry, 40*, 353–364.

Critchely, M. (1964b). The problem of visual agnosia. *Journal of Neurological Sciences, 1*, 274–290.

Cutting, J. E. (1974). Two left hemisphere mechanisms in speech perception. *Perception and Psychophysics, 16*, 601–612.

De Boysson-Bardies, B., Bacri, N., Sagart, L., & Poizat, M. (1980). Timing in late babbling. *Journal of Child Language, 8*, 525–539.

d'Elia, G., & Perris, C. (1974). Cerebral functional dominance and memory functioning. *Acta Psychiatrica Scandinavica, 255*, 143–157.

Denes, G., & Semenza, C. (1975). Auditory modality-specific anomia. Evidence from a case of pure word deafness. *Cortex, 11*, 401–411.

De Renzi, E., & Vignolo, L. A. (1962). The Token test. *Brain, 85*, 665–678.

DeRenzi, E., Zambolini, A., & Crisi, G. (1987). The pattern of neuropsychological impairment associated with left posterior cerebral artery infarcts. *Brain, 110*, 1099–1116.

Efron, R. (1963). The effect of handedness on the perception of simultaneity and temporal order. *Brain, 86*, 261–284.

Ellis, A. W. (1982). Spelling and writing (and reading and speaking). In A. W. Ellis (Ed.), *Normality and pathology in cognitive functions.* London: Academic Press.

Faaborg-Anderson, K. C. (1957). Electromyographic investigation of intrinsic laryngeal muscles in humans. *Acta Physiologica Scandinavica, 140*, 1–148.

Faber, R., Abrams, R., Taylor, M., Kasprisin, A., Morris, C., & Weisz, R. (1983). Comparison of schizophrenic patients with formal thought disorder and neurologically impaired patients with aphasia. *American Journal of Psychiatry, 140*, 1348–1351.

Flor-Henry, P. (1983). *Cerebral basis of psychopathology.* Boston: John Wright.

Freud, S. (1900). *The interpretation of dreams.* (Vol. 5.) London: Hogarth Press.

Friderici, A. D., Schoenle, P. W., & Goodglass, H. (1981). Mechanisms underlying writing and speech in aphasia. *Brain and Language, 13*, 212–222.

Galin, D., Diamond, D. R., & Braff, D. (1977). Lateralization of conversion symptoms: More frequent on the left. *American Journal of Psychiatry, 134*, 578–580.

Galin, D., Diamond, R., & Herron, J. (1979a). Development of crossed and uncrossed tactile localization on the fingers. *Brain and Language, 4*, 588–590.

Gallagher, R. E., & Joseph, R. (1982). Non-linguistic knowledge, hemispheric laterality, and the conservaton of inequivalence. *Journal of General Psychology, 107*, 31–40.

Gardner, H. (1975). *The shattered mind.* New York: Vintage Books.

Gerstmann, J. (1930). Syndrome of finger agnosia, disorientation for right and left, agraphia and acalculia. *Archives of Neurology and Psychiatry, 44*, 398–408.

Geschwind, N., Quadfasel, F. A., & Segarra, J. M. (1968). Isolation of the speech area. *Neuropsychologia, 6*, 327–340.

Gloning, I., Gloning, K., Hoff, H. (1968). *Neuropsychological symptoms and syndromes in lesions of the occipial lobe and the adjacent areas.* Paris: Gauthier-Villars.

Goldstein, K. (1942). *After effects of brain injuries in war.* New York: Grune & Stratton.

Goldstein, K. (1948). *Language and language disturbances*. New York: Grune & Stratton.

Goodglass, H., & Berko, J. (1960). Agrammatism and inflectional morphology in English. *Journal of Speech and Hearing Research, 3*, 257–267.

Goodglass, H., & Kaplan, E. (1972). *Boston diagnostic aphasia examination*. Philadelphia: Lea & Febiger.

Graff-Radford, N. R., Cooper, W. E., Colsher, P. L., & Damasio, A. R. (1986). An unlearned foreign "accent" in a patient with aphasia. *Brain and Language, 28*, 86–94.

Green, P., & Kontenko, V. (1980). Superior speech comprehension in schizophrenics under monaural versus binaural listening conditions. *Journal of Abnormal Psychology, 89*, 339–408.

Greenblatt, S. H. (1973). Alexia without agraphia or hemianopia. *Brain, 96*, 307–316.

Gross, C. G., Rocha-Miranda, C. E., & Bender, D. B. (1972). Visual properties of neurons in inferotemporal cortex of the macaque. *Journal of Neurophysiology, 35*, 96–111.

Halperin, Y., Nachshon, I., & Carmon, A. (1973). Shift of ear superiority in dichotic listening to temporally patterned nonverbal stimuli. *Journal of Experimental Psychology, 101*, 46–54.

Hecaen, H., & Albert, M. L. (1978). *Human neuropsychology*. New York: John Wiley & Sons.

Hecaen, H., & Kremin, H. (1976). Neurolinguistic research on reading disorders from left hemisphere lesions. In H. A. Whitkaer & H. Whitaker (Eds.), *Studies in neurolinguistics* (pp. 47–63). New York: Academic Press.

Heilman, K. M. (1979). Neglect and related disorders. In K. M. Heilman & E. Valenstein (Eds.), *Clinical neuropsychology*. New York: Oxford University Press.

Heilman, K. M., Rothi, L., & Kertesz, A. (1983). Localization of apraxia-producing lesions. In A. Kertesz (Ed.), *Localization in neuropsychology*. New York: Academic Press.

Heilman, K. M., Rothi, L. J., & Valenstein, E. (1982). Two forms of ideomotor apraxia. *Neurology (New York), 32*, 342–346.

Heilman, K., & Scholes, R. J. (1976). The nature of comprehension errors in Broca's conduction, and Wernicke's aphasia. *Cortex, 12*, 258–265.

Heilman, K., Scholes, R., & Watson, R. T. (1975). Auditory affective agnosia. *Journal of Neurology, Neurosurgery and Psychiatry, 38*, 69–72.

Hicks, R. E. (1975). Intrahemispheric resposne competition between voal and unimanual performance in normal adult humann males. *Journal of Comparative and Physiological Psychology, 89*, 50–60.

Hoff-Ginsberg, E., & Shatz, M. (1982). Linguistic input and the child's acquisition of language.

Hoffman, R. E. (1986). Verbal hallucinations and language production processes in schizophrenia. *Behavioral and Brain Sciences, 9*, 503–548.

Hoffman, R., Stopek, S., & Andreasen, N. (1986). A discourse analysis comparing manic versus schizophrenic speech disorganization. *Archives of General Psychiatry, 43*, 831–838.

Hrbek, V. (1977). Pathophysiologic interpretation of Gerstmann's syndrome. *Neuropsychologia, 11*, 377–388.

Jacobsen, E. (1932). Electrophysiology of mental activities. *American Journal of Psychology, 44*, 677–694.

James, W. (1961). *Psychology*. New York: Harper & Row.

Joseph, R. (1980). Awareness, the origin of thought, and the role of conscious self-deception in resistance and repression. *Psychological Reports, 46*, 767–781.

Joseph, R. (1982). The neuropsychology of development: Hemispheric laterality, limbic language and the origin of thought. *Journal of Clinical Psychology, 38*, 4–33.

Joseph, R. (1986). Confabulation and delusional denial: Frontal lobe and lateralized influences. *Journal of Clinical Psychology, 42*, 507–518.

Joseph, R. (1988a). The right cerebral hemisphere: Neuropsychiatry, neuropsychology, neurodynamics. *Journal of Clinical Psychology, 44*, 630–673.

Joseph, R. (1988b). Dual mental functioning in a split-brain patient. *Journal of Clinical Psychology, 44*, 770–779.

Joseph, R. (1989). The limbic system: Emotion, laterality, unconscious mind. *Psychoanalytic Review*, in press.

Joseph, R., Gallagher, R. E., Holloway, W., & Kahn, J. (1984). Two brains—one child. Interhemispheric transfer deficits and confabulation in children aged 3,7,10. *Cortex, 20*, 317–331.

Jung, C. (1954). *Experimental researches, Collected Works, II*. New Jersey: Princeton University Press.

Jung, C. G. (1964). *Man and his symbols*. New York: Dell.

Kay, J., & Ellis, A. (1987). A cognitive neuropsychological case study of anomia. *Brain, 110*, 613–629.

Kertesz, A. (1983a). Localization of lesions in Wernicke's aphasia. In A. Kertesz (Ed.), *Localization in neuropsychology* (pp. 150–170). New York: Academic Press.

Kertesz, A. (1983b). Right-hemisphere lesions in constructional apraxia and visuospatial deficit. In A. Kertesz (Ed.), *Localization in neuropsychology* (301–318). New York: Academic Press.

Kimura, D. (1961). Cerebral dominance and the perception of verbal stimuli. *Canadian Journal of Psychology, 15,* 156–171.

Kimura, D. (1963). Right temporal lobe damage: Perception of unfamiliar stimuli after damage. *Archives of Neurology, 18,* 264–271.

Kimura, D. (1976). The neural basis of language qua gesture. In H. Whitaker & H. A. Whitaker (Eds.), *Studies in neurolinguistics.* (Vol. 2.) New York: Academic Press.

Kimura, D. (1977). Acquisition of a motor skill after left-hemisphere damage. *Brain, 100,* 527–542.

Kimura, D. (1979). Neuromotor mechanisms in the evolution of human communication. In H. D. Steklis & M. J. Raleigh (Eds.), *Neurobiology of social communication in primates.* New York: Academic Press.

Kimura, D. (1982). Left-hemisphere control of oral and brachial movement and their relation to communication. *Philosophical Transactions of the Royal Society of London, 298,* 135–149.

Kimura, D., & Archibald, Y. (1974). Motor functions of the left hemisphere, *Brain, 97,* 337–350.

Kimura, D., & Folb, S. (1968). Neural processing of backward speech sounds. *Science, 161,* 395–396.

Kinsbourne, M., & Cook, J. (1971). Generalized and lateralized effect of concurrent verbalization on a unimanual skill. *Quarterly Journal of Experimental Psychology, 23,* 341–345.

Kinsbourne, M., & Warrington, E. K. (1962). A variety of reading disabilities associated with right hemisphere lesions. *Journal of Neurology, Neurosurgery and Psychiatry, 25,* 339–344.

Kinsbourne, M., & Warrington, E. K. (1964). Disorders of spelling. *Journal of Neurology, Neurosurgery, and Psychiatry, 27,* 224–228.

Lackner, J. L., & Teuber, H.-L. (1973). Alterations in auditory fusion thresholds after cerebral injury in man. *Neuropsychologia, 11,* 409–415.

Landis, T., Graves, R., & Goodglass, H. (1982). Aphasic reading and writing: Possible evidence for right hemisphere participation. *Cortex, 18* 105–112.

Lebrun, Y. (1987). Anosognosia in aphasics. *Cortex, 23,* 251–263.

Lecours, A. R. (1975). Myelogenetic correlates of the development of speech and language. In E. Lenneberg & E. Lenneberg (Eds.), *Foundations of language development.* New York: Academic Press.

Legatt, A. D., Rubin, M. J., Kaplan, L. R., Healton, G. P., & Brust, A. L. (1987). Global aphasia without hemiparesis. *Neurology (New York), 37,* 201–205.

Lenneberg, E. (1967). *Biological foundations of language.* New York: John Wiley & Sons.

Leopold, W. E. (1947). *Speech development of a binlingual child.* (Vol. 2.) Evanston, IL: Northwestern University Press.

Levine, D. N., & Sweet, E. (1983). Localization of lesions in Broca's motor aphasia. In A. Kertesz (Ed). *Localization in neuropsychology* (pp. 185–207). New York: Academic Press.

Levy, J. (1974). Psychological implications of bilateral asymmetry. In S. Diomond & J. G. Beaumont (Eds.), *Hemisphere function in the human brain* (pp. 121–132). London: Paul Elek, Ltd.

Lomas, J., & Kimura, D. (1976). Intrahemispheric interactions between speaking and sequential manual activity. *Neuropsychologia, 14,* 23–33.

Luria, A. (1980). *Higher cortical functions in man.* New York. Basic Books.

MacNeilage, P. F., Studdert-Kennedy, M. G., & Lindblom, B. (1987). Primate handedness reconsidered. *Behavioral Brain Science, 10,* 247–303.

Marcie, P., & Hecaen, H. (1979). Agraphia. In K. M. Heilman & E. Valenstein (Eds.), *Clinical neuropsychology* (pp. 92–126). New York: Oxford University Press.

Marshall, J. C., & Newcombe, F. (1966). Syntactic and semantic errors in paralexia. Neuropsychologia, 4, 169–176.

Mateer, C. A. (1983). Motor and perceptual functions of the left hemisphere and their interaction. In S. J. Segalowitz (Ed.), *Language functions and brain organization* (pp. 80–110). New York: Academic Press.

Mateer, C., & Kimura, D. (1976). Impairment of nonverbal oral movements in aphasia. *Brain and Language, 4,* 262–276.

McFie, J., & Zangwill, O. L. (1960). Visual–constructive disabilities associated with lesions of the left cerebral hemisphere. *Brain, 83,* 243–260.

McGuigan, F. J. (1978). Imagery and thinking. Covert functioning of the motor system. In G. E. Schwartz & D. Shapiro (Eds.), *Conscousness and self regulation.* (Vol. 2.) (pp. 210–240). New York: Plenum Press.

Miller, G. A., Galanter, E., & Pribram, K. H. (1960). *Plans and the structure of behavior.* New York: Holt.

Mills, L., & Rollman, G. B. (1980). Hemispheric asymmetry for auditory perception of temporal order. *Neuropsychologia, 18*, 41–47.

Milner, B. (1964). Some effects of frontal lobectomy in man. In J. M. Warren & K. Akert (Eds.), *The frontal granular cortext and behavior* (pp. 313–334). New York: McGraw-Hill.

Milner, B. (1970). Memory and the medial temporal regions of the brain. In K. Pribram & D. E. Broadbent (Eds.) *Biology of memory*. New York: Academic Press.

Milner, B., & Teuber, H. L. (1968). Alteration of perception and memory in man. In L. Weiskrantz (Ed.), *Analysis of behavioral changes*. New York: Harper & Row.

Milner, E. (1967). *Human neural and behavioral development*. Springfield, IL: Charles C Thomas.

Moscovitch, M. (1973). Language and the cerebral hemispheres. In P. Pliner, et al. (Eds.), *Communication and affect: Language and thought* (pp. 107–170). New York: Academic Press.

Njiokiktjien, C. (1988). *Pediatric behavioural neurology*. Amsterdam: Suyi Publications.

O'Leary, D. S. (1980). A developmental study of interhemispheric transfer in children aged 5 to 10. *Child Development, 51*, 743–750.

Papcun, G., Krashen, S., Terbeek, D., *et al.* (1974). Is the left hemisphere specialized for speech, language and-or something else? *Journal of the Acoustical Society of America, 55*, 319–327.

Penfield, W., & Roberts, L. (1959). *Speech and brain mechanisms*. Princeton, NJ: Princeton University Press.

Perris, C. (1974). Averaged evoked responses (AER) in patients with affective disorders. *Acta Psychiatrica Scandinavica, 255*, 1–107.

Piaget, J. (1952). *The origins of intelligence in children*. New York: Norton.

Piaget, J. (1962). *Play, dreams and imitations in childhood*. New York: Norton.

Piaget, J. (1974). *The child and reality*. New York. Viking Press.

Rizzo, M., & Hurtig, R. (1987). Looking but not seeing. *Neurology (New York), 37*, 1642–1646.

Robinson, B. W. (1967). Vocalization evoked from forebrain in *Macaca mulatta*. *Physiology and behavior, 2*, 345–354.

Robinson, R. G., & Benson, D. F. (1981). Depression in aphasic patients: Frequency, severity, and clinical–pathological correlations. *Brain and Language, 14*, 282–291.

Robinson, R. R., & Szetela, B. (1981). Mood change following left hemisphere brain injury. *Annals of Neurology, 9*, 447–453.

Roeltgen, D. P., Sevush, S., & Heilman, K. M. (1983). Pure Gerstmann's syndrome from a focal lesion. *Archives of Neurology, 40*, 46–47.

Rothi, L. J. G., Mack, L., & Heilman, K. M. (1986). Pantomime agnosia. *Journal of Neurology, Neurosurgery and Psychiatry, 49*, 451–454.

Rubens, A. B. (1979). Agnosia. In K. M. Heilman & E. Valenstein (Eds.), *Clinical neuropsychology* (pp. 233–267). New York: Oxford University Press.

Rutter, D. (1979). The reconstruction of schizphrenic speech. *British Journal of Psychiatry, 134*, 356–359.

Salamy, A. (1978). Commissural transmission: Maturational changes in humans. *Science, 200*, 1409–1411.

Samuels, J. A., & Benson, D. F. (1979). Some aspects of language comprehension in anterior aphasia. *Brain and Language, 8*, 275–286.

Sauguet, J., Benton, A. L., & Hecaen, H. (1971). Disturbances of the body schema in relation to language impairment and hemispheric locus of lesion. *Journal of Neurology, Neurosurgery and Psychiatry, 34*, 496–501.

Schilder, P. (1951). On the development of thoughts. In D. Rappaport (Ed.), *Organization and pathology of thought*. New York: Columbia University Press.

Shankweiler, D., & Studdert-Kennedy, M. (1966). Lateral differences in perception of dichotically presented synthetic consonant–vowel syllables and steady-state vowels. *Journal of the Society of America, 39*, 1256A.

Shankweiler, D., & Studdert-Kennedy, M. (1967). Identification of consonants and vowels presented to left and right ears. *Quarterly Journal of Experimental Psychology, 19*, 59–63.

Smith, A. (1966). Speech and other functions after left (dominant) hemispherectomy. *Journal of Neurology, Neurosurgery and Psychiatry, 29*, 467–471.

Smith, A., & Burklund, C. W. (1966). Dominant hemispherectomy. *Science, 153*, 1280–1282.

Spitz, R. A., & Wolf, K. M. (1946). The smiling response: A contribution to the ontogenesis of social relations. *Genetic Psychology Monographs, 34*, 57–125.

Strub, R. L., & Geschwind, N. (1983). Localization in Gerstmann syndrome. In A. Kertesz (Ed.), *Localization in neuropsychology* (pp. 173–190). New York: Academic Press.

Studdert-Kennedy, M., & Shankweiler, D. (1970). Hemispheric specialization for speech perception. *Journal of the Acoustical Society of America, 48,* 579–594.

Tanaka, Y., Yamadori, A., & Mori, E. (1987). Pure word deafness following bilateral lesions. *Brain, 110,* 381–403.

Teuber, H. L. (1968). Disorders of memory following penetrating missile wounds of the brain. *Neurology (New York), 18,* 287–288.

Vignolo, L. A. (1983). Modality-specific disorders of written language in A. Kertesz (Ed.), *Localization in neuropsychology.* New York: Academic Press.

Vygotsky, L. S. (1962). *Thought and language.* Cambridge: MIT Press.

Weinberger, D. R., Berman, K. F., & Zek, R. F. (1986). Physiological dysfunction of dorsolarteral cortex in schizophrenia. *Archives of General Psychiatry, 114,* 114–125.

Wyke, M. (1968). The effects of lesions in the performance of an arm–hand precision task. *Neuropsychologia, 6,* 125–134.

Yakovlev, P. I., & Lecours, A. (1967). The myelogenetic cycles of regional maturation of the brain. In A. Minkowski (Ed.), *Regional development of the brain in early life.* London: Blackwell.

Yamadori, A., Osumi, U., Mashuara, S., & Okuto, M. (1977). Preservation of singing in Broca's aphasia. *Journal of Neurology, Neurosurgery and Psychiatry, 40,* 221–224.

Zaidel, E. (1977). Unilateral auditory language comprehension on the token test following cerebral commissurotomy and hemispherectomy. *Neuropsychologia, 15,* 1–13.

Zurif, E. B., Caramazza, A., & Myerson, R. (1972). Grammatical judgments on agrammatic aphasics. *Neuropsychologia, 10,* 405–417.

Zurif, E. B., & Carson, G. (1970). Dyslexia in relation to cerebral dominance and temporal analysis. *Neuropsychologia, 8,* 239–244.

The Limbic System
Emotion, Laterality, and Unconscious Mind

Many members of Western civilization experience emotion as a potentially overwhelming force that warrants and yet resists control—as something irrational that can happen to you ("you make me so angry"). Perhaps in part, this schism between the rational and the emotional is attributable to the raw energy of emotion having its source in the nuclei of the ancient limbic lobe—what some have referred to as the reptilian brain, a series of nuclei that first made their phylogenetic appearance long before man walked upon this earth. Although over the course of evolution a new brain (neocortex) has developed, we remain creatures of emotion. We have not completely emerged from the phylogenetic swamps of our original psychic existence. The old limbic brain has not been replaced.

Buried within the depths of the cerebrum are several large aggregates of limbic neurons that are preeminent in the mediation and expression of emotional, motivational, sexual, and social behavior and that control and monitor internal homeostasis and basic needs, such as hunger and thirst. These regions include the hypothalamus, amygdala, hippocampus, septal nuclei, cingulate, various thalamic nuclei, portions of the reticular activating system, the orbital frontal lobes, certain nuclei of the cerebellum, and other structures that together form the limbic system.

Of specific concern in this chapter are the hypothalamus, amygdala, hippocampus, and septal nuclei, the social—emotional and psychic functions they mediate, and the neural circuitry that supports their activity. Limbic laterality, temporal lobe epilepsy, hallucinations and memory, and select aspects of psychological and unconscious development, including the pleasure principle and primary process, are also briefly discussed (Fig. 18).

AFFECTIVE ORIGINS: OLFACTION AND SOMESTHESIS

Emotionality serves a protective function, either to promote survival of the individual (e.g., fight or flight) of that of the species (e.g., sexual activity). The first and most primitive manifestations of emotion are elicited in response to olfactory (e.g., pher-

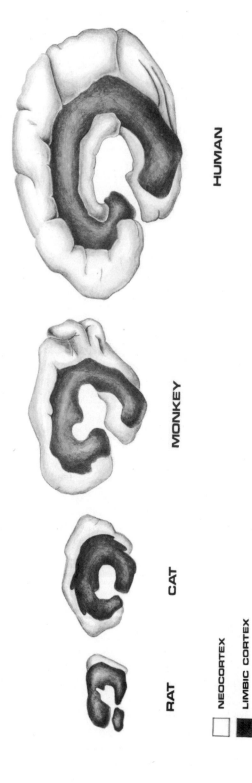

RAT

CAT

MONKEY

HUMAN

NEOCORTEX

LIMBIC CORTEX

FIGURE 18. Schematic diagram of the limbic cortex across four species. Note relative similarities in size and location.

omones and other externally secreted chemical messengers) and tactile sensory stimulation. These primitive emotions are expressed as withdrawal (fear) or approach reactions to pain or threat and are elicited in response to motivational needs, such as the seeking of a sexual partner or for the procurement of food (prey) and nourishment (Graeber, 1980; Michael & Keverne, 1974; Savage, 1980; Wilson, 1962).

Olfaction was originally crucial to evolutionary and phylogenetic development, as it informed the organism about the environment at a distance, without the necessity of physical contact. By means of olfactory cues and the detection of pheromones, the organism is able to detect and track food, determine the intent and social–emotional status of conspecies, as well as signal its own intent, motivation, social position, and/or sexual availability (Michael & Keverne, 1974; Wilson, 1962).

For example, consider pheromones, substances secreted by the skin through specialized glands or found in urine and feces. Chemical communication through pheromones is used by moths, social insects, dogs, cats, and primates, as well as amphibia, sharks, and reptiles. Although detection of pheromones among insects is often accomplished through specialized chemoreceptors located on various parts of the body (Wilson, 1962), mammals and primates rely on olfactory receptors within the nostrils that transmit this information to the olfactory bulb (or lobe in some species) and the telencephalon (Graeber, 1980; Savage, 1980).

Among mammals, olfactory cues are also used for marking possessions and one's territory. For example, dogs will urinate on trees and bushes, whereas a stallion might urinate on the feces of his mare. Prosimian primates will actually urinate on their hands, rub the secretions over their body, and thus mark everything they come into contact with. It has also been shown that male primates, as well as other mammals, rendered anosmic (through the cutting of the olfactory nerves) completely lose interest in sexually available females because of the inability to detect olfactory (pheromone) cues indicating sexual readiness (Michael & Kaverne, 1974). Thus, olfaction is a crucial mode of communication; among some species, the olfactory bulb is so highly developed that it is considered a lobe of the brain.

Among humans olfaction appears to have lost its leading role in signaling motivationally significant information. However, olfactory cues are still employed for indicating sexuality (e.g., perfume), and odor exerts a powerful influence on what is considered socially acceptable, hence the abundance of artificial chemicals designed to eliminate various body fragrances. Moreover, one need only suffer a severe cold to appreciate the dominant function of smell in the ability to detect and appreciate fully the flavor of food and thereby experience pleasure in eating (Fig. 19). Odors also affect learning and memory and have the capability of triggering vivid recollections of some far away and past event.

Ontogenetically, although influenced by olfactory cues, humans first experience or express emotionality in relationship to the body and in response to tactile sensations or rapid changes in position (Emde & Koenig, 1969; Spitz & Wolf, 1946). Pain is also first experienced in relationship to the body, and is somesthetically rooted, although some have argued that pain is not an emotion.

Among human infants, the earliest smiles are induced through tactile stimulation (e.g., light stroking or even blowing on the skin), whereas loss of support is the most powerful stimulus for triggering an emotional reaction in the newborn (Emde & Koenig,

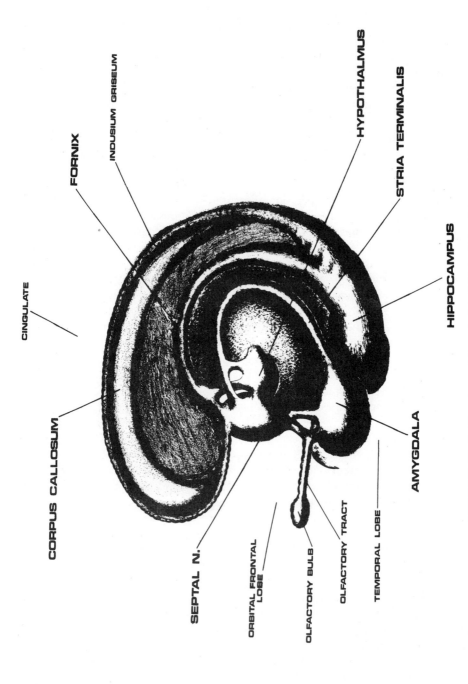

FIGURE 19. The limbic system and the major interlinking pathways between nuclei.

1969; Spitz & Wolf, 1946). The earliest and most consistent manifestation of emotion in the infant consists of screaming and crying, whereas positive affect is limited to an attitude of acceptance and quiescence (Spitz & Wolf, 1946), emotions first mediated by the hypothalamus that may or may not be true emotions at all.

In their journey from the external to the internal environment, olfactory and tactile input are transmitted to various limbic nuclei, such as the lateral hypothalamus and entorhinal area of the hippocampus (olfactory only) and the amygdala (olfaction and somesthesis). Indeed, it is through nuclei such as the amygdala (as opposed to the hypothalamus) that the first true (or rather, felt) aspects of emotion appear to be generated. It is also because of the tremendous input of olfactory information to various limbic nuclei that this part of the brain was at one time referred to as the rhinencephalon, literally "nose brain."

HYPOTHALAMUS

The hypothalamus is a very ancient structure. Unlike most other brain regions, it has maintained a striking similarity in structure throughout phylogeny and apparently over the course of evolution (Crosby, DeJonge, & Schneider, 1966). Located in the most medial aspect of the brain, along the walls and floor of the third ventricle, this nucleus is fully functional at birth and is the central core from which all emotions derive their motive force.

The hypothalamus is highly involved in all aspects of endocrine, hormonal, visceral, and autonomic functions; it mediates or exerts controlling influences on eating, drinking, the experience of pleasure, rage, and aversion. The hypothalamus is also sexually dimorphic; i.e., both structurally and functionally, the hypothalamus of men and women is sexually dissimilar.

Sexual Dimorphism in the Hypothalamus

As is well known, sexual differentiation is strongly influenced by the presence or absence of gonadal steroid hormones during certain critical periods of prenatal development in many species, including humans. However, not only are the external genitalia and other physical features sexually differentiated, but certain regions of the brain have also been found to be sexually dimorphic and differentially sensitive to steroids, particularly the preoptic area and ventromedial nucleus of the hypothalamus, as well as the amygdala (Bleier, Byne, & Siggelkow, 1982; Dorner, 1976; Gorski, Gordon, Shyrne, & Southam, 1978; Rainbow, Parsons, & McEwen, 1982; Raisman & Field, 1971, 1973).

Specifically, the presence or absence of the male hormone testosterone, during this critical neonatal period, directly affects and determines the pattern of interconnections between the amygdala and hypothalamus and between axons and dendrites in these nuclei, and thereby the organization of specific neural circuits. In the absence of testosterone, the female pattern of neuronal development occurs.

For example, if the testes are removed before differentiation, or if a chemical blocker of testosterone is administered, preventing this hormone from reaching target cells in the limbic system, not only does the female pattern of neuronal development occur, but males so treated behave and process information in a manner similar to that of females (e.g., Joseph, Hess, & Birecree, 1978); i.e., they develop female brains. Conversely, if females are administered testosterone during this critical period, the male pattern of differentiation and behavior results.

That the preoptic and other hypothalamic regions are sexually dimorphic is not surprising, in that it has long been known that this area is critical in controlling the basal output of gonadotropins in females before ovulation and is heavily involved in mediating cyclic changes in hormone levels, such as follicle-stimulating estrogen, hormone (FSH), luteinizing hormone (LH), and progesterone. Chemical and electrical stimulation of the preoptic and ventromedial thalamic nuclei also triggers sexual behavior and even sexual posturing in females and males (Lisk, 1967, 1971).

In primates, electrical stimulation of the preoptic area increases sexual behavior in males and significantly increases the frequency of erections, copulations, and ejaculations, we well as pelvic thrusting followed by an explosive discharge of semen even in the absence of a mate (Maclean, 1973). Conversely, lesions to the preoptic and posterior hypothalamus eliminates male sexual behavior and results in gonadal atrophy.

Lateral and Ventromedial Hypothalamic Nuclei

Although consisting of several nuclear subgroups, the lateral and medial (ventromedial) hypothalamic nuclei play particularly important roles in the control of the autonomic nervous system, the experience of pleasure and aversion, eating and drinking, and raw (undirected) emotionality. These nuclei also appear to share a somewhat antagonistic relationship (Fig. 20).

For example, the medial hypothalamus controls parasympathetic activities (e.g., reduction in heart rate, increased peripheral circulation) and exerts a dampening effect on certain forms of emotional/motivational arousal. The lateral hypothalamus mediates sympathetic activity (increasing heart rate, elevating blood pressure) and is involved in controlling the metabolic and somatic correlates of heightened emotionality. In this regard, the lateral and medial region act to exert counterbalancing influences on each other.

Hunger and Thirst

The lateral and medial region are highly involved in monitoring internal homeostasis and motivating the organism to respond to internal needs such as hunger and thirst. For example, both nuclei appear to contain receptors that are sensitive to the body's fat content (lipostatic receptors) and to circulating metabolites (e.g., glucose), which together indicate the need for food and nourishment. The lateral hypothalamus also appears to contain osmoreceptors (Joynt, 1966) that determine whether water intake should be altered.

Electrophysiologically, it has been determined that the hypothalamus not only becomes highly active immediately before and while the organism is eating or drinking, but the lateral region alters its activity when the subject is hungry and is simply looking at food (Hamburg, 1971; Rolls, Burton, & Mora, 1976). In fact, if the lateral hypothalamus is electrically stimulated, a compulsion to eat and drink results (Delgado & Anand, 1953). Conversely, if the lateral area is destroyed bilaterally, aphagia and adipsia are so severe that animals will die unless force fed (Teitelbaum & Epstein, 1962).

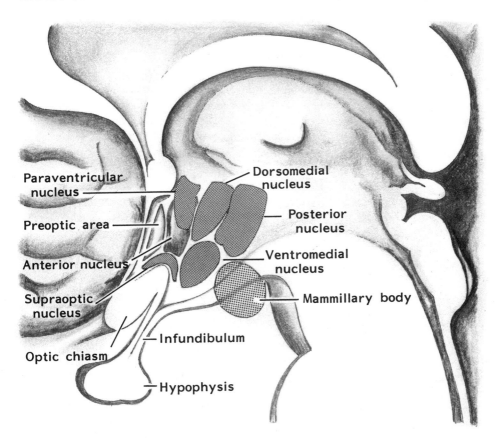

FIGURE 20. Schematic diagram of the nuclei of the medial hypothalamus and adjacent structures. From *Human neuroanatomy* by R. C. Truex & M. B. Carpenter, 1969. Courtesy of The Williams & Wilkins Co., Baltimore, MD.

If the medial hypothalamus is surgically destroyed, inhibitory influences on the lateral region appear to be abolished such that hypothalamic hyperphagia and severe obesity result (Teitelbaum, 1961). Thus, the medial area seems to act as a satiety center but as a center that can be overridden.

Overall, it appears that the lateral hypothalamus is involved in the initiation of eating and acts to maintain a lower weight limit such that when the limit is reached the organism is stimulated to eat. Conversely, the medial regions seems to be involved in setting a higher weight limit such that when these levels are approached, it triggers the cessation of eating. In part, these nuclei exert these differential influences on eating and drinking by means of motivational/emotional influences they exert on other brain nuclei (e.g., by reward or punishment).

Pleasure and Reward

In 1952, Heath (cited by Maclean, 1969) reported what was then considered remarkable. Electrical stimulation near the septal nuclei elicited feelings of pleasure in human subjects: "I have a glowing feeling. I feel good!" Subsequently, Olds and Milner (1954) reported that rats would tirelessly perform operants to receive electrical stimulation in this same region and concluded that stimulation "has an effect that is apparently equivalent to that of a conventional primary reward." Even hungry animals would demonstrate a preference for self-stimulation over food.

Feelings of pleasure (as demonstrated by self-stimulation) have been obtained following excitation to a number of diverse limbic areas, including the olfactory bulbs, amygdala, hippocampus, cingulate, substantia nigra (a major source of dopamine), locus coeruleus (a major source of norepinephrine), raphe nucleus (serotonin), caudate, putamen, thalamus, reticular formation, medial forebrain bundle, and orbital frontal lobes (Brady, 1960; Lilly, 1960; Olds & Forbes, 1981; Stein & Ray, 1959; Waraczynski & Stellar, 1987).

In mapping the brain for positive loci for self-stimulation, Olds (1956) found that the medial forebrain bundle (MFB) was a major pathway that supported this activity. Although the MFB interconnects the hippocampus, hypothalamus, septum, amygdala, and orbital frontal lobes (areas that give rise to self-stimulation), Olds discovered that in its course up to the lateral hypothalamus, reward sites become more densely packed. Moreover, the greatest area of concentration and the highest rates of self-stimulatory activity were found to occur not in the MFB but in the lateral hypothalamus (Olds, 1956; Olds & Forbes, 1981). Indeed, animals "would continue to stimulate as rapidly as possible until physical fatigue forced them to slow or to sleep" (Olds, 1956).

Electrophysiological studies of single lateral hypothalamic neurons have also indicated that these cells become highly active in response to rewarding food items (Nakamura & Ono, 1986). In fact, many of these cells will become aroused by neutral stimuli repeatedly associated with rewards such as a cue tone—even in the absence of the actual reward (Nakamura & Ono, 1986; Nishino, Sasaki, Fukuda, & Muramoto, 1980). However, this ability to form associations appears to be secondary to amygdaloid and other source of input (Fukuda, Ono, & Nakamura, 1987).

Nevertheless, if the lateral region is destroyed, the experience of pleasure and emotional responsiveness is almost completely attenuated. For example, in primates, faces become blank and expressionless, whereas if the lesion is unilateral, marked neglect and indifference regarding all sensory events occurring on the contralateral side occur (Marshall & Teitelbaum, 1974). Animals will in fact cease to eat and will die.

Aversion

In contrast to the lateral hypothalamus and its involvement in pleasurable self-stimulation, activation of the medial hypothalamus is apparently so aversive that subjects will work to reduce it (Olds & Forbes, 1981). Thus, electrical stimulation of the medial region leads to behavior that terminates the stimulation—apparently so as to obtain relief (e.g., active avoidance). In this regard, when considering behavior such as eating, it might be postulated that when upper weight limits (or nutritional requirements) are met, the medial region becomes activated, which in turn leads to behavior (e.g., cessation of eating) that terminates its activation.

It is possible, however, that medial hypothalamic activity may also lead to a state of quiescence such that the organism is motivated simply to cease to respond. In some instances, this quiescent state may be physiologically neutral, whereas in other situations the result may be highly aversive. Nevertheless, quiescence is associated with parasympathetic activity, which is also mediated by the medial area.

Hypothalamic Damage and Emotional Incontinence: Laughter and Rage

When electrically stimulated, the hypothalamus responds by triggering two seemingly oppositional feeling states: pleasure and unpleasure/aversion. The generation of these emotional reactions in turn influences the organism to respond so as to increase or decrease what is being experienced. Through its rich interconnections with other limbic regions, including the neocortex and frontal lobes, the hypothalamus is able to mobilize and motivate the organism either to cease or to continue to behave. Nevertheless, at the level of the hypothalamus, the emotional states elicited are very primitive, diffuse, undirected and unrefined. The organism feels pleasure in general, or aversion/unpleasure in general. Higher-order emotional reactions (e.g., desire, love, hate) require the involvement of other limbic regions as well as neocortical participation.

Emotional functioning at the level of the hypothalamus is not only quite limited and primitive, it is also largely reflexive. For example, when induced by stimulation, the moment the electrical stimulus is turned off, the emotion elicited is immediately abolished. By contrast, true emotions (which require other limbic interactions) are not simply turned on or off but can last from minutes to hours to days and weeks before completely dissipating.

Nevertheless, in humans, disturbances of hypothalamic functioning (e.g., caused by an irritating lesion such as tumor) can give rise to seemingly complex, higher-order behavioral—emotional reactions, such as pathological uncontrollable laughter and crying. However, in some cases, when patients are questioned, they may deny having any feelings that correspond to the emotion displayed (Davison & Kelman, 1939; Ironside, 1956; Martin, 1950). In part, these reactions are sometimes due to disinhibitory release of brainstem structures involved in respiration, whereas in other instances the resulting behavior is caused by hypothalamic triggering of other limbic nuclei.

Uncontrolled Laughter

Pathological laughter has frequently been reported to occur with hypophyseal and midline tumors involving the hypothalamus, aneurysm in this vicinity, hemorrhage, astrocytoma, or papilloma of the third ventricle (resulting in hypothalamic compression), as well as surgical manipulation of this nucleus (Davison & Kelman, 1939; Dott, 1938; Foerster & Gagel, 1933; Martin, 1950; Money & Hosta, 1967; Ironside, 1956; List, Downman, & Bagheiv, 1958).

For example, Martin (1950) describes a man who, while "attending his mother's funeral was seized at the graveside with an attack of uncontrollable laughter which embarrassed and distressed him considerably" (p. 455). Although this particular attack dissipated, it was soon accompanied by several further fits of laughter and he died soon thereafter. At postmortem examination, a large ruptured aneurysm was found compressing the mamillary bodies and hypothalamus.

In a similar case (Anderson, 1936, cited by Martin, 1950), a patient literally died laughing following the eruption of the posterior communicating artery that resulted in compression (by hemorrhage) of the hypothalamus. "She was shaken by laughter and could not stop: short expirations followed each other in spasms, without the patient being able to make an adequate inspiration of air, she became cyanosed and nothing could stop the spasm of laughter which eventually became noiseless and little more than a grimace. After 24 hours of profound coma, she died."

Because laughter in these instances has not been accompanied by corresponding feeling states, this pseudoemotional condition has been referred to as sham mirth (Martin, 1950). However, in some cases, abnormal stimulation in this region (such as due to compression effects from neoplasm) has triggered corresponding emotions and behaviors—presumably due to activation of other limbic nuclei.

For example, laughter has been noted to occur with hilarious or obscene speech—usually as a prelude to stupor or death—in cases in which tumor has infiltrated the hypothalamus (Ironside, 1956). In several instances, it has been reported by one group of neurosurgeons (Foerster & Gagel, 1933) that while swabbing the blood from the floor of the third ventricle, patients "became lively, talkative, joking, and whistling each time the infundibular region of the hypothalamus was manipulated." In one case, the patient became excited and began to sing.

Hypothalamic Rage

Stimulation of the lateral hypothalamus can induce extremes in emotionality, including intense attacks of rage accompanied by biting and attack upon any moving object (Flynn, Edwards, & Bandler, 1971; Gunne & Lewander, 1966; Wasman & Flynn, 1962). If this nucleus is destroyed, aggressive and attack behavior is abolished (Karli & Vergness, 1969). Thus, the lateral hypothalamus is responsible for rage and for aggressive behavior.

The lateral hypothalamus maintains an oppositional relationship with the medial hypothalamus. Thus, stimulation of the medial region counters the lateral area such that rage reactions are reduced or eliminated (Ingram, 1952; Wheatley, 1944), whereas if the medial is destroyed. There results lateral hypothalamic release and the triggering of extreme savagery.

In man, inflammation, neoplasm, and compression of the hypothalamus have also been noted to give rise to rage attacks (Pilleri & Poeck, 1965), and surgical manipulations or tumors within the hypothalamus have been observed to elicit manic and ragelike outbursts (Alpers, 1940). These appear to be release phenomenon, however. That is, rage, attack, aggressive, and related behaviors associated with the hypothalamus appears to be under the inhibitory influence of higher order limbic nuclei such as the amygdala and septum (Siegel & Skog, 1970). When the controlling pathways between these areas are damaged (i.e., disconnection) these behaviors are sometimes elicited.

For example, Pilleri and Poeck (1965) described a man with severe damage throughout the cerebrum, including the amygdala, hippocampus, and cingulate, but with complete sparing of the hypothalamus, who continually reacted with howling, growling, and baring of teeth in response to noise or a slight touch or if approached. Hence, the hypothalamus, being released, responds reflexively in an aggressive nonspecific manner to any stimulus. Lesions of the frontal—hypothalamic pathways have been noted to result in severe rage reactions as well (Fulton & Ingraham, 1929; Kennard, 1945).

Nevertheless, like sham mirth, rage reactions elicited in response to direct electrical activation of the hypothalamus immediately and completely dissipate when the stimulation is removed. These outbursts have been referred to as sham rage.

Lateralization

Although scant, there is some evidence to suggest that the right hypothalamus may be more heavily involved in the control of neuroendocrine functioning, particularly in females. Greater right hypothalamic concentration of substances such as LHRH (luteinizing hormone) has also been reported (see Gerendai, 1984, for review).

Psychic Manifestations of Hypothalamic Activity

Phylogenetically and from an evolutionary perspective, the appearance and development of the hypothalamus predate the emergence and differentiation of all other limbic nuclei, e.g., amygdala, septal nucleus, and hippocampus (Andy & Stephan, 1961; Brown, 1983; Herrick, 1925; Humphrey, 1972). It constitutes the most primitive, archaic, reflexive, and purely biological aspect of the psyche.

Biologically, the hypothalamus serves the body tissues by attempting to maintain internal homeostasis and by providing for the immediate discharge of tenions in an almost reflexive manner. Studies of lateral and medial hypothalamic functioning indicate that it appears to act reflexively, in an almost on/off manner so as to seek or maintain the experience of pleasure and escape or avoid unpleasant noxious conditions.

Emotions elicited by the hypothalamus are largely undirected, short-lived, and unconnected with events occurring within the external environment, being triggered reflexively and without concern or understanding regarding consequences. Direct contact with the real world is quite limited and almost entirely indirect as the hypothalamus is largely concerned with the internal environment of the organism. It has no sense of morals, danger, values, logic, and so forth, and can neither feel nor express love or hate. Although quite powerful, hypothalamic emotions are largely undifferentiated, consisting of such feelings as pleasure, unpleasure, aversion, rage, hunger, and thirst.

As the hypothalamus is concerned with the internal environment, much of its activity occurs outside conscious-awareness. Moreover, being involved in maintaining internal homeostasis, through, for example, its ability to reward or punish the organism with feelings of pleasure or aversion, it tends to serve what Freud (1911) described as the pleasure principle.

The Pleasure Principle

The lateral and medial nuclei exert counterbalancing influences that serve to modulate activity occurring in the other. As described by Freud (1911), the pleasure principle not only serves to maximize pleasant experiences, but acts to keep the psyche as a whole free from high levels of excitation (be they pleasurable or unpleasant).

Like the hypothalamus, the pleasure principle is present from birth and for some time thereafter the search for pleasure is manifested in an unrestricted manner and with great intensity, as there are no oppositional forces (except those between the lateral and medial regions) to counter it's strivings. Indeed, higher order limbic nuclei have yet to mature.

Functionally isolated, the hypothalamus at birth has no way of reducing tension or of mobilizing the organism for any form of effective action. It is helpless. When tensions associated with immediate needs (e.g., hunger or thirst) become unpleasant the only response available to the hypothalamus is to cry and make ragelike vocalizations. When satiated, the hypothalamus can only respond with a feeling state suggesting pleasure or at least quiescence. Indeed, as is well known, for the first few months of life, the infant's awareness largely consists of a very restricted matrix involving tactile, visceral (hunger), and kinesthetic sensations, whereas emotionally the infant is capable of screaming, crying, or demonstrating very rudimentary features of pleasure, i.e., an attitude of acceptance of quiescence (McGraw, 1969; Milner, 1967; Piaget, 1952; Spitz & Wolf, 1946). It is only with the further differentiation and maturation of higher-order limbic nuclei (e.g., amygdala, septal nucleus, hippocampus) that the infant begins to achieve some awareness of external reality and begins to form memories as well as differentiate and associate externally occurring events and individuals.

AMYGDALA

In contrast to the primitive hypothalamus, the more recently developed amygdala is preeminent in the control and mediation of all higher order emotional and motivational activities. Through its rich interconnections with various neocortical and subcortical regions, amygdaloid neurons are able to monitor and abstract from the sensory array stimuli that are of motivational significance to the organism (Steklis & Kling, 1985). This includes the ability to discern and express even subtle social—emotional nuances such as friendliness, fear, love, affection, distrust, and anger, and at a more basic level, determine whether something might be good to eat. In fact, amygdaloid neurons respond selectively to the flavor of certain preferred foods, as well as to the sight or sound of something that might be especially desirable to eat (Fukuda *et al.*, 1987; O'Keefe & Bouma, 1969; Ono *et al.*, 1980).

Single amygdaloid neurons receive considerable topographic input, and are predominantly polymodal, responding to a variety of stimuli from different modalities simultaneously (O'Keefe & Bouma, 1969; Perryman, Kling, & Lloyd, 1987; Sawa & Delgado, 1963; Schutze, Knuepfer, Eismann, Stumpf, & Stock, 1987; Turner, Mishkin, & Knapp, 1980; Ursin & Kaasa, 1960; Van Hoesen, 1981). The amygdala is also very sensitive to somesthetic input and physical contact such that even a slight touch in a very circumscribed area of the body can produce amygdaloid excitation. Overall, in addition to emotional and motivational functioning, because multimodal assimilation of various sensory impressions occurs in this region, it is also involved in attention, learning, and memory.

Medial and Lateral Amygdaloid Nuclei

The amygdala is buried within the depths of the anterior—inferior temporal lobe and consists of two major nuclear groups. These are a phylogenetically ancient anteromedial group (or medial amygdala) involved in olfaction and motor activity, as well as a relatively newer basolateral division (lateral amygdala) that first appears in primates (Herrick,

1925; Humphrey, 1972). Like the lateral and medial hypothalamus, these two amygdaloid nuclei subserve different functions and maintain different anatomical interconnections.

Emybryologically, the medial amygdala is the first portion of the basal ganglia striatal complex to appear during development, being formed through neuroblast migration from the epithilium of the lateral ventricle (Humphrey, 1972). As it circles in an arc from the frontal to temporal lobe, the tail of the caudate nucleus actually terminates and merges with the amygdala. This portion of the amygdala is in fact part of the basal ganglia and is heavily involved in motivating and coordinating gross, or whole-body, motor activity.

The medial amygdala receives fibers from the olfactory tract and through a rope of fibers called the stria terminalis, projects directly to and receives fibers from the medial hypothalamus (through which it exerts inhibitory influences) as well as the septal nucleus (Carlsen, De Olmos, & Heimer, 1982; Gloor, 1955; Russchen, 1982; Swanson & Cowan, 1979). In addition, the medial (and lateral) regions are rich in cells containing enkephalins, and opiate receptors can be found throughout the amygdala (Atweh & Kuhar, 1977; Uhl, Kudar, & Snyder, 1978).

Sexuality

Portions of the hypothalamus and amygdala are sexually dimorphic; i.e., there are male and female amygdaloid nuclei. Thus, at a very basic and primitive level, emotional and motivational perceptual/behavioral functioning becomes influenced and guided by the neuroanatomical sexual bias of the host. Electrical stimulation of the amygdala, the medial division in particular, results in sex-related behavior and activity. In females this includes ovulation, uterine contractions and lactogenetic responses, and in males penile erections (Robinson & Mishkin, 1968; Shealy & Peele, 1957).

Damage to the amygdala bilaterally often results in heightened and indiscriminant sexual activity. For example, primates and other animals (while in captivity) will engage in excessive maturbation and genital manipulation and will repeatedly attempt to copulate even with species other than their own (e.g., a cat with a dog, a dog with a turtle) regardless of their sex. With bilateral destruction, animals are not only overly active sexually but are unable to identify appropriate partners (Brown & Schaefer, 1888; Kluver & Bucy, 1939). This abnormality is one aspect of a complex of symptoms sometimes referred to as the Kluver—Bucy syndrome (to be discussed in more detail below).

Lateral Amygdala

With the evolutionary ascent of primates, the relatively new lateral division of the amygdala progressively expands and differentiates. The lateral amygdala contributes fibers to the stria terminalis and gives rise to the amygdalofugal pathway, through which it projects to the lateral and medial hypothalamus (upon which it exerts inhibitory and excitatory influences, respectively), the dorsal medial thalamus (which is involved in memory, attention, and arousal), olfactory tubercle, as well as other subcortical regions (Aggleton, Burton, & Passingham, 1980; Carlsen, *et al.*, 1982; Dreifuss *et al.,* 1968; Gloor, 1955, 1960; Klinger & Gloor, 1960; Mehler, 1980; Russchen, 1982). It also receives fibers from the medial forebrain bundle, which in turn has its site of origin in the lateral hypothalamus (Mehler, 1980).

In general, whereas the medial amygdala is highly involved in motor, olfactory and sexual functioning, the lateral division is intimately involved in all aspects of higher order emotional activity; hence its rich interconnections with the lateral and medial hypothalamus, and the neocortex. The lateral amygdala maintains rich interconnections with the inferior, middle, and superior temporal lobes, as well as the insular temporal region, which in turn allows it to sample and influence the auditory, somesthetic, and visual information being received and processed in these areas, as well as to scrutinize this information for motivational and emotional significance (Herzog & Van Hoesen 1976; Kling *et al.*, 1987; Machne & Segundo, 1956; Mesulam & Mufson, 1982; O'Keefe & Bouma, 1969; Steklis & Kling, 1985; Turner *et al.*, 1980; Van Hoesen, 1981). Gustatory and respiratory sense are also rerepresented in this vicinity (Fukuda *et al.*, 1987; Maclean, 1949; Ono *et al.*, 1980), and the lateral division maintains rich interconnections with cingulated gyrus, orbital frontal lobes (Pandya, Van Hoesen, Domeskick, 1973), and the parietal cortex (O'Keefe & Bouma, 1969), through which it receives complex somesthetic information.

The lateral amygdala is highly important in analyzing information received and transferring information back to the neocortex so that further elaboration may be carried out at the cortical level. It is through the lateral division that emotional meaning and significance can be assigned to as well as extracted from that which is experienced.

The amygdala, overall, maintains a functionally interdependent relationship with the hypothalamus. It is able to modulate and even control rudimentary emotional forces governed by the hypothalamic nucleus. However, it also acts at the behest of hypothalamically induced drives. For example, if certain nutritional requirements need to be met, the hypothalamus signals the amygdala, which then surveys the external environment for something good to eat. By contrast, when, via environmental surveilance, the amygdala discovers a potentially threatening stimulus, it acts to excite and drive the hypothalamus so that the organism is mobilized to take appropriate action. Thus, when the hypothalamus is activated by the amygdala, instead of responding in an on—off manner, cellular activity continues for an appreciably longer time period (Dreifuss *et al.*, 1968). The amygdala can tap into the reservoir of emotional energy mediated by the hypothalamus to achieve certain ends.

Attention

The amygdala acts to perform environmental surveillance and can trigger orienting responses as well as mediate the maintenance of attention if something of interest or importance were to appear (Gloor, 1955, 1960; Kaada, 1951; Ursin & Kaasa, 1960). Electrical stimulation of the lateral division can initiate quick and/or anxious glancing and searching movements of the eyes and head, such that the organism appears aroused and highly alert as if in expectation of something that is going to happen (Ursin & Kaada, 1960). The EEG becomes desynchronized (indicating arousal), heart rate becomes depressed, respiration patterns change, and the galvanic skin response significantly alters (Bagshaw & Benzies, 1968; Ursin & Kaada, 1960)—reactions that characteristically accompany the orienting response of most species. Once a stimulus of potential interest is detected, the amygdala acts to analyze its emotional–motivational importance and will act to alert other nuclei such as the hypothalamus so that appropriate action may take place.

Fear, Rage, and Aggression

Initially, electrical stimulation of the amygdala produces sustained attention and orienting reactions. If the stimulation continues fear and/or rage reactions are elicited (Ursin & Kaada, 1960). When fear follows the attention response, the pupils dilate and the subject will cringe, withdraw, and cower. This cowering reaction in turn may give way to extreme fear and/or panic such that the animal will attempt to take flight.

Among humans, the fear response is one of the most common manifestations of amygdaloid electrical stimulation. Moreover, unlike hypothalamic on/off emotional reactions, attention and fear reactions can last up to several minutes after the withdrawal of stimulation.

In addition to behavioral manifestations of heightened emotionality, amygdaloid stimulation can result in intense changes in emotional facial expression. This includes facial contortions, baring of the teeth, dilation of the pupils, widening or narrowing of the eyelids, flaring of the nostrils, tearing, as well as sniffing, licking, and chewing (Anand & Dua, 1955; Ursin & Kaada, 1960). Indeed, some of the behavioral manifestations of a seizure in this vicinity (i.e., temporal lobe epilepsy) typically include chewing, smacking of the lips, and licking.

In many instances, rather than fear, there instead results anger, irritation, and rage, which seems to build up gradually, until finally the animal or human attacks (Egger & Flynn, 1963; Gunne & Lewander, 1966; Ursin & Kaada, 1960; Zbrozyna, 1963). Unlike hypothalamic sham rage, amygdaloid activation results in attacks directed at something real or, in the absence of an actual stimulus, at something imaginary. Moreover, rage and attack will persist well beyond the termination of the electrical stimulation of the amygdala. In fact, the amygdala remains electrophysiologically active for long periods, even after a stimulus has been removed (be it external—perceptual, or internal—electrical), such that is appears to continue to process—in the abstract—information even when that information is no longer observable (O'Keefe & Bouma, 1969).

In addition to permitting sustained electrophysiological activity, the amygdala has been shown to be heavily involved in the maintenance of behavioral responsiveness even in the absence of an immediately tangible or visible objective or stimulus (O'Keefe & Bouma, 1969). This includes motivating the organism to engage in the seeking of hidden objects or continuing a certain activity in anticipation of achieving some particular long-term goal. At a more immediate level, the amygdala is probably very important in object permanence (i.e., keeping an object in mind when it is no longer visible) and concrete or abstract anticipation. Anticipation is, of course, very important in the prolongation of emotional states such as fear or anger, as well as the generation of more complex emotions such as anxiety. In this regard, the amygdala is probably important not only in regard to emotion, but in maintaining mood states.

Fear and rage reactions have also been triggered in humans following depth electrode stimulation of the amygdala (Chapman, 1960; Chapman, Schroeder, Geyer, Brazier, Fager, Poppen, Soloman, & Yakovlev, 1954; Heath, Monroe, & Mickle, 1955; Mark, Ervin, & Sweet, 1972). Mark *et al.* (1972) describe one female patient who following amygdaloid stimulation became irritable and angry, and then enraged. Her lips retracted, there was extreme facial grimacing, threatening behavior, and then rage and attack—all of which persisted well beyond stimulus termination.

Similarly, Schiff *et al.* (1982) described a man who developed intractable aggression following a head injury and damage (determined via depth electrode) to the amygdala (i.e., abnormal electrical activity). Subsequently, he became easily enraged, sexually preoccupied (although sexually hypoactive), and developed hyperreligiosity and psue-domystical ideas. Tumors invading the amygdala have been reported to trigger rage attacks (Sweet, Ervin, & Mark, 1960; Vonderache, 1940).

The amygdala appears capable of not only triggering and steering hypothalamic activity but acting on higher level neocortical processes so that individuals form emotional ideas. Indeed, the amygdala is able to overwhelm the neocortex and the rest of the brain so that the person not only forms emotional ideas but responds to them. A famous example of this is Charles Whitman, who in 1966 climbed a tower at the University of Texas and began to indiscriminately kill people with a rifle.

Whitman had initially consulted a psychiatrist about his periodic and uncontrollable violent impulses but was unable to obtain relief. Prior to climbing the tower, he wrote himself a letter (Sweet *et al.*, 1969):

> I don't really understand myself these days. Lately I have been a victim of many unusual and irrational thoughts. These thoughts constantly recur, and it requires a tremendous mental effort to concentrate. I talked to a doctor once for about two hours and tried to convey to him my fears that I felt overcome by overwhelming violent impulses. After one session I never saw the Doctor again, and since then I have been fighting my mental turmoil alone. After my death I wish that an autopsy would be performed to see if there is any visible physical disorder. I have had tremendous headaches in the past.

Later he wrote:

> It was after much thought that I decided to kill my wife, Kathy, tonight after I pick her up from work. . . . I love her dearly, and she has been a fine wife to me as any man could ever hope to have. I cannot rationally pinpoint any specific reason for doing this. . . .

That evening, he killed his wife and mother and wrote:

> I imagine it appears that I brutally killed both of my loved ones. I was only trying to do a good thorough job. . . .

The following morning, he climbed the University tower carrying a high-powered hunting rifle and for the next 90 min he shot at everything that moved, killing 14 and wounding 38. Postmortem autopsy of his brain demonstrated a glioblastoma multiforme tumor the size of a walnut compressing the amygdaloid nucleus (Sweet *et al.*, 1969).

Docility and Amygdaloid Destruction

Bilateral destruction of the amygdala usually results in increased tameness, docility, and reduced aggressiveness in cats, monkeys and other animals (Schreiner & Kling, 1956; Weiskrantz, 1956; Vochteloo & Koolhaas, 1987), including purportedly ferocious crea-tures such as the agouti and lynx (Schreiner & Kling, 1956). In man, bilateral amygdala destruction (by neurosurgery) has been reported to reduce and/or eliminate paroxysmal aggressive and violent behavior (Terzian & Ore, 1955).

In some creatures, however, bilateral ablation of the amygdala has been reported to at least initially result in increased aggressive responding (Bard & Mountcastle, 1948) and, if sufficiently aroused or irritated, even the most placid of amygdalectomized animals can be induced to fight fiercely (Fuller, Rosvold, & Pribram, 1957). However, these aggressive responses are very short-lived and appear to be reflexively mediated by the hypothalamus. Thus, these findings (and the data reviewed above) suggest that true aggressive feelings are dependent on the functional integrity of the amygdala (versus the hypothalamus).

Social–Emotional Agnosia

Among primates and mammals, bilateral destruction of the amygdala significantly disturbs the ability to determine and identify the motivational and emotional significance of externally occurring events, to discern social–emotional nuances conveyed by others, or to select what behavior is appropriate for a specific social context (Bunnel, 1966; Fuller, Rosvold & Pribram, 1957; Gloor, 1960; Kluver & Bucy, 1939). Bilateral lesions lower responsiveness to aversive and social stimuli, reduce aggressiveness, fearfulness, competitiveness, dominance, and social interest (Rosvold, Mirsky, & Pribram, 1954). Indeed, this condition is so pervasive that subjects seem to have tremendous difficulty discerning the meaning or recognizing the significance of even common objects—a condition sometimes referred to as psychic blindness or the Kluver–Bucy syndrome.

Thus, animals with bilateral amygdaloid destruction, although able to see and interact with their environment, respond in an emotionally blunted manner and seem unable to recognize what they see, feel, and experience. Things seem stripped of meaning. Like an infant (who similarly is without a fully functional amygdala), patients with this condition engage in extreme orality and will indiscriminantly pick up various objects and place them in their mouth regardless of its appropriateness. There is a repetitive quality to this behavior, for once they put it down they seem to have forgotten that they had just explored it, and will immediately pick it up and place it again in their mouth as if it were a completely unfamiliar object.

Although ostensibly exploratory, there is thus a failure to learn, to remember, to discern motivational significance, to habituate with repeated contact, or to discriminate between appropriate and inappropriate stimuli. Rather, when the amygdala has been removed bilaterally, the organism reverts to the most basic and primitive modes of object interaction such that everything that is seen and touched is placed in the mouth (Brown & Schaffer, 1888; Gloor, 1960; Kluver & Bucy, 1939). This condition pervades all aspects of higher-level social–emotional functioning, including the ability to interact appropriately with loved ones.

For example, Terzian and Ore (1955) described a young man who, following bilateral removal of the amygdala, subsequently demonstrated an inability to recognize anyone, including close friends, relatives, and his mother. He ceased to respond in an emotional manner to his environment and seemed unable to recognize feelings expressed by others. He also exhibited many features of the Kluver–Bucy syndrome (perserverative oral "exploratory" behavior and psychic blindness), as well as an insatiable appetite. In addition, he became extremely socially unresponsive such that he preferred to sit in isolation, well away from others.

Among primates who have undergone bilateral amygdaloid removal, once they are released from captivity and allowed to return to their social group, a social–emotional agnosia becomes readily apparent, as they no longer respond to or seem able to appreciate or understand emotional or social nuances. Indeed, they appear to have little or no interest in social activity and persistently attempt to avoid contact with others (Dicks, Myers, & Kling, 1969; Jonason & Enloe, 1971; Jonason, Enloe, Contrucci, & Meyer, 1973). If approached they withdraw, and if followed they flee. Indeed, they behave as if they have no understanding of what is expected of them or what others intend or are attempting to convey, even when the behavior is quite friendly and concerned. Among adults with bilateral lesions, total isolation seems to be preferred.

In addition, they no longer display appropriate social or emotional behaviors, and if kept in captivity will fall in dominance in a group or competitive situation—even when formerly dominant (Bunnel, 1966; Dicks *et al.*, 1969; Fuller *et al.*, 1957; Jonason & Enloe, 1971; Jonason *et al.*, 1973; Rosvold, Mirsky, & Pribram, 1954). As might be expected, maternal behavior is severely affected. According to Kling (1972), mothers will behave as if their "infant were a strange object to be mouthed, bitten, and tossed around as though it were a rubber ball."

Laterality and the Amygdala

Limbic Language

Although language is usually discussed in regard to grammar and vocabulary, there is a third major feature to expression and comprehension through which a speaker may convey, and a listener determine, intent, attitude, feeling, and meaning. Language is both descriptive and emotional. A listener comprehends not only what is said, but how it is said—what a speaker feels.

Feeling and attitude is generally communicated via vocal inflection, intonation, and melody such that anger, happiness, sadness, sarcasm, and so forth, are indicated by such cues as variations in pitch, timbre, and stress contours—vocal capacities associated with the functional integrity of the right cerebral hemisphere, and the right frontal and temporal regions in particular (Joseph, 1988a; see also Chapter 1, The Right Cerebral Hemisphere). For example, studies using dichotic listening have repeatedly shown that the right hemisphere is superior in distinguishing stress and pitch contours, determining frequency, amplitude, melody, duration, processing inflectional contours, and even decoding contextual information in the absence of denotative speech.

Conversely, patients who have undergone right temporal lobe neurosurgery or who have suffered damage involving this area, often demonstrate impairments in regard to many aspects of prosodic–melodic perception, such that nonverbal environmental sounds and musical stimuli fail to be adequately recognized. People who have suffered deep right frontal or temporal lobe damage also have difficulty controlling the pitch and inflection of their voice, whereas patients undergoing sodium amytal anesthetization of the right hemisphere speak in a bland monotone.

It has been argued in detail (Joseph, 1982, 1988a) that the superior capacity of the right hemisphere in processing and expressing melodic–prosodic–emotional information is directly related to lateralized limbic functioning, and in particular, a greater abundance of neuronal interconnections with various limbic nuclei such as the amygdala. Emotional vocalizations are limbic in origin and are hierarchically rerepresented, processed, and expressed by various neocortical regions within the frontal and temporal lobes.

In fact, the major fiber pathway that links the language axis (Wernicke's and Broca's areas) of the left hemisphere and the melodic–prosodic–emotional Axis of the right, i.e., the arcuate fasciculus, extends from the left frontal convexity (Broca's area) through the inferior parietal lobule, and after giving off major fibers to Wernicke's region continues down into the depths of the inferior temporal lobe where it establishes contact with the amygdala. In this way, the amygdala has a significant influence on emotional speech (Figs. 21–23).

Indeed, both phylogenetically and ontogenetically, the original impetus to vocalize springs forth from roots buried within the depths of the ancient limbic lobes (e.g., amygdala, hypothalamus, septum). For example, although nonhumans do not have the capacity to speak, they still vocalize, and these vocalizations are primarily limbic in origin, being evoked in situations involving sexual arousal, terror, anger, flight, helplessness, and separation from the primary caretaker when young. The first vocalizations of human infants are similarly emotional in origin and limbically mediated (Joseph, 1982).

Although cries and vocalizations indicative of rage or pleasure have been elicited through hypothalamic stimulation, of all limbic nuclei the amygdala is the most vocally active—particularly the lateral division (Robinson, 1967). In humans and animals, a wide range of emotional sounds have been evoked through amygdala activation, such as sounds indicative of pleasure, sadness, happiness, and anger (Robinson, 1967; Ursin & Kaada, 1960). Conversely, in man, destruction limited to the amygdala (Freeman & Williams, 1952, 1963), the right amygdala, in particular, has abolished the ability to sing, convey melodic information, or properly enunciate by vocal inflection. Similar disturbances occur with right hemisphere damage (Joseph, 1988a). Indeed, when the right temporal region (including the amygdala) has been grossly damaged or surgically removed, the ability to perceive, process, or even vocally reproduce most aspects of musical and emotional auditory input is significantly curtailed. (See Chapter 1, The Right Cerebral Hemisphere.)

Emotion and Temporal Lobe Seizures

The amygdala is buried within the depths of the anterior–inferior temporal lobe and maintains rich interconnections with areas throughout the temporal neocortex. Because of their intimate association, damage to the temporal lobe, particularly the anterior regions, often involves and disrupts amygdaloid functioning. In fact, because the amygdala and inferior–anterior temporal lobe have, of all brain regions, the lowest seizure threshold, and are minimally resistant, and are therefore maximally vulnerable to developing abnormal seizure activity, even mild injuries may result in kindling (i.e., abnormal activation), and therefore disruption of their functional integrity. Indeed, damage to adjacent tissue has been known to spread, by kindling, to the amygdala and inferior regions. One consequence is temporal lobe epilepsy.

Personality, emotional, and sexual disturbances are a frequent complication of temporal lobe seizures in a significant minority of patients. Such patients may develop

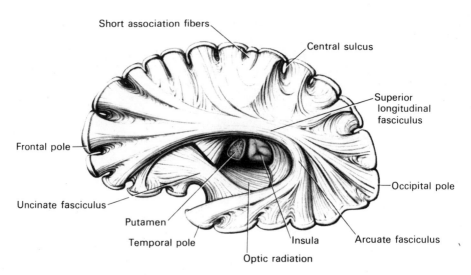

FIGURE 21. Dissection of the lateral surface of the left hemisphere so as to display the long and short association fibers. Note extension of the arcuate fasciculus from the temporal pole as it courses beneath Wernicke's area, the inferior parietal lobule, and Broca's area. From *The core text of neuroanatomy* by M. Carpenter, 1972. Courtesy of the Williams & Wilkins Co., Baltimore, MD.

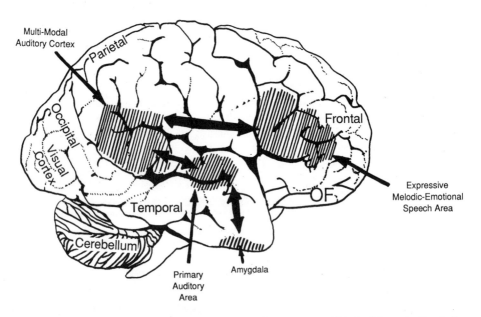

FIGURE 22. Schematic representation of melodic–emotional language areas within the right cerebral hemisphere. Auditory information is received in the primary auditory area as well as within the amygdala (and other limbic areas). Emotional and other characteristic are discerned, comprehended, and/or assigned to the sounds perceived by limbic structures as well as the multimodal auditory cortex, which extends into the inferior parietal region. This information is transferred from the temporal–parietal and limbic areas to the right frontal convexity, which mediates its vocal expression.

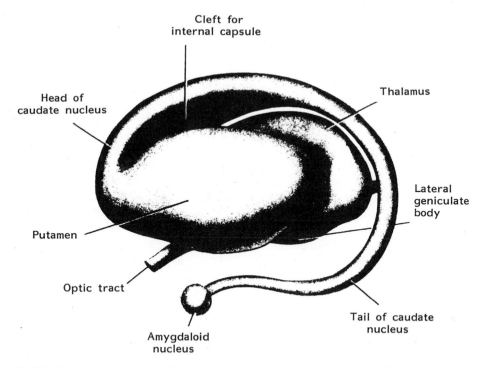

FIGURE 23. Schematic drawing of the striatum, thalamus, and amygdaloid nucleus. Note continuity of the putamen and caudate and that of the caudate nucleus and the amygdala. From *Human neuroanatomy* by R. C. Truex & M. B. Carpenter, 1969. Courtesy of the Williams & Wilkins Co., Baltimore, MD.

paranoid, hysterical, or depressive tendencies, deepening of mood, hyposexuality, and other characteristics suggestive of affective disorders (Bear, Leven, Blumer, Chetam, & Ryder, 1982; Gibbs, 1951; Herman & Chambria, 1980; Strauss, Risser, & Jones, 1982; Williams, 1956). Immediately following or during the course of a seizure 10% or more of such patients experience a change in emotionality (Herman & Chambria, 1980; Strauss *et al.,* 1982; Williams, 1956).

In part, because the highest incidence of psychiatric disorder occurs in cases in which the EEG spike focus is in the anterior temporal area (Gibbs, 1951), and because limbic nuclei such as the amygdala are frequently involved, it has been postulated that seizure activity sometimes hyperactivates these nuclei (Bear, 1979), which in turn distorts the affective meaning applied to afferent streams of visual, auditory, and somesthetic information (Gibbs, 1951).

Thus, during a seizure, these patients may be temporarily overwhelmed by feelings such as fear, or things they see or hear seem to become abnormally invested with emotional significance (Bear *et al.,* 1979; Gibbs, 1951; Gloor *et al.,* 1982), presumably due to abnormal amygdala activation. Interestingly, one common symptom of temporal lobe epilepsy is an aura of tastes, and more often odors, that are usually quite unpleasant (e.g., like burning wire, burning feces, burning rubber or tires.)

Seizure induced emotional changes tend to predominantly involve feelings of depression, pleasure, displeasure, or fear—with fear being one of the most common emotional experiences (Gloor *et al.*, 1982; Williams, 1956). More rarely, seizures involving sexual behavior, crying, laughing, or ragelike responses have been associated with temporal lobe epilepsy.

There is some evidence to suggest that certain emotional changes are more frequently associated with seizure originating in the right temporal lobe and/or amygdala, whereas disturbances involving thought (e.g., psychosis, schizophrenia) characterize left temporal lobe abnormalities (Flor-Henry, 1969, 1983; Offen, Davidoff, Troost, & Richey, 1976; Joseph, 1988; Sherwin, 1981; Schiff *et al.*, 1982; Taylor, 1975; Weil, 1956).

For example, in their depth electrode study of five patients with seizure disorders, Gloor *et al.* (1982) found that all feelings of fear and displeasure were associated with right temporal, right amygdala, or right hippocampal activation. These findings are consistent with the observations of Slater, Beard, and Glithero (1969), Bear and Fedio (1977), Flor-Henry (1969), and others, who have noted an association between right temporal seizures and affective disorders.

Other reports, however, have been less clear cut—presumably because seizure originating in the amygdala/temporal lobe can quickly spread from one hemisphere to another (through the anterior commissure) and because of the failure to employ depth electrodes to pinpoint the seizure foci. Thus, in some instances, emotions such as fear seem to arise regardless of which hemisphere is involved (Strauss *et al.*, 1982). Nevertheless, even in these cases, an emotional dichotomy is apparent. For example, Herman and Chambria (1980) described cases with right temporal foci in whom free-floating fears developed that were not tied to something specific but that encompassed terrifying, "death-like" and "nightmarish" feelings, whereas a patient with a left temporal foci developed specific fears of certain individuals and situations. Similarly, Weil (1956) reports that most of his patients with right-sided foci developed intense fears but were unable to describe what they were afraid of.

Stimulation of the amygdala can significantly alter facial emotional expression, including tearing. In a small minority of cases, right temporal seizures have been reported to cause paroxysmal attacks of weeping, with lacrimation, the making of mournful sounds, including sobbing and crying (Offen *et al.*, 1976). However, crying as well as laughing seizures have also been noted to occur with left-sided involvement (Chen & Forster, 1973; Sethi & Rao, 1976). Nevertheless, without the benefit of depth electrodes, such as employed by Gloor and colleagues (1982), it is difficult to determine in which amygdal and/or temprol lobe a seizure actually originates.

The amygdala and regions of the hypothalamus are sexually dimorphic, and stimulation of either area can trigger sexual behavior. Similarly, sensations of sexual excitement, sometimes leading to orgasm, may also occur as a function of seizures originating in the temporal lobe (Currier, Little, Suess, & Andy, 1971; Freemon & Nevis, 1969; Remillard *et al.*, 1983) and in the frontal lobe (Spencer, Spencer, Williamson, & Mattson, 1983). Of interest, 7 of 10 patients with sexual seizures described by Remillard *et al.* (1983) had foci originating in the right hemisphere. Similar findings have been reported by Freemon and Nevis (1969), Penfield and Rasmussen (1950, p. 27), and Spencer *et al.* (1983).

Sexual seizures caused by temporal lobe abnormalities are often accompanied by actual sexual behavior. "The patient was sitting at the kitchen table with her daughter making out a shopping list. She stopped, appeared dazed, slumped to the floor on her back, lifted her skirt, spread her knees, and elevated her pelvis rhythmically. She made appropriate vocalizations for sexual intercourse, such as "it feels so good" and "further, further" (Currier *et al.*, 1971, p. 260).

Frontal Lobe Sexual Seizures

The frontal lobes, the orbital region in particular, maintain rich interconnections with the amygdala (Nauta, 1964), and receives olfactory projections as well (Tanabe, 1975). Epileptiform activity arising in the deep frontal (orbital) regions has also been associated with the development of sexual seizures, including exhibitionism, genital manipulation, and masturbatory activity (Spencer *et al.*, 1983).

Similar to that described regarding right temporal emotional and sexual disturbances, Spencer *et al.* (1983) found that three of their four patients with sexual automatism had seizures originating in the right frontal area, whereas the remaining patient had bifrontal disturbances. Other investigators have also noted that peculiar disturbances in emotion and personality are far more likely to arise following right versus left frontal damage (Joseph, 1986, 1988; Hillbom, 1960; Lishman, 1968).

Presumably, at least in part, emotional and sexual disturbances associated with right temporal and right frontal (orbital) dysfunction are caused by activation of the limbic structures, with which they are intimately interconnected. However, there is also much evidence to indicate that in some respects, inferior temporal and orbital frontal areas are in fact outgrowths of and thus part of the limbic system.

Summary

Over the course of early evolutionary development, the hypothalamus reigned supreme in the control and expression of raw and reflexive emotionality, i.e., pleasure, displeasure, aversion, and rage. Largely, however, it has acted as an eye turned inward, monitoring internal homeostasis and concerned with basic needs. With the development of the amygdala, the organism was now equipped with an eye turned outward, so that the external emotional features of reality could be tested and ascertained. When signaled by the hypothalamus the amygdala begins to search the sensory array for appropriate emotional—motivational stimuli, until what is desired is discovered and attended to.

However, with the differentiation of the amygdala, emotional functioning also became differentiated and highly refined. The amygdala hierarchically wrested control of emotion from the hypothalamus. The amygdala is primary in regard to the perception and expression of most aspects of emotionality, including fear, aggression, pleasure, happiness, and sadness, and in fact assigns emotional or motivational significance to that which is experienced. It can thus induce the organism to act on something seen, felt, heard, or anticipated. The integrity of the amygdala is essential in regard to the analysis of social–emotional nuances, the organization and mobilization of the person's internal motivational status regarding these cues, as well as the mediation of higher-order emotional expression and impulse control. When damaged or functionally compromised, social–emotional functioning becomes grossly disturbed.

Through its rich interconnections with other brain regions, the amygdaloid nucleus is able to sample and influence activity that occurs in other parts of the cerebrum and add emotional color to one's perceptions. As such, it is highly involved in the assimilation and association of divergent emotional, motivational, somesthetic, visceral, auditory, visual, motor, olfactory, and gustatory stimuli. Thus, it is very much involved with learning, memory, and attention and can generate reinforcement for certain behaviors (Douglas, 1967). Moreover, through reward or punishment, it can promote the encoding, storage, and later retrieval of particular types of information. That is, learning often involves reward, and it is through the amygdala (in concert with other nuclei) that emotional consequences can be attributed to certain events, actions, or experiences, as well as extracted from the world of possibility, so that it can be attended to and remembered.

Lastly, as is evident from studies of patients displaying abnormal activity or seizures originating in or involving this nuclei, the amygdala is able to overwhelm the neocortex and gain control over behavior. As based on electrophysiological studies, the amygdala seems to be capable of literally turning off the neocortex (such as occurs during a seizure), at least for brief time periods. That is, the amygdala can induce electrophysiological slow-wave theta activity in the neocortex, which indicates low levels of arousal as well as high-voltage fast activity. In the normal brain, it probably exerts similar influences such that at times people (i.e., their neocortex) lose control over themselves and respond in a highly emotionally charged manner.

HIPPOCAMPUS

The hippocampus is an elongated structure located within the inferior medial wall of the temporal lobe (posterior to the amygdala); it surrounds, in part, the lateral ventricle. In humans, the hippocampus consists of an anterior and posterior region and is shaped somewhat like a telephone receiver.

There are three major neural pathways leading to and from the hippocampus. These include the fornix–fimbrial fiber system, a supracallosal pathway (i.e., the indusium griseum), which passes through the cingulate, and through the entorhinal area, sometimes referred to as the gateway to the hippocampus.

It is through the entorhinal area that the hippocampus receives olfactory and amygdaloid projections (Carlsen et al., 1982; Gloor, 1955; Krettek & Price, 1976a; Steward, 1977) and fibers from the orbital frontal and temporal lobes (Van Hoesen et al., 1972). It is through the fornix and fimbrial pathways that the hippocampus makes major interconnections with the thalamus, septal nuclei, medial hypothalamus, and through which it exerts either inhibitory or excitatory influences on these nuclei (Feldman, Saphier, & Conforti, 1987; Guillary, 1957; Poletti & Sujatanon, 1980).

Septal interactions: The hippocampus maintains a particularly intimate relationship with the septal nuclei (sometimes referred to as the septum—not to be confused with the septum pelucidum). The septal nucleus partly serves as in interactional relay center as it channels hippocampal influences to other structures such as the hypothalamus and reticular formation (and vice versa) and as a major link through which the hippocampus and amygdala sometimes interact (Hagino & Yamaoka, 1976).

Amygdala interactions: The hippocampus is greatly influenced by the amygdala, which in turn monitors and responds to hippocampal activity (Gloor, 1955; Green & Adey, 1956; Steriade, 1964) (Figs. 23–25). The amygdala also acts to relay certain forms of information from the hippocampus to the hypothalamus (Poletti & Sajatanon, 1980).

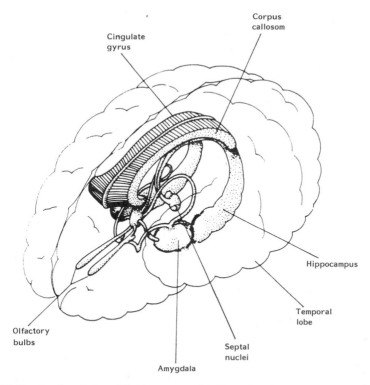

FIGURE 24. Superior–lateral view of limbic system nuclei. From *Physiological psychology* by M. Schwartz, 1978. Reprinted by permission of Prentice-Hall, Inc., Englewood Cliffs, NJ.

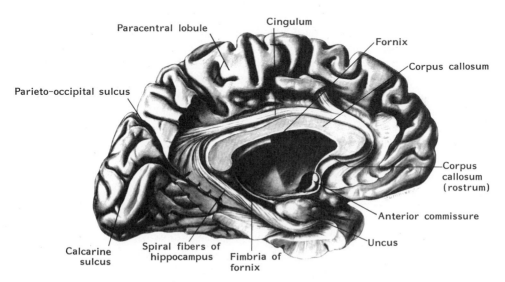

FIGURE 25. Dissection of the medial surface of the left cerebral hemisphere. Reproduced by permission from *Neuroanatomy,* 2nd Ed., by F. A. Mettler, 1948, C. V. Mosby Company, St. Louis, MO.

Together the hippocampus and amygdala complement and interact in regard to attention, the generation of emotional and other types of imagery, as well as learning and memory.

Hippocampal Arousal, Attention, and Inhibitory Influences

Various investigators have assigned a major role to the hippocampus in information processing, including memory, new learning, cognitive mapping of the environment, voluntary movement toward a goal, as well as attention, behavioral arousal, and orienting reactions (Douglas, 1967; Grastayan *et al.,* 1959; Green & Arduini, 1954; Isaacson, 1982; Milner, 1966, 1970, 1971; Olton, Branch, & Best, 1978; Routtenberg, 1968). For example, hippocampal cells alter their activity greatly in response to certain spatial correlates, particularly as an animal moves about in its environment (Olton *et al.,* 1978). It develops slow-wave theta activity during arousal (Green & Arduini, 1954) or when presented with noxious or novel stimuli (Adey, Dunlop, & Hendrix, 1960). However, few studies have implicated this nucleus as important in emotional functioning per se, although responses such as "anxiety" or "bewilderment" have been observed when directly electrically stimulated (Kaada, Jansen, & Andersen, 1954).

Hippocampal–Neocortical Interactions

Desynchronization of the cortical EEG is associated with high levels of arousal and information input. As the level of input increases, the greater the level of cortical arousal (Como, Joseph, Fiducia, & Siegel, 1979; Joseph, Como, Forrest, Fiducia, & Siegel, 1981). However, when arousal levels become too great, efficiency in information processing, memory, new learning, and attention becomes compromised, as the brain becomes overwhelmed.

When the neocortex becomes desynchronized (indicating cortical arousal), the hippocampus often (but not always) develops slow-wave theta activity (Grastyan *et al.,* 1959; Green & Arduini, 1954) such that it appears to be functioning at a much lower level of arousal. Conversely, when cortical arousal is reduced to a low level (indicated by EEG synchrony), the hippocampal EEG often becomes desynchronized.

These findings suggest when the neocortex is highly stimulated, the hippocampus functions at a much lower level in order to monitor what is being received and processed so as not to become overwhelmed. When the neocortex is not highly aroused, the hippocampus presumably compensates by increasing its own level of arousal so as to tune into information that is being processed at a low level of intensity.

In situations in which both the cortex and the hippocampus become desynchronized, distractability and hyperresponsiveness result and the subject becomes overwhelmed and confused and may orient to and approach several stimuli (Grastyan *et al.,* 1959). Attention, learning, and memory functioning are decreased. Such situations sometimes occur when one is highly anxious.

There is also evidence to suggest that the hippocampus may act to reduce extremes in cortical arousal. For example, whereas stimulation of the reticular activating system augments cortical arousal and EEG-evoked potentials, hippocampal stimulation reduces or inhibits these potentials such that cortical responsiveness and arousal are dampened

(Feldman, 1962; Redding, 1967). If cortical arousal is at a low level, hippocampal stimulation often leads to augmentation of the cortical evoked potential (Redding, 1967).

The hippocampus also exerts desynchronizing or synchronizing influences on various thalamic nuclei, in turn augmenting or decreasing activity in this region (Green & Adey, 1956; Guillary, 1955; Nauta, 1956, 1958). As the thalamus is the major relay nucleus to the neocortex, the hippocampus appears to be able to block or enhance information transfer to various neocortical areas.

It is likely that the hippocampus may act to influence information reception at the neocortical level as well as possibly reduce extremes in cortical arousal (be they too low or high) via inhibition or excitation, and/or it may act so that the neocortex is neither over- nor underwhelmed when engaged in the reception and processing of information. That is, very high or very low states of excitation are incompatible with alertness and selective attention and with the ability to learn and retain information (Joseph et al., 1981).

Aversion and Punishment

In many ways, the hippocampus appears to act in concert with the medial hypothalamus and septal nuclei (with which it maintains rich interconnections) so as to prevent extremes in arousal and thus maintain a state of quiet alertness (or quiescence). Moreover, as with the medial hypothalamus, it has been reported that the subjective components of aversive emotion in humans is correlated with electrophysiological alternations in the hippocampus and septal area (Heath, 1976).

The hippocampus also appears to be heavily involved in the modulation of reactions to frustrations or punishment (Gray, 1970), particularly in regard to learning. For example, the hippocampus responds with trains of slow theta waves when presented with noxious stimuli but habituates with repeated presentation. Moreover, there is some evidence to suggest that this nucleus in conjunction with the amygdala and septal nuclei is important in generating negative cognitive-mood states such as anxiety.

Attention and Inhibition

The hippocampus participates in the elicitation of orienting reactions and the maintenance of an aroused state of attention (Foreman & Stevens, 1987; Grastayan et al., 1959; Green & Arduini, 1954; Routtenberg, 1968). When exposed to novel stimuli or when engaged in active searching of the environment, hippocampal theta appears (Adey et al., 1960). However, with repeated presentations of a novel stimulus, the hippocampus habituates and theta disappears (Adey et al., 1960). Thus, as information is attended to, recognized, and presumably learned and/or stored in memory, hippocampal participation diminishes. Theta also appears during the early stages of learning as well as when engaged in selective attention and the making of discriminant responses (Grastyan et al., 1959).

When the hippocampus is damaged or destroyed, animals have great difficulty inhibiting behavioral responsiveness or shifting attention. For example, Clark and Issacson (1965) found that animals with hippocampal lesions could not learn to wait 20 sec between bar presses, if first trained to respond to a continuous schedule. There is an inability to switch from a continuous to a discontinuous pattern, such that a marked degree of perseveration and inability to change sets or inhibit a pattern of behavior once initiated occurs (Douglas, 1967; Ellen, Wilson, & Powell, 1964). Habituation is largely abolished, and the ability to think or respond divergently is disrupted.

In part, this finding suggests that hippocampal damage disrupts the ability to learn and thus remember—findings that have been repeatedly demonstrated in humans. In animals, disinhibition caused by hippocampal damage can even prevent the learning of a passive-avoidance task, such as simple ceasing to move (Kimura, 1958).

When coupled with the evidence presented above, it appears that the hippocampus acts to enhance or diminish areas of neural excitation selectively, which in turn allows for differential selective attention and differential responding. When damaged, the ability to shift from one set of perceptions to another or to change behavioral patterns is disrupted, and the organism becomes overwhelmed by a particular mode of input. Learning, memory, as well as attention are greatly compromised.

Learning and Memory

The hippocampus is most usually associated with learning and memory encoding (e.g., long-term storage and retrieval of newly learned information), particularly the anterior regions (Fedio & Van Buren, 1974; Milner, 1966; 1970; Penfield & Milner, 1958; Rawlins, 1985; Scoville & Milner, 1957). Many other brain areas, such as the mamillary bodies and dorsal–medial nucleus of the thalamus, are also important in memory functioning.

Bilateral destruction of the anterior hippocampus results in striking and profound disturbances involving memory and new learning (i.e., anterograde amnesia). For example, one such patient who underwent bilateral destruction of this nuclei (H.M.), was subsequently found to have almost completely lost the ability to recall anything experienced after surgery. If you introduced yourself to him, left the room, and then returned a few minutes later, he would have no recall of having met or spoken to you. Dr. Brenda Milner has worked with H.M. for almost 20 years, and yet she is an utter stranger to him.

H.M. is in fact so amnesic for everything that has occurred since his surgery (although memory for events prior to his surgery is comparatively exceedingly well preserved), that every time he rediscovers that his favorite uncle died (years after his surgery) he suffers the same grief as if he had just been informed for the first time.

Despite his lack of memory for new (nonmotor) information, Henry (or H.M.), has adequate intelligence, is painfully aware of his deficit, and constantly apologizes for his problem. "Right now, I'm wondering" he once said, "Have I done or said anything amiss?" You see, at this moment everything looks clear to me, but what happened just before? That's what worries me. It's like waking from a dream. I just don't remember. . . . Every day is alone in itself, whatever enjoyment I've had, and whatever sorrow I've had. . . . I just don't remember" (Blakemore, 1977, p. 96).

Presumably the hippocampus acts to protect memory and the encoding of new information during the storage and consolidation phase via the gating of afferent streams of information and the filtering/exclusion (or dampening) of irrelevant and interfering stimuli. When the hippocampus is damaged, input overload results, the neuroaxis is overwhelmed by neural noise, and the consolidation phase of memory is disrupted such that relevant information is not properly stored or even attended to. Consequently, the ability to form associations (e.g., between stimulus and response) or to alter preexisting schemas (such as occurs during learning) is attenuated (Douglas, 1967).

Hippocampal and Amygdaloid Interactions: Memory

It has been argued that significant impairments involving memory (in man) cannot be produced by lesions restricted to the hippocampus (cf. Horel, 1978). Thus, in some instances with restricted lesions, good recall of new information is possible for at least several minutes (Horel, 1978; Penfield & Milner, 1958). Rather, there is evidence that strongly suggests that the hippocampus plays an interdependent role with the amygdala in regard to memory (Kesner & Andrus, 1982; Mishkin, 1978; Sarter & Markowitsch, 1985). Interestingly, nuclei such as the dorsal–medial region of the thalamus, which have also been shown to be important in memory (Squire & Moore, 1979), maintain rich interconnections with the amygdala (Krettek & Price, 1977b; Nauta, 1971).

Nevertheless, although psychic blindness is produced by damage to the amygdala, striking anterograde deficits in recall do not seem to occur (Horel, 1978; Scoville & Milner, 1957). Rather, the role of the amygdala in memory and learning seems to involve activities related to reward, orientation, and attention, as well as emotional arousal (Sarter & Markowitsch, 1985). If some event is associated with positive or negative emotional states, it is more likely to be learned and remembered.

The amygdala seems to reinforce and maintain hippocampal activity through the identification of motivationally significant information and the generation of pleasurable rewards (through action on the lateral hypothalamus). That is, reward increases the probability of attention being paid to a particular stimulus or consequence as a function of its association with reinforcement (Douglas, 1967; Kesner & Andrus, 1982).

However, the amygdala and hippocampus may act differentially in regard to the effects of positive versus negative reinforcement on learning and memory. For example, whereas the hippocampus produces theta in response to noxious stimuli, the amygdala increases its activity following the reception of a reward (Norton, 1970). Thus, if errors are made during acquisition (negative emotional state), possibly the hippocampus modulates the appropriate reaction, whereas when presented with a reward, the amygdala reinforces the organism's response.

Thus, the hippocampus acts to reduce or enhance extremes in arousal associated with information reception and storage in memory, whereas the amygdala acts to identify the social–emotional–motivational characteristics of the stimuli as well as to generate (in conjunction with the hippocampus) appropriate emotional rewards to reinforce learning and memory. We find that when both the amygdala and hippocampus are damaged, striking and profound disturbances in memory functioning result (Kesner & Andrus, 1982; Mishkin, 1978).

Laterality

It is now very well known that lesions involving the mesial–inferior temporal lobes (i.e., destruction or damage to the amygdala/hippocampus) of the left cerebral hemisphere typically produce significant disturbances involving verbal memory—particularly as contrasted with patients with right-sided destruction. Left-sided damage disrupts the ability to recall simple sentences and complex verbal narrative passages or to learn verbal paired associates or a series of digits (B. Milner, 1966, 1970, 1971).

By contrast, right temporal destruction typically produces deficits involving visual memory, such as the learning and recall of geometric patterns, visual mazes, or human faces (Corkin, 1965; Milner, 1966; Kimura, 1963). Right-sided damage also disrupts the ability to recognize (through recall) olfactory stimuli (Rausch, Serafetinides, & Crandall, 1977), emotional sounds and passages (Wechsler, 1973), sounds from the environment, as well as tactile mazes (Joseph, 1988a; Chapter 1, The Right Cerebral Hemisphere).

It appears, therefore, that the left amygdala/hippocampus is highly involved in processing and/or attending to verbal information, whereas the right amygdala/hippocampus is more involved in the learning, memory and recollection of nonverbal, visual–spatial, environmental, emotional, motivational, tactile, olfactory, and facial information.

THE PRIMARY PROCESS

Amygdaloid–Hippocampal Interactions during Infancy

Hallucinations

The amygdala--hippocampus complex, particularly that of the right hemisphere, is very important in the production and recollection of nonlinguistic images associated with past experience. In fact, direct electrical stimulation of this region within the temporal lobes results not only in the recollection of images but in the creation of fully formed visual and auditory hallucinations (Halgren *et al.,* 1978; Horowitz *et al.,* 1968; Malh *et al.,* 1964; Penfield & Perot, 1963), as well as feelings of familiarity (e.g., dé jà vu).

Indeed, it has long been known that tumors invading specific regions of the brain can trigger the formation of hallucinations that range from the simple (flashing lights) to the complex. The most complex forms of hallucination, however, are associated with tumors within the most anterior portion of the temporal lobe (Critchley, 1939; Gibbs, 1951; Horowitz *et al.,* 1968; Tarachow, 1941), i.e., the region containing the amygdala and anterior hippocampus.

Similarly, electrical stimulation of the anterior lateral temporal cortical surface results in visual hallucinations of people, objects, faces, and various sounds (Horowitz *et al.,* 1968)—particularly the right temporal lobe (Halgren *et al.,* 1978). Depth electrode stimulation and thus direct activation of the amygdala and/or hippocampus is especially effective.

For example, stimulation of the right amygdala produces visual hallucinations, body sensations, *dé jà vu,* illusions, as well as gustatory and alimentary experiences (Weingarten *et al.,* 1977). Conversely, Freeman and Williams (1963) reported that the surgical removal of the right amygdala in one patient abolished hallucinations. Stimulation of the right hippocampus has also been associated with the production of dejà-vu-, memory-, and dreamlike hallucinations (Halgren *et al.,* 1978), and in fact, hallucinations seem to occur most frequently following hippocampal activation (Horowitz *et al.,* 1968).

As is well known, LSD can elicit profound hallucinations involving all spheres of experience. Following the administration of LSD, high-amplitude slow waves (theta) and bursts of paroxysmal spike discharges occur in the hippocampus and amygdala (Chapman & Walter, 1965; Chapman, Walter, Ross *et al.*, 1963), but with little cortical abnormal activity. In both humans and chimpanzees in whom the temporal lobes, amygdala, and hippocampus have been removed, LSD ceases to produce hallucinatory phenomena (Baldwin *et al.*, 1959; Serafetinides, 1965). Moreover, LSD-induced hallucinations are significantly reduced when the right versus left temporal lobe has been surgically ablated (Serafetinides, 1965). Overall, it appears that the amygdala, hippocampus, and the neocortex of the temporal lobe are highly interactionally involved in the production of hallucinatory experiences. Presumably, it is the neocortex of the temporal lobe that acts to interpret this material (Penfield & Perot, 1963) as perceptual phenomena.

Dreaming

When hallucinations follow depth electrode or cortical stimulation, much of the material experienced is very dreamlike (Halgren *et al.*, 1978; Malh *et al.*, 1964) and consists of recent perceptions, ideas, feelings, and other emotions that are similarly illusionary and dreamlike. Indeed, the right hippocampus, and the right hemisphere in general (Broughton, 1982; Goldstein *et al.*, 1972; Hodoba, 1986; Humphrey & Zangwill, 1961; Kerr & Foulkes, 1978; Meyer, Ishikawa, Hata, & Karacan, 1987), also appear to be involved in the production of dream imagery as well as REM (at least in part) during sleep.

For example, there have been reports of patients with right cerebral damage, hypoplasia, and abnormalities in the corpus callosum who have ceased to dream altogether, suffer a loss of hypnotic imagery, or tend to dream only in words (Botez, Olivier, Vezina, Botez, & Kaufman, 1985; Humphrey & Zangwill, 1951; Kerr & Foulkes, 1981; Murri, Arena, Siciliano, Mazzotta, & Muratorio, 1984). However, there have also been some reports that when the left hemisphere has been damaged, particularly the posterior portions (i.e., aphasic patients), the ability to verbally report and recall dreams also is greatly attenuated (e.g., Murri *et al.*, 1984). Of course, aphasics have difficulty describing much of anything, let alone their dreams.

Electrophysiologically, the right hemisphere also becomes highly active during REM, whereas, conversely, the left brain becomes more active during NREM (Goldstein *et al.*, 1972; Hodoba, 1986). Similarly, measurements of cerebral blood flow have shown an increase in the right temporal regions during REM sleep and in subjects who upon wakening report visual, hypnagogic, hallucinatory, and auditory dreaming (J. S. Meyer *et al.*, 1987). Interestingly, abnormal and enhanced activity in the right temporal and temporal—occipital area acts to increase dreaming and REM sleep for an atypically long time period (Hodoba, 1986). Thus, it appears that there is a specific complementary relationship between REM sleep and right temporal electrophysiological activity.

In addition, during REM, the hippocampus begins to produce slow wave, theta activity (Jouvet, 1967; Olmstead, Best, & Mays, 1973; Robinson, Kramis, & Vanderwolf, 1977). Presumably, during REM, the hippocampus acts as a reservoir from which various images, words, and ideas are drawn and incorporated into the matrix of dreamlike activity being woven by the right hemisphere. It is probably just as likely that the hippocampus serves as a source from which material is drawn during the course of a daydream.

Interestingly, daydreams appear to follow the same 90- to 120-min cycle that characterize the fluctuation between REM and NREM periods, as well as fluctuations in mental capabilities associated with the right and left hemisphere (Broughton, 1982; Kripke & Sonneschein 1973). That is, the cerebral hemispheres tend to oscillate in activity every 90–120 min—a cycle that appears to correspond to the REM–NREM cycle and the appearance of day and night dreams.

Dreams and Infancy

In the newborn, and up until approximately 6–9 months, there are two distinct stages of sleep which correspond to REM and N-REM periods demonstrated by adults (Berg & Berg, 1978; Dreyfus-Brisac & Monod, 1975; Parmelee, Wenner, Akiyama, Schults, & Stern, 1967). Among infants, however, REM occur during wakefulness as well as during sleep. In fact, REM can be observed when the eyes are open, when the infant is crying, fussing, eating, or sucking (Emde & Metcalf, 1970). Moreover, REM is also observed to occur within a few moments after an infant begins to engage in nutritional sucking and appears identical to that which occurs during sleep (Emde & Metcalf, 1970).

The production of REM during waking in some respects seems paradoxical and a number of different mechanism are no doubt responsible. Nevertheless, it might be safe to assume that like an adult, when the infant is in REM, he or she is dreaming, or at least, in a dreamlike state. This state might correspond to what Freud described as the primary process. That is, when produced when the infant is crying or fussing, it is dreaming of whatever relief it seeks. Correspondingly, REM that occurs while eating or sucking may have to do with the limbic structures involved not only in the production of dreamlike activity, but the identification, learning, and retention of motivationally significant information (i.e., the amygdala and hippocampus).

The Primary Process

The hypothalamus, our exceedingly ancient and primitive Id, has an "eye" that only sees inward. It can tell if the body needs nourishment but cannot determine what might be good to eat. It can feel thirst, but has no way of slaking this desire. The hypothalamus can only say: "I want," "I need," and can only signal pleasure and displeasure. However, as the seat of pleasure, the hypothalamus can be exceedingly gracious in rewarding the organism when its needs are met. Conversely, when its needs go unmet, it can respond not only with displeasure and feelings of aversion, but with undirected fury and rage. It can cause the organism to cry out. However, the cry does not produce the immediately desired relief or reduction in tension. Pressure is exerted on the limbic system and the organism to engage in environmental surveillance so as to meet the needs monitored by the hypothalamus.

Over the course of the first months of life, as the amygdala and then the hippocampus develop, the organism begins to develop an eye that not only sees outward but that can register and recall events, objects, people, and so forth associated with tension reduction, pleasure, and the satiety of the infants internal needs (e.g., the taste, smell, feeling of mother's breast and milk, the experience of sucking and relief). This is called learning.

With the maturation of these two limbic nuclei, the infant is increasingly able to differentiate what occurs in the external environment based on hypothalamically monitored needs and the emotional/motivational significance of that which is experienced. The infant can now orient, selectively attend, determine what brings satisfaction, and store this information in memory.

Primary Imagery

Although admittedly we have no direct knowledge as to the psychic interactions in the neonate, it does seem reasonable to assume that as the neocortex and underlying structures and fiber pathways mature, neural "programs" are formed that correspond to the repeated registration of experiences which are deemed significant (e.g., pleasurable). That is, neural pathways that are repetitively fired, deactivated, or activated in response to specific sensory and affective activities and experiences, become associated with that activity, such that an associated neural circuit is formed (Joseph, 1982; Penfield, 1954; Spinelli, 1970); i.e., a memory is created. Eventually, if this circuit is reactivated, the "learned" pattern is reexperienced; i.e., the organism remembers.

Thus, when the amygdala/hippocampus is stimulated by a hungry hypothalamus, the events and images associated with past experiences of pleasure not only can be searched out externally but can be recalled in imaginal form. For example, as an infant experiences hunger and stomach contractions as well as its own cries of displeasure, these states become associated with the sound, smell, taste, and other cues of mother and her associated movement, as well as other stimuli that accompany being fed (cf. Piaget, 1952, pp. 37, 407–408). Repetitively experienced, the sequence from hunger to satiety evokes and becomes associated with the activation of certain neural pathways.

Eventually, when the infant becomes hungry and that hunger is prolonged, the entire neural sequence associated with hunger and feeding (i.e., hunger, mother, food, satiety) may become involuntarily triggered and activated (through association) such that an "image" of being fed is experienced. The activation of these rudimentary and infantile memory images is probably what constitutes, at least in part, the primary process.

Behaviorally, this is manifested by REM and by sucking and tongue movements as if eating, when in fact no food is present (cf. Piaget, 1952). When hungry, the infant will begin to cry and REM might be observed; the infant will then stop crying and smack its lips and make sucking movements (mediated by the amygdala) as if it were being fed. The infant experiences being fed in the form of a dream (Joseph, 1982) or hallucination.

The brain of the human infant is quite immature for several years, in turn restricting information reception and processing (Joseph, 1982; Joseph, Gallagher, Holloway, & Kahn, 1984); also, given the limited amount of reality contact infants are able to achieve, these rudimentary memories and images (even when they occur during waking, i.e., REM) are probably indistinguishable from actual experience simply because they are experience.

Like a dream, when replayed, the infant presumably reexperiences to some degree the sensations, emotions, and so forth originally linked to tension reduction. Thus, the young infant, still unable to distinguish between representation and reality, responds to the image as reality (Freud, 1911), even while awake—as manifested by REM. When hunger is prolonged, the associations linked to feeding are triggered, and for a brief period the infant behaves as if its hunger has been sated. Reality is replaced by an image, or rather, a "dream." This is the primary process.

Since the hypothalamus (which monitors internal homeostasis) is not conscious that the dream images experienced are not real, it initially accepts the memory/dream images transmitted from the amygdala and hippocampus and ceases to cry, i.e., it responds to the imagined sources of nourishment just as it responds to a cue tone associated with a food reward (Nakamura & Ono, 1986; Ono et al., 1980). However, the hypothalamus is not long fooled, for the primary process does not offer effective long-lasting relief from tension. As the pain of hunger remains and increases, limbic activity is increased, and the image falls away, to be replaced by a cry of hunger (Joseph, 1982). The amygdala and hippocampus are thus forced to renew their surveillance of the environment in search of sources of tension reduction. Cognitive development is thus promoted (Freud, 1911):

> Whatever was thought of (desired) was simply imagined in an hallucinatory form, as still happens today with our dream-thoughts every night. This attempt at satisfaction by means of hallucination was abandoned only in consequence of the absence of the expected gratification, because of the disappointment experienced. Instead, the mental apparatus had to decide to form a conception of the real circumstances in the outer world and to exert itself to alter them. . . . The increased significance of external reality heightened the significance also of the sense-organs directed towards the outer word, and of the consciousness attached to them; the later now learned to comprehend the qualities of sense in addition to the qualities of pleasure and "pain" which hitherto had alone been of interest to it. A special function was instituted which had periodically to search the outer word in order that its data might be already familiar if an urgent need should arise; this function was attention. Its activity meets the sense-impressions halfway, instead of awaiting their appearance. At the same time there was probably introduced a system of notation, whose task was to deposit the results of this periodical activity of consciousness—a part of that which we call memory. (pp. 410–411)

SEPTAL NUCLEI

Phylogenetically, the septal nuclei develops following the appearance of the amygdala, at about the same time and rate as the hippocampus (Andy & Stephan, 1976; Brown, 1983; Humphrey, 1972). It also increases in relative size and complexity as we ascend the ancestral tree, attaining its greatest degree of development in humans.

Specifically, the septal nuclei lie in the medial portions of the hemispheres, just anterior to the third ventricle near the hypothalamus. The septum projects heavily throughout the hypothalamus and maintains rich interconnections with all regions of the hippocampus (Mesulam, Mufson, Levey, & Wainer, 1983; Siegel & Edinger, 1976). It also contributes to and receives fibers from the amygdala via the stria terminalis (Swanson & Cowan, 1979) and receives and gives rise to one of the most massive roots of the medial forebrain bundle through which it receives olfactory and ascending brainstem (reticular formation) fibers (Nauta, 1956).

Aversion and Internal Inhibition

In general, the septal nucleus appears to act in conjunction with the medial hypothalamus and hippocampus, particularly as related to internal inhibition and the exertion of quieting and dampening influences on arousal and limbic system functioning. In this regard, the septum appears to counterbalance some aspects of amygdaloid and lateral hypothalamic activity while stimultaneously facilitating the actions of the hippocampus and media hypothalamus (Kolb & Whishaw, 1977; Mogenson, 1976; Petsche, Gogolack, & Van Zwieten, 1965; Petsche, Stumpf, & Gogolack, 1962).

Specifically, depending on the level of hypothalamic arousal, the septum exerts facilitatory or inhibitory influences on this nuclei (Mogenson, 1976) and from impulses it receives and relays from the reticular activating system, mediates and greatly influences hippocampal activity as well (Kolb & Whishaw, 1977; Petsche et al., 1962, 1965). The septal region (along with that of the hippocampus and medial hypothalamus) has also been reported in humans to show electrophysiological alterations in activity that correspond to subjective feelings of aversion (Heath, 1976).

The septum and amygdala appear to enjoy largely an antagonistic relationship, particularly in regard to influencing the hypothalamus. For example, the amygdala acts either to facilitate or to inhibit septal functioning, whereas septal influences on the amygdala are largely inhibitory. However, in large part, the amygdala and septal nuclei appear to exert most of their counterbalancing influences at the level of the hypothalamus, particularly in regard to emotionality.

Quiescence

A primary activity of the septal nucleus appears to be that of reducing extremes in emotionality and arousal and maintaining the organism in state of quiescence and readiness to respond. Stimulation of the septum acts to reduce blood pressure and heart rate and to induce adrenocortical secretion (Endroczi, Schreiberg, & Lissak, 1963; Kaada, 1951; Ranson, Kabat, & Magoun, 1935). It also counters lateral hypothalamic self-stimulatory activity (Mogenson, 1976).

Rage

Electrical stimulation of the septum counters and inhibits aggressive behavior (Rubenstein & Delgado, 1963) and suppresses the expression of rage reactions following hypothalamic stimulation (Siegel & Edinger, 1976).

If the septal nucleus is destroyed, these counterbalancing influences are removed such that initially dramatic increases in aggressive behavior, including rage (Ahmad & Harvey, 1968; Blanchard & Blanchard, 1968; Brady & Nauta, 1953; King, 1958), results. Bilateral lesions in fact give rise to explosive emotional reactivity to tactile, visual, or auditory stimulation, which can take the form of attack (fight) or flight. If the amygdala is subsequently lesioned, the septal rage and emotional reactivity are completely attenuated (King & Meyer, 1958). Thus, septal lesions appear to result in a loss of modulatory and inhibitory restraint.

Septal Social Functioning

Eventually, within a few weeks or months, rage and aggressiveness due to septal lesions subside and/or completely disappear. However, a generalized tendency to overrespond and a generalized failure to inhibit emotional responsiveness persist (McClary,

1961; 1966; Poplawsky, 1987). In particular, rather than rage or irritability, septal lesions produce indiscriminant socializing and an extreme need for social and physical contact (Jonason & Enloe, 1971; Jonason *et al.*, 1973; McClary, 1961, 1966; Meyer, Ruth, & Lavond, 1978).

Socialization and Contact Comfort

In contrast with amygdaloid lesions, which produce a severe social–emotional agnosia and social avoidance, septal lesions produce a dramatic and persistent increase in social cohesiveness (Jonason & Enloe, 1971; Jonason *et al.*, 1973; D. R. Meyer *et al.*, 1978). Thus, the normal intact amygdala appears to promote social behavior, whereas the septal nucleus seems to counter socializing tendencies.

With complete bilateral destruction of the septum in animals, the drive for social contact appears to be irresistible such that persistent attempts to make physical contact occur—even with species quite unlike their own. This occurs because the amygdala (as well as other nuclei) are no longer opposed by the septal nucleus.

Ritchie (1975, cited by D. R. Meyer *et al.*, 1978) reported that septally lesioned rats, unlike normals, will readily seek out mice (to which they are normally indifferent) or rabbits (which they usually avoid). If presented with a choice of an empty (i.e., safe) chamber or one containing a cat, septally lesioned rats persistently attempt to huddle and crawl upon this normally feared creature, even when the cat is acting perturbed. If a group of septally lesioned animals are placed together, extreme huddling results. So intense is this need for contact comfort following septal lesions that if other animals are not available they will seek out blocks of wood, old rags, bare wire frames, or walls.

Among humans with right-sided or bilateral disturbances in septal functioning (such as due to seizure activity generated in this region), a behavior referred to as stickiness is sometimes observed. Such individuals seek to make repeated, prolonged, and often inappropriate contact with anyone who is available or who happens to be nearby so as to tell them stories or jokes or merely pass the time. They seem to have little actual concern regarding the feelings of others or how interested they might be in interacting. Indeed, they do not readily take a hint and are difficult to get rid of. In hospital situations, they can be found intruding on other patients and their families, hanging out by the nurse's station, or incessantly visiting other rooms to chat.

Attachment and Amygdaloid–Septal Developmental Interactions

Broadly considered, the various nuclei comprising the limbic system demonstrate functional maturity at different rates. Correspondingly, certain behaviors and capacities appear at various time periods, overlay previous capacities, become differentiated, and/or in turn become suppressed or eliminated.

At birth the hypothalamus reins supreme in regard to emotion. The infant freely expresses feelings of aversion and rage or pleasure or quiescence and demonstrates extreme orality and other behaviors similar to a state in which the amygdala is functionally nonexistent.

As the amygdala and hippocampus begin to develop and mature, the organism becomes more reality oriented and more social as the ability to attend selectively to externally occurring events and to store this information in memory becomes more pronounced. The pleasure principle (although still dominant) begins to be served by the reality principle (Freud, 1911).

Since the development of the amygdala precedes that of the septal nuclei, social–emotional activities mediated by the amygdala are expressed in an uninhibited fashion. That is, when the counterbalancing influences of the septum are absent (as a result of surgical removal or functional immaturity), the behavior expressed is in many respects similar to that expressed by infants, for example, indiscriminant contact seeking (e.g., attachment behavior).

Attachment

Attachment is not the same as dependency. Necessarily, the infant is dependent on its caretaker (e.g., mother). However, until the child is 6–7 months of age, it will smile at the approach of anyone, even complete strangers, and will vigorously protest any form of separation from these unknown people (e.g., if they leave the room). This stage corresponds to the amygdaloid development period, during which septal influences are largely nil.

At about 7 months of age, the infant becomes more discriminant in its interactions and it is during this time period that a very real and specific attachment is formed, e.g., to one's mother—an attachment that becomes progressively more intense and stable. This period represents initial septal developmental influences such that global contact seeking becomes increasingly narrowed and restricted.

After these specific attachments have been formed, children begin to show anxiety, fear, and even flight reactions at the approach of a stranger (Spitz & Wolf, 1946). By 9 months, 70% of children respond aversively, whereas by 10 months they might cry out if a stranger were to appear (Schaffer, 1966; Waters, Matas, & Sroufe, 1975). By 1 year of age, 90% of children respond aversively to strangers (Schaffer, 1966).

Thus, during the amygdaloid phase there is indiscriminant approach and contact seeking. During the septal stage, indiscriminant social contact seeking is inhibited, whereas the specific attachments already formed are strengthened, reinforced, and maintained. The differential rates of amygdala and septal development are thus crucial in promoting survival and social interaction with significant others.

Their differential maturation rates also represent critical time periods, which in turn require specific interactional social–physical forms of stimulation, such as the presence and care of a primary caretaker. If these interactional needs are not met during the critical development period, gross abnormalities can result.

Indeed, if contact with others is restricted during these early phases, the ability to socially interact successfully at a later stage of development is retarded. This is even true among the so-called lower animals. For example, kittens that are not exposed to humans grow up to be wild and unapproachable. The phenomena of imprinting probably also requires that similar interactions take place.

Contact Comfort

As is well known, for the first 6–8 months of life, physical and social interaction with others is critical in regard to psychological, neurological, and physical development. During this period (which corresponds to the amygdaloid phase of maturation), contact seeking is indiscriminant. However, indiscriminant contact seeking and attachment during early development maximizes opportunities for physical–social interaction. So intense is the need for physical and social contact that young animals will form attachments to bare wire frames (Harlow, 1962), to television sets, to dogs that might maul them, and to creatures that might kill them (Cairn, 1966). Young human children will form attachments to mothers who might abuse them. With removal of the septum, animals will even seek contact with creatures that might eat them.

So pervasive is this need for physical interaction (especially among humans) that, when grossly reduced or denied, the result is often death. For example, in several well-known studies of children raised in foundling homes during the early 1900s, when the need for contact was not well recognized, morbidity rates for children under 1 year of age were more than 70%. Of 10,272 children admitted to the Dublin Foundling home during a single 25-year period, only 45 survived (Langmeier & Matejcek, 1975, for review).

Of those who have survived an infancy spent in institutions in which mothering and contact comfort were minimized, signs of low intelligence, extreme passivity, apathy, as well as severe attentional deficits are often characteristic (Dennis, 1960; Langmeier & Matejcek, 1975; Spitz, 1945). Such individuals have difficulty forming attachment or maintaining social interactions later in life.

In his famous series of experiments with monkeys, Harlow (1962) also showed that even those raised with surrogate terry cloth mothers develop extremely bizarre behaviors:

> The laboratory monkeys sit in their cages and stare fixedly into space, circle their cages in a repetitive stereotyped manner and clasp their heads in their hands or arms and rock for long periods of time. They often develop compulsive habits, such as pinching precisely the same patch of skin on their chest between the same fingers hundreds of times a day; occasionally such behavior may become punitive and the animal may chew and tear at its body until it bleeds. (p. 138)

it is noteworthy that the maternal behavior of chimpanzees raised in isolation is also quite abnormal and in fact similar to that of mothers who have had their amygdalas destroyed. As described by Harlow (1965):

> After the birth of her baby, the first of these unmothered mothers ignored the infant and sat relatively motionless at one side of the cage, staring fixedly into space hour after hour. As the infant matured desperate attempts to effect maternal contact were consistently repulsed. . . . Other motherless monkeys were indifferent to their babies or brutalized them, biting off their fingers or toes, pounding them, and nearly killing them until caretakers intervened. One of the most interesting findings was that despite the consistent punishment, the babies persisted in their attempts to make maternal contact. (pp. 256–257, 259)

Deprivation and Amygdaloid–Septal Functioning

In addition to mediating all aspects of higher-order emotional functioning, the amygdala is particularly responsive to tactual stimulation such that single cells may respond to touch, regardless of where on the body the person was stimulated. When there is inadequate tactile and physical–social interaction during early development, the ability of these cells to develop and function adequately is significantly reduced. That is, the amygdala (as well as other nuclei) becomes environmentally damaged.

As has been repeatedly demonstrated in studies of the visual system as well as on cerebral development, one consequence of reduced environmental input during certain critical periods of development is cell death, atrophy, and functional retardation, as well as inhibition by competing neuronal cell assemblies (Casagrande & Joseph, 1980; Green-ough, 1976; Rosenzweig, 1971). Consequently, gross behavioral and perceptual abnor-malities result (Harlow, 1962; Joseph & Casagrande, 1980; Joseph & Gallagher, 1982).

For example, if the lids of one eye are surgically sutured shut, patterned visual input is prevented from reaching target cells in the lateral geniculate nucleus of the thalamus. When this occurs target neurons become smaller, fewer in number, and functionally suppressed by adjacent cells receiving normal input. If the sutures are reversed such that the formerly deprived eye is opened, the subject responds as if blind. However, if the normal eye is surgically removed, some vision returns to the formerly deprived eye, and some functional neuronal recovery is observed (Casagrande & Joseph, 1980), presumably because of the removal of inhibitory influences. This deprivation effect is only noted to occur during the first few months after birth in primates.

Given the similarity in social unresponsiveness and disturbances in maternal behav-ior demonstrated by amygdalectomized and socially–maternally deprived primates, it is likely that like the visual system, abnormalities in cellular development and function also occur within the amygdala and septum secondary to deprivation. Unfortunately, few researchers have explored this line of inquiry.

Nevertheless, it has been demonstrated that the right amygdala is larger than the left in animals reared in enriched and normal environments, whereas these differences are nonsignificant in animals reared in a restricted setting (Diamond, 1985), suggesting that deprivation differentially reduces right amygdaloid growth. This finding is significant because among humans, the right cerebral hemisphere has been shown to be dominant in regard to most aspects of social–emotional functioning. (See Chapter 1, The Right Cere-bral hemisphere.)

Heath (1972) also noted that the monkeys reared without mothers develop abnormal spiking in the septal region. Similarly, Heath (1954) found abnormal seizurelike dis-charges in the septum of withdrawn schizophrenics, noting that the severity of the abnor-mality was correlated with the severity of the psychosis.

Among those with normal limbic systems, it is presumably the interaction of these same nuclei that gives rise to attachment and bonding behavior in adults. Moreover, it is probably through the interactions mediated by these nuclei that emotions such as jealousy are generated. That some individuals respond with considerable grief, anger, and even uncontrollable rage when a "loved one" has ended a relationship probably can also be explained from a limbic perspective.

THE UNCONSCIOUS MIND

The limbic system, as defined in this chapter, provides the foundations for the development of not only emotion, but social–psychological functioning as well as the more rudimentary aspects of unconscious mental activity. The limbic system, however, represents the most primitive features of the unconscious. A second, more highly devel-oped, unconscious (i.e., nonlinguistic) mind is maintained via the functional interactions of the right cerebral hemisphere (Joseph, 1988a,b); however this mental realm only seems to be unconscious from the perspective of the left cerebral hemisphere. Nevertheless, because the interaction of various limbic nuclei is also important in learning and memory, as well as social–emotional functioning, it is likely that a variety of neurotic disturbances, needs, desires, and insecurities have as their foundation events differentially experienced and attended to by the limbic system.

This seems particularly true regarding events experienced during infancy and early development. For example, it is well known that most events experienced before age 4 are extremely difficult to recall. In part this is because of the different modes of information processing and coding employed by adults versus children (Joseph, 1988a). That is, much of what was experienced, learned, and stored in memory during early childhood occurred before the development of language. Thus, adults, relying on language, can no longer access the code in which this early information was stored. The key no longer fits the lock.

Nevertheless, because the limbic system of both an adult and infant uses non-linguistic social–tactual–emotional–visual forms of information processing and expression, much of what occurs at this level falls outside the immediate jurisdiction of the conscious mind, which relies predominantly on language and rational, temporal–sequential linguistic thought for understanding.

Because of this, we may feel angry or sad and not consciously (i.e., linguistically) know why. However, at a limbic level, we may feel anxious or angry because something was seen, heard, or even smelled, which called forth old limbic memories of some unpleasant event—memories that are not accessible to the linguistic mind.

Take, for example, a young child, who, like many infants, at times manipulated her genitalia. Unfortunately, this little girl's mother (being very repressed and rigid) responded with shock and disgust when she discovered her daughter's action. Resolving to put an end to this "repulsive behavior," the mother shouted "No" in an angry voice and slapped the child every time her daughter touched herself.

Soon the behavior was abolished through simple stimulus–response learning. This is because, at a limbic level, every time the urge to touch the genitalia arose, the behavior was severely punished. The child's urge to touch became associated with physical pain, and later with the anxiety of anticipated pain. Only three nuclei are necessary to form this circuit—the hypothalamus, amygdala, and hippocampus—as it is purely emotional and without thought. Indeed, much of this learning can probably occur without amygdaloid or hippocampal involvement.

Nevertheless, as an adult, this young woman now has difficulty associating with men, as sometimes their mere presence brings forth terrible feelings of anxiety. She has one failed relationship after another, and soon discovers herself to be frigid. She hates sex, she hates to be touched, and men repell her.

Consciously, she may be able to generate a panoply of explanations, all of which, at some level, are believable, albeit erroneous. Consciously, she has no true idea as to the source of her difficulties. Nevertheless, at the limbic level, the explanation is very basic. Certain men trigger the onset of amorous feelings. Unfortunately, the woman never feels sexually aroused. The first inklings of arousal immediately generate feelings of anxiety and limbic memories of physical pain. This is what she experiences and responds to.

CONCLUSION

A variety of nuclei and brain regions are important in emotional functioning. In this chapter, only a few of these regions are discussed. In some respects, many might argue that such structures as the hippocampus should not be considered part of the limbic system because of its involvement with memory. Indeed, it has become increasingly fashionable to decry even the use of the term limbic system, as there are simply so many diverse cerebral regions involved in the control and mediation of emotional functioning. Even by the most liberal of anatomical definitions there can be no structural basis for the concept when all such nuclei are considered. This is not the case, however, in regard to the highly interactional anatomical and functional system maintained by the amygdala, hypothalamus, hippocampus, and septal nuclei. Therefore, I encourage continued use of the term, particularly in that to most people limbic system implies that part of the "old" brain concerned with emotional functioning.

REFERENCES

Adey, W. R., Dunlop, C. W., & Hendrix, C. E. (1960). Hippocampal slow waves: Distribution and phase relations in the course of approach learning. *Archives of Neurology, 3,* 74–90.

Adey, W. R., Dunlop, C. W., & Sunderland, S. (1958). A survey of rhinencephalic interconnections with the brainstem. *Journal of Comparative Neurology, 110,* 173–204.

Aggleton, J. P., Burton, M. J., & Passingham, R. E. (1980). Cortical and subcortical afferents to the amygdala of the rhesus monkey. *Brain Research, 190,* 347–368.

Ahmad, S. S., & Harvey, J. A. (1968). Long-term effect of septal lesions and social experience on shock-elicited fighting in rats. *Journal of Comparative and Physiological Psychology, 66,* 596–602.

Alpers, N. (1940). Personality and emotional disorders associated with hypothalamic lesions. *Association of Researchers in Nervous and Mental Disease, 20,* 725–752.

Anand, B. K., & Dua, S. (1956). Electrical stimulation of the limbic system of brain ("visceral brain") in the waking animal. *Indian Journal of Medical Research, 44,* 107–119.

Andy, O. J., & Stephan, H. (1961). Septal nuclei in the soricidae (insectivores). *Journal of Comparative Neurology, 117,* 251–273.

Atweh, S. F., & Kuhar, M. J. (1977). Autoradiographic localization of opiate receptors in rat brain. *Brain Research, 129,* 1-12.

Bagshaw, M., & Benzies, S. (1968). Multiple measures of the orienting reaction and their dissociation after amygdalectomy in monkeys. *Experimental Neurology, 27,* 31–40.

Baldwin, M., Lewis, S. A., & Bach, S. A. (1959). The effects of lysergic acid after cerebral ablation. *Neurology (New York), 9,* 469–474.

Bard, P., & Mountcastle, V. B. (1948). Some forebrain mechanisms involved in expression of rage with special reference to suppression of angry behavior. *Journal of Nervous and Mental Disease, 27,* 362–404.

Bear, D. M., & Fedio, P. (1977). Quantitative analysis of interictal behavior in temporal lobe epilepsy. *Archives of Neurology, 34,* 454–467.

Bear, D. M. (1979). Temporal lobe epilepsy: a syndrome of sensory–limbic hyperconnexion. *Cortex, 15,* 357–384.

Bear, D. M., Leven, K., Blumer, D., Chetam, D., & Ryder, J. (1982). Interictal behavior in hospitalized temporal lobe epileptics: relationship to idiopathic psychiatric syndromes. *Journal of Neurology, Neurosurgery and Psychiatry, 45,* 481–488.

Berg, W. K., & Berg, K. M. (1978). Psychophysiological development in infancy. State, sensory function, and attention. *Psychological Bulletin, 47,* 103–170.

Blakemore, C. (1977). *Mechanics of the mind.* New York: Cambridge University Press.

Blanchard, R. J., & Blanchard, D. C. (1968). Limbic lesions and reflexive fighting. *Journal of Comparative and Physiological Psychology, 66,* 603–605.

Bleier, R., Byne, W., & Siggelkow, I. (1982). Cytoarchitectonic sexual dimorphisms of the medial preoptic and anterior hypothalamic area in guinea pig, rat, hamster, and mouse. *Journal of Comparative Neurology, 212,* 118–130.

Botez, M. I., Olivier, M., Vezina, J-I., Botez, T., Kaufman, B. (1985). Deffective revisualization: Dissociation between cognitive and imagistic thought. Case report and short review of the literature, *Cortex, 21,* 375–389.

Brady, J. V. (1960). Temporal and emotional effects related to intracranial electrical self-stimulation. In E. Ramsey & D. O. Doherty (Eds.), *Electrical studies on the unanesthetized brain* (pp. 301–333). New York: Hoeber.

Brady, J. V., & Nauta, W. J. H. (1953). Subcortical mechanisms in emotional behavior: Affective changes following septal lesions in the rat. *Journal of Comparative and Physiological Psychology, 46,* 339–346.

Broughton, R. (1982). Human consciousness and sleep/waking rhythms: A review of some neuropsychological considerations. *Journal of Clinical Neuropsychology, 4,* 193–218.

Brown, J. W. (1983). Early prenatal development of the human precommissural septum. *Journal of Comparative Neurology, 215,* 331–350.

Brown, S., & Schaefer, A. E. (1888). An investigation into the functions of the occipital and temporal lobe of the monkey's brain. *Philadelphia Transactions of the Royal Society of Britain, 179,* 303–327.

Bunnell, B. N. (1966). Amygdaloid lesions and social dominance in the hooded rat. *Psychonomic Science, 6,* 93–94.

Carpenter, M. B. (1977). *Human Neuroanatomy.* New York: Williams & Wilkins,

Carlsen, J., De Olmos, J., & Heimer, L. (1982). Tracing of two-neuron pathways in the olfactory system by the aid of transneuronal degeneration: Projection to the amygdaloid body and hippocampal formation. *Journal of Comparative Neurology, 208,* 196–208.

Casagrande, V. A., & Joseph, R. (1980). Morphological effects of monocular deprivation and recovery on the dorsal lateral geniculate nucleus in galago. *Journal of Comparative Neurology, 194,* 413–426.

Cairns, R. B. (1967). The attachment behavior of mammals. *Psychological Review, 73,* 409–426.

Chapman, L. F., & Walter, R. D. (1965). Actions of lysergic acid dienthalamid on averaged human cortical evoked responses to light flash. *Recent Advances in Biological Psychiatry, 7,* 23–36.

Chapman, L. F., Walter, R. D., Ross, W., *et al.* (1963). Altered electrical activity of human hippocampus and amygdala induced by LSD-25. *Physiologist, 5,* 118.

Chapman, W. P. (1960). Depth electrode studies in patients with temporal lobe epilepsy. In E. R. Ramey & D. S. O'Doherty (Eds.), *Electrical studies on the unanesthetized brain* (pp. 334–350). New York: Hoeber.

Chapman, W. P., Schroeder, H. R., Geyer, G., Brazier, M. A. B., Fager, C., Poppen, T. L., Soloman, H. C., & Yakovlev, P. I. (1954). Physiological evidence concerning importance of the amygdaloid nuclear region in the integration of circulatory functioning and emotion and man. *Science, 177,* 949–951.

Chen, R., & Forster, F. M. (1973). Cursive and gelastic epilepsy. *Neurology (New York), 23,* 1019–1029.

Clark, C. V. H., & Isaacson, R. L. (1965). Effects of bilateral hippocampal ablation on DRL performance. *Journal of Comparative and Physiological Psychology, 59,* 137–140.

Como, P., Joseph, R., Fiducis, D., & Siegel, J. (1979). Visually evoked potentials and after-discharge as a function of arousal and frontal lesion in rats. *Proceedings of the Society for Neuroscience, 5,* 542.

Corking, S. (1965). Tactually-guided maze learning in man: Effects of unilateral cortical excisions and bilateral hippocampal lesions. *Neuropsychologia, 3,* 339–351.

Critchley, M. (1939). Neurogical aspects of visual and auditory hallucinations. *British Medical Journal, 107,* 634–639.

Crosby, E. C., DeJonge, B. D., & Schneider, R. C. (1966). Evidence for some of the trends in the phylogenetic development of the vertebrate telencephalon. In R. Hassler & H. Stephan (Eds.), *Evolution of the Forebrain* (pp. 333–371). Stuttgart: G. T. Verlag.

Currier, R. D., Little, S. C., Suess, J. F., & Andy, O. J. (1971). Sexual seizures. *Archives of Neurology, 25,* 260–264.

Cushing, H. (1932). *Papers relating to the pituitary body, hypothalamus and parasympathetic nervous system.* Springfield, IL: Charles C. Thomas.

Daly, D., & Moulder, D. (1957). Gelastic epilepsy. *Neurology (New York), 7,* 26–36.

Davison, C., & Kelman, H. (1939). Pathological laughing and crying. *Archives of Neurology and Psychiatry, 42,* 595–643.

Delgado, J. (1955). Cerebral structures involved in transmission and elaboration of noxious stimulation. *Journal of Neurophysiology, 18,* 261–275.

Delgado, J., & Anand, B. K. (1953). Increase of food intake induced by electrical stimulation of the laterial hypothalamus. *American Journal of Physiology, 172,* 162–168.

Dennis, W. (1960). Causes of retardation among institutional children. Iran. *Journal of Genetic Psychology, 96,* 47–59.

Diamond, M. C. (1985). Rat forebrain morphology: Right–left; male–female; young–old; enriched–improvished. In S. D. Glick (Ed.), *Cerebral lateralization in nonhuman primates* (pp. 181–201). Orlando, FL: Academic Press.

Dicks, D., Myers, R. E., & Kling, A. (1969). Uncus and amygdaloid lesions on social behavior in free ranging rhesus monkey. *Science, 160,* 69–71.

Dott, N. M. (1938). Surgical aspects of the hypothalamus. In W. E. LeGross Clark (Ed.), *The hypothalamus* (pp. 77–103). Edinburgh: Oliver & Boyd.

Douglas, R. J. (1967). The hippocampus and behavior. *Psychological Bulletin, 67,* 416–442.

Dorner, G. (1976). *Hormones and brain differentiation* Amsterdam: Elsevier/North- Holland.

Dreifuss, J. J., Murphy, J. T., & Gloor, P. (1968). Contrasting effects of two identified amygdaloid efferent pathways on single hypothalamic neurons. *Journal of Neurophysiology, 31,* 237–248.

Drefus-Brisac, C. (1970). Sleep ontogenesis in human prematures after 32 weeks of age. *Developmental Psychobiology, 3,* 91–121.

Dreyfus-Brisac, C., & Monod, N. (1975). The electroencephalogram of full-term newborns and premature infants. In C. Drefus-Brisac (Ed.), *Handbook of electroencephalography and clinical neurophysiology* (Vol. 6b) (pp. 240–260). Amsterdam: Elsevier.

Egger, M. D., & Flynn, J. P. (1963). Effect of electrical stimulation of the amygdala on hypothalamically elicited attach behavior. *Journal of Neurophysiology, 26,* 705–720.

Ellen, P., Wilson, A. S., & Powell, E. W. (1964). Septal inhibition and timing behavior in the rat. *Journal of Comparative Neurology, 10,* 120–132.

Emde, R. N., & Koenig, K. L. (1969). Neonatal smiling and rapid eye movement states. *American Academy of Child Psychiatry, 8,* 57–67.

Emde, R. N., & Metcalf, D. R. (1970), An electroencephalographic study of behavior and rapid eye movement states in the human newborn. *Journal of Nervous and Mental Disease, 150,* 376–386.

Endroczi, E., Schreiberg, G., & Lissak, K. (1963). The role of central nervous activating and inhibitory structures in the control of pituitary–adrenocortical function. *Acta Physiologica, 24,* 211–221.

Erickson, T. (1945). Erotomanis (nymphomania) as an expression of cortical epileptiform discharge. *Archives of Neurology and Psychiatry, 53,* 226–231.

Fedio, P., & Van Buren, J. (1974). Memory deficits during electrical stimulation of the speech cortex in conscious man. *Brain and Language, 1,* 29–42.

Feldman, S. (1962). Neurophysiological mechanisms modifying afferent hypothalamic–hippocampal condition. *Experimental Neurology, 5,* 269–291.

Feldman, S., Saphier, D., & Conforti, N. (1987). Hypothalamic afferent connections mediating adrenocortical responses that follow hippocampal stimulation. *Experimental Neurology, 98,* 103–109.

Flor-Henry, P. (1969). Psychosis and temporal lobe epilepsy: a controlled investigation. *Epilepsia, 10,* 363–395.

Flor-Henry, P. (1983). *Cerebral basis of psychopathology.* Boston: John Wright.

Flynn, J. P., Edwards, S. B., & Bandler, R. J. (1971). Changes in sensory and motor systems during critically elicited attack. *Behavioral Science, 16,* 1–19.

Foerster, O. O., & Gagel, O. (1932). Die Vorderseitenstrangdurschschneidun biem Menschen (English summary). *Z. Neurology and Psychiatry, 138,* 1–92.

Foreman, N., & Stevens, R. (1987). Relationships between the superior colliculus and hippocampus: Neural and behavioral considerations. *Behavioral and Brain Sciences, 10,* 101–152.

Freemon, F. R., & Nevis, A. H. (1969). Temporal lobe sexual seizures. *Neurology, (New York), 19,* 87–90.

Freeman, W., & Williams, J. (1952). Human sonar. *Journal of Nervous and Mental Disease, 32,* 456–462.

Freeman, W., & Williams, J. (1963). Hallucinations in Braille. *Archives of Neurology and Psychiatry, 70,* 630–634.

Freud, S. (1911). Formulations regarding the two principals in mental functioning. *A general selection from the works of Sigmund Freud.* London: Hogarth Press.

Fukuda, M., Ono, T., & Nakamura, K. (1987). Functional relation among inferotemporal cortex, amygdala and lateral hypothalamus in monkey operant feeding behavior. *Journal of Neurophysiology, 57,* 1060–1077.

Fuller, J. L., Rosvold, H. E., & Pribram, K. H. (1957). Effect on affective and cognitive behavior in the dog of lesions of the pyriform–amygdaloid–hippocampal complex. *Journal of Comparative and Physiological Psychology, 50,* 89–96.

Fulton, J. F., & Ingraham, F. D. (1929). Emotional disturbances following experimental lesions of the base of the brain. *Journal of Physiology, 67,* 47–90.

Gerendai, I. (1984). Lateralization of neuroendocrine control. In N. Geschwind & A. M. Galaburda (Eds.), *Cerebral dominance* (pp. 137–150). Cambridge: Harvard University Press.

Gibbs, A. F. (1951). Ictal and non-ictal psychiatric disorders in temporal lobe epilepsy. *Journal of Nervous and Mental Disease, 113,* 522–528.

Gloor, P. (1955). Electrophysiological studies on the connections of the amygdaloid nucleus of the cat. I & II. *Electroencephalography and Clinical Neurophysiology, 7,* 223–242, 243–262.

Gloor, P. (1960). Amygdala. In J. Field (Ed.), *Handbook of physiology* (pp. 300–370). Washington, DC: American Physiological Society.

Gloor, P., Olivier, A. Quesney, L. F., Andermann, F., & Horowitz, S. (1982). The role of the limbic system in experimental phenomena of temporal lobe epilepsy. *Annals of Neurology, 12,* 129–144.

Goldstein, L., Stolzfus, N., & Gardocki, J. (1959). Changes in interhemispheric amplitude relationships in the EEG during sleep. *Physiology and Behavior, 59,* 811–815.

Gorski, R. A., Gordon, J. H., Shryne, J. E., & Southam, A. M. (1978). Evidence for a morphological sex difference within the medial preoptic area of the rat brain. *Brain Research, 148,* 333–346.

Graeber, R. C. (1980). Telencephalic function in elasmobranchs. A behavioral perspective. In S. O. E. Ebbesson (Ed.), *Comparative neurology of the telencephalon* (pp. 301–327). New York: Plenum Press.

Grastyan, E., Lissak, K., Madarasz, I., & Donhoffer, H. (1959). Hippocampal electrical activity during the development of conditioned reflexes. *Electroencephalography and Clinical Neurophysiology, 11,* 409–430.

Gray, J. A. (1970). Sodium amobarbital, the hippocampal theta rhythm and the partial reinforcement extinction effect. *Psychological Review, 77,* 465–480.

Green, J. D., & Adey, W. R. (1956). Electrophysiological studies of hippocampal connections and excitability. *Electroencephalography and Clinical Neurophysiology, 8,* 245–262.

Green, J. E., & Arduini, A. (1954). Hippocampal electrical activity in arousal. *Journal of Neurophysiology, 17,* 533–557.

Greenough, W. (1976). Enduring effects of differential experience and training. In M. R. Rosenzweig & E. L. Bennett (Eds.), *Neural mechanisms of learning and memory* (pp. 170–240). Cambridge, MA: MIT Press.

Guillery, R. W. (1957). Degeneration in the hypothalamic connexions of the albinorat. *Journal of Anatomy, 91,* 403–419.

Gunne, L. M., & Lewander, T. (1966). Monoamine in brain and adrenal glands of cats after electrically induced defense reactions. *Acta Physiologica Scandinavica, 67,* 405–410.

Hagino, N., & Yamoaka, S. (1976). A neuroendocrinological approach to the investigation of the septum. In J. F. DeFrance (Ed.), *The septal nuclei.* New York: Plenum Press.

Harlow, H. F. (1962). The heterosexual affectional system in monkeys. *American Psychologist, 17,* 1–9.

Harlow, H. F. (1965). Sexual behavior in the rhesus monkey. In F. Beach (Ed.), *Sex and behavior* (pp. 220–235). New York: John Wiley & Sons.

Halgren, E., Babb, T. L., & Crandall, P. H. (1978). Activity of human hippocampal formation and amygdala neurons during memory tests. *Electroencephalography and Clinical Neurophysiology, 45,* 585–601.

Heath, R. G. (1954). *Studies in schizophrenia.* Cambridge, MA: Harvard University Press.

Heath, R. G. (1972). Physiological basis of emotional expression. *Biological Psychiatry, 5,* 172–184.

Heath, R. G. (1976). Brain function in epilepsy: Midbrain, medullary and cerebellar interaction with the rostral forebrain. *Journal of Neurology, Neurosurgery and Psychiatry, 39,* 1037–1051.

Health, R. G., Monroe, R., & Mickle, W. (1955). Stimulation of the amygdaloid nucleus in schizophrenic patients. *American Journal of Psychiatry, 111,* 862–863.

Hermann, B. P., & Chambria, S. (1980). Interictal psychopathology in patients with ictal fear. *Archives of Neurology, 37,* 667–668.

Herrick, C. J. (1925). The amphibian forebrain. *Journal of Comparative Neurology, 39,* 400–489.

Herzog, A. G., & Van Hoesen, G. W. (1976). Temporal neocortical afferent connections to the amygdala in thesus monkey. *Brain Research, 115,* 57–59.

Hillbom, E. (1960). After-effects of brain injuries. *Acta Psychiatrica Scandinavica (Suppl.), 142,* 1–180.

Hodoba, D. (1986). Paradoxic sleep facilitation by interictal epileptic activity of right temporal origin. *Biological Psychiatry, 21,* 1267–1278.

Horel, J. A. (1978). The neuroanatomy of amnesia. *Brain, 101,* 403–445.

Horowitz, M. J., Adams, J. E., & Rutkin, B. B. (1968). Visual imagery on brain stimulation. *Archives of General Psychiatry, 19,* 469–486.

Humphrey, M. E., & Zangwill, O. L. (1951). Cessation of dreaming after brain injury. *Journal of Neurology, Neurosurgery, and Psychiatry, 14,* 322–240.

Humphrey, T. (1972). The development of the human amygdaloid complex. In B. E. Elefterhiou (Ed.) *The neurobiology of the amygdala.* New York: Plenum Press.

Ingram, W. R. (1952). Brainstem mechanisms and behavior. *Electroencephalography and Clinical Neurophysiology, 4,* 395–406.

Ironside, R. (1956). Disorders of laughter due to brain lesions. *Brain, 79,* 589–609.

Isaacson, R. L. (1982). *The limbic system.* New York: Plenum Press.

Isaacson, R. L., Douglas, R. J., & Moore, R. Y. (1961). The effect of radical hippocampal ablation on acquisition of avoidance responses. *Journal of Comparative and Physiological Psychology, 54,* 625–628.

Jonason, K. R., & Enloe, L. J. (1972). Alterations in social behavior following septal and amygdaloid lesions in the rat. *Journal of Comparative and Physiological Psychology, 75,* 280–301.

Jonason, K. R., Enloe, L. J., Contrucci, J., & Meyer, P. M. (1973). Effects of stimulation and successive septal and amygdaloid lesions on social behavior in the rat. *Journal of Comparative and Physiological Psychology, 83,* 54–61.

Joseph, R. (1982). The neuropsychology of development: Hemispheric laterality, limbic language and the origin of thought. *Journal of Clinical Psychology, 38,* 4–33.

Joseph, R. (1986a). Confabulation and delusional denial: Frontal lobe and lateralized influences. *Journal of Clinical Psychology, 42,* 507–519.

Joseph, R. (1986b). Reversal of cerebral dominance for language and emotion in a corpus callosotomy patient. *Journal of Neurology, Neurosurgery, and Psychiatry, 49,* 628–634.

Joseph, R. (1988a). The right cerebral hemisphere: Neuropsychiatry, neuropsychology, neurodynamics. *Journal of Clinical Psychology,*

Joseph, R. (1988b). Dual mental functioning in a split-brain patient. *Journal of Clinical Psychology,*

Joseph, R., & Casagrande, V. A. (1980). Visual field defects and recovery following lid closure in a prosimian primate. *Behavioral Brain Research 1,* 150–178.

Joseph, R., Forrest, N., Fiducis, D., Como, P., & Siegel, J. (1981). Behavioral and electrophysiological correlates of arousal. *Physiological Psychology, 9,* 90–95.

Joseph, R., & Gallagher, R. E. (1980). Gender and early environment influences on activity, arousal, overresponsiveness, and exploration. *Developmental Psycobiology, 13,* 527–544.

Joseph, R., Gallagher, R. E., Holloway, W., & Kahn, J. (1984). Two brains, one child: interhemispheric information transfer deficits and confabulatory responding in children ages 4, 7, 10. *Cortex, 20,* 317–331.

Joseph, R., Hess, S., & Birecree, E. (1978). Effects of sex hormone manipulations and exploration on sex differences in learning. *Behavioral Biology, 24,* 364–377.

Jouvent, M. (1967). Neurophysiology of the states of sleep. *Physiological Review, 47,* 117–177.

Joynt, R. J. (1966). Verney's concept of the osmoreceptor. *Archives of Neurology, 14,* 331–334.

Kaada, B. R. (1951). Somato-motor, autonomic and electrocortical responses to electrical stimulation of "rhinencephalon" and other structures in primates, cat, and dog. *Acta Physiologica Scandinavica, (Suppl.), 24,* 1–170.

Kaada, B. R., Andersen, P., & Jensen, J. (1954). Stimulation of the amygdaloid nuclear complex in unanesthetized cats. *Neurology (New York), 4,* 48–64.

Kaada, B. R., Jansen, J., & Andersen, P. (1953). Stimulation of hippocampus and medial cortical areas in unanesthetized cats. *Neurology (New York), 3,* 844–857.

Karli, P., & Vergnes, M. (1969). Interspecific aggressive behavior and its manipulation by brain ablation and stimulation. In S. Garattini & E. B. Sigg (Eds.), *Aggressive behavior* (pp. 270–302). Amsterdam: Excepta Medica.

Kennard, M. A. (1945). Focal autonomic representation in the cortex and its relation to sham rage. *Journal of Neuropathology and Experimental Neurology, 4,* 295–304.

Kerr, N. H., & Foulkes, D. (1978). Reported absence of visual dream imagery in a normally sighted subject with Turners syndrome. *Journal of Mental Imagery, 2,* 247–264.

Kerr, N. H., & Foulkes, D. (1978). Reported absence of visual dream imagery in a normally sighted subject with Turner's syndrome. *Journal of Mental Imagery, 2,* 247–264.

Kesner, R. B., & Andrus, R. G. (1982). Amygdala stimulation disrupts the magnitude of reinforcement contribution to long-term memory. *Physiological Psychology, 10,* 55–59.

Kimura, D. (1963). Effects of selective hippocampal damage on avoidance behavior in the rat. *Canadian Journal of Psychology, 12,* 213–218.

Kimura, D. (1963). Right temporal lobe damage: Perception of unfamiliar stimuli after damage. *Archives of Neurology, 8,* 264–271.

King, F. A. (1958). Effects of septal and amygdaloid lesions on emotional behavior and conditioned avoidance responses in the rat. *Science, 128,* 655–656.

Kling, A. (1972). Effects of amygdalectomy on social-affective behavior in non-human primates. In B. E. Eleftheriou (Ed.), *The neurobiology of the amygdala* (pp. 127–170). New York: Plenum Press.

Kling, A. S., Lloyd, R. L., & Perryman, K. M. (1987). Slow wave changes in amygdala to visual, auditory and social stimuli following lesions of the inferior temporal cortex in squirrel monkey. *Behavioral and Neural Biology, 47,* 54–72.

Klinger, J., & Gloor, P. (1960). The connections of the amygdala and of the anterior temporal cortex in the human brain. *Journal of Comparative Neurology, 115,* 333–352.

Kluver, H., & Bucy, P. C. (1939). Preliminary analysis of functions of the temporal lobes in monkeys. *Archives of Neurology and Psychiatry, 42,* 979–1000.

Kolb, B., & Whishaw, W. (1977). IQ effects of brain lesions and atropine on hippocampal and neocortical EEG in the rat. *Experimental Neurology, 56,* 1–22.

Krettek, J. E., & Price, J. L. (1977a). Projections from the amygdaloid complex and adjacent olfactory structures to the entorhinal cortex and to the subiculum in rat and cat. *Journal of Comparative Neurology, 172,* 723–752.

Krettek, J. E., & Price, J. L. (1977b). Projections from the amygdaloid complex to the cerebral cortex and thalamus in the rat and cat. *Journal of Comparative Neurology, 172,* 687–722.

Kripke, D. F., & Sonnenschein, (1973). A 90-minute daydream cycle. *Sleep Research, 2,* 187–190.

Langmeier, J., & Matejcek, Z. (1975). *Psychological deprivation in childhood.* New York: John Wiley & Sons.

Lilly, J. C. (1960). Learning motivated by subcortical stimulation. In E. Ramsey & E. O'Doherty (Eds.), *Electrical studies on the unanesthetized brain* (pp. 67–103). New York: Hoeber.

Lishman, W. A. (1968). Brain damage in relation to psychiatric disability after head injury. *British Journal of Psychiatry, 114,* 373–410.

Lisk, W. G. (1967). Neural localization for androgen activation of copulatory behavior in the male rat. *Endocrinology, 80,* 754–780.

Lisk, W. G. (1971). Diencephalic placement of estradiol and sexual receptivity in the female rat. *American Journal of Physiology, 203,* 493–500.

List, C. F., Dowman, C. E., & Bagheiv, R. (1958). Posterior hypothalamic hermatomas and gangliomas causing precious puberty. *Neurology (New York), 8,* 164–174.

Loiseau, P., Cohandon, F., & Cohandon, S. (1971). Gelastic epilepsy. A review and report of five cases. *Epilepsia, 12,* 313–320.

Machne, X., & Segundo, J. (1956). Unitary responses to afferent volleys in amygdaloid complex. *Journal of Neurophysiology, 19,* 232–240.

Maclean, P. D. (1949). Psychosomatic disease and the "visceral brain." Recent developments bearing on the Papex theory of emotion. *Psychosomatic Medicine, 11,* 338–353.

Maclean, P. D. (1952). Some psychiatric implications of physiological studies of fronto-temporal portion of limbic system (visceral brain). *Electroencephalography and Clinical Neurophysiology, 4,* 407–414.

Maclean, P. D. (1969). The hypothalamus and emotional behavior. In W. Haymaker (Ed.), *The hypothalamus* (pp. 127–167). Springfield, IL: Charles C Thomas.

Maclean, P. D. (1973). New findings of brain function and sociosexual behavior. In J. Zubin & J. Money (Eds.), *Contemporary sexual behavior* (pp. 90–117). Baltimore: John Hopkins Press.

Mahl, G. F., Rothenberg, A., Delgado, J. M. R., & Hamlin, H. (1964). Psychological response in the human to intracerebral electrical stimulation. *Psychosomatic Medicine, 26,* 337–368.

Mark, V. H., Ervin, F. R., & Sweet, W. H. (1972). Deep temporal lobe stimulation in man. In B. E. Eleftheriou (Ed.), *The neurobiology of the amygdala* (pp. 207–240). New York: Plenum Press.

Marshall, J. F., & Teitelbaum, P. (1974). Further analysis of sensory inattention following lateral hypothalamic damage in rats. *Journal of Comparative and Physiological Psychology, 86,* 375–395.

Martin, J. P. (1950). Fits of laughter (sham mirth) in organic cerebral disease. *Brain 73,* 453–464.

McClary, R. A. Response specificity in the behavioral effect of limbic system lesions in the cat. *Journal of Comparative and Physiological Psychology, 54,* 605–613.

McClary, R. A. (1966). Response-modulating functions of the limbic system. In E. Stellar & J. M. Sprague (Eds.), *Progress in physiological psychology,* New York: Academic Press.

McGraw, M. B. (1969). *The neuromuscular maturation of the human infant.* New York: Hafner.

Mehler, W. R. (1980). Subcortical afferent connections of the amygdala in the monkey. *Journal of Comparative Neurology, 190,* 733–762.

Mesulam, M.-M., & Mufson, E. J. (1982). Insula of the old world monkey. III. *Journal of Comparative Neurology, 212,* 38–52.

Mesulam, M.-M., Mufson, E. J., Levey, A. I., & Wainer, B. H. (1983). Cholinergic innervation of the cortex by the basal forebrain. *Journal of Comparative Neurology, 214,* 170–197.

Meyer, D. R., Ruth, R. A., & Lavond, D. G. (1978). The septal social cohesiveness effect. *Physiology & Behavior, 21,* 1027–1029.

Meyer, J. S., Ishikawa, Y., Hata, T., & Karacan, I. (1987). Cerebral blood flow in normal and abnormal sleep and dreaming. *Brain and Cognition, 6,* 266–294.

Michael, R. P., & Kaverne, E. B. (1974). Pheramones in the communication of sexual status in primates. In W. Ver der Kloot, C. Walcott, & B. Dane (Eds.), *Readings in behavior* (pp. 202–247). New York: Holt, Rinehart & Winston.

Milner, B. (1966). Amnesia following operations on the temporal lobes. In C. W. M. Whitt and O. L. Zangwill (Eds.), *Amnesia* (pp. 75–89). London: Butterworths.

Milner, B. (1970). Memory and the medial temporal regions of the brain. In K. Pribram and D. E. Broadbent (Eds.), *Biology of memory* (pp. 37–52). Orlando, FL: Academic Press.

Milner, B. (1971). Interhemispheric differences in the localization of psychological processes in man. *British Medical Bulletin, 71,* 272–275.

Milner, E. (1967). *Human neural and behavioral development.* Springfield, IL: Charles C. Thomas.

Mishkin, M. (1978). Memory in monkeys severely impaired by combined but not be separate removal of amygdala and hippocampus. *Nature (London), 273,* 297–299.

Mogenson, G. (1976). Septal–hypothalamic relationships. In J. F. DeFrance (Ed.), *The septal nuclei.* New York: Plenum Press.

Money, J., & Hosta G. (1967). Laughing seizures and sexual precocity. *John Hopkins Medical Journal, 120,* 326–330.

Murri, L., Arena, R., Siciliano, G., Mazzotta, R., & Muratorio, A. (1984). Dream recall in patients with focal cerebral lesions. *Archives of Neurology, 41,* 183–185.

Nakamura, K., & Ono, T. (1986). Lateral hypothalamus neuron involvement in integration of natural and artificial rewards and cue signals. *Journal of Neurophysiology, 55,* 163–181.

Nauta, W. J. H. (1956). An experimental study of the fornix in the rat. *Journal of Comparative Neurology, 104,* 247–272.

Nauta, W. J. H. (1958). Hippocampal projections and related neural pathways to the midbrain in cat. *Brain, 81,* 319–340.

Nauta, W. J. H. (1964). Some efferent connections of the prefrontal cortex in the monkey. In J. M. Warren & K. Akert (Eds.), *The frontal granular cortex and behavior* (pp. 397–407). New York: McGraw-Hill.

Nauta, W. J. H. (1971). The problem of the frontal lobe: A reinterpretation. *Journal of Psychiatric Research, 8,* 167–187.

Offen, M. L., Davidoff, R. A., Troost, B. T., & Richey, E. T. (1976). Dacrystic epilepsy. *Journal of Neurology, Neurosurgery and Psychiatry, 39,* 829–834.

O'Keefe, J., & Bouma, H. (1969). Complex sensory properties of certain amygdala units in the freely moving cat. *Experimental Neurology, 23,* 384–398.

Olds, J. A. (1956). A preliminary mapping of electrical reinforcing effects in rat brain. *Journal of Comparative and Physiological Psychology, 49,* 281–285.

Olds, J., & Milner, P. (1954). Positive reinforcement produced by electrical stimulation of septal areas and other regions of the rat brain. *Journal of Comparative and Physiological Psychology, 47,* 419–427.

Olds, M. E., & Forbes, J. L. (1981). The central basis of motivation: Intracranial self-stimulation studies. *Annual Review of Psychology, 32,* 523–574.

Olmstead, C. E., Best, P. J., & Mays, L. W. (1973). Neural activity in the dorsal hippocampus during paradoxical sleep, slow wave sleep and waking. *Brain Research, 60,* 381–391.

Olton, D. S., Branch, M., & Best, P. J. (1978). Spatial correlates of hippocampal unit activity. *Experimental Neurology, 58,* 397–409.

Ono, T., Nishino, H. Sasaki, K., Fukuda, M., & Muramoto, K. (1980). Role of the lateral hypothalamus and the amygdala in feeding behavior. *Brain Research Bulletin, 5,* 143–149.

Oppler, W. (1950). Manic psychosis in a case of parasagittal meningioma. *Archives of Neurology and Psychiatry, 47,* 417–430.

Pandya, D. N., Van Hoesen, G. W., & Domeskick, V. B. (1973). A cinguloamygdaloid projection in the rhesus monkey. *Brain Research, 61,* 369–373.

Parmelee, A. H., Wenner, W. H., Akiyama, Y., Schultz, M. A., & Stern, E. (1967). Sleep states in premature infants. *Developmental Medicine and Child Neurology, 14,* 70–77.

Penfield, W. (1954). The permanent records of the stream of consciousness. *Acta Psychologica, 11,* 47–69.

Penfield, W., & Milner, B. (1958). Memory deficit produced by bilateral lesions in the hippocampal zone. *Archives of Neurology and Psychiatry, 79,* 475–497.

Penfield, W., & Perot, A. (1963). The brain's record of auditory and visual experience. A final summary and discussion. *Brain 86,* 595–696.

Penfield, W., & Rasmussen, T. (1950). *The cerebral cortex of man.* New York: Macmillan.

Perryman, K. M., Kling, A. S., & Lloyd, R. L. (1987). Differential effects of inferior temporal cortex lesions upon visual and auditory-evoked potentials in the amygdala of the squirrel monkey. *Behavioral and Neural biology, 47,* 73–79.

Petsche, H., Gogolack, G., & Van Zwieten, P. A. (1965). Rhythmicity of septal cell discharges at various levels of reticular excitation. *Electroencephalography and Clinical Neurophysiology, 19,* 25–33.

Petsche, H., Stumpf, C. H. & Gogolack, G. (1962). The significance of the rabbit's septum as a relay station between midbrain and hippocampus. *Electroencephalography and Clinical Neurophysiology, 14,* 202–211.

Piaget, J. (1952). *The origins of intelligence.* New York: International University Press.

Pilleri, G., & Poeck, K. (1965). Sham rage-like behavior in a case of traumatic decerebration. *Confina Neurologica, 25,* 156–166.

Poletti, C. E., & Sujatanond, M. (1980). Evidence for a second hippocampal efferent pathway to hypothalamus and basal forebrain comparable to fornix system: A unit study in the monkey. *Journal of Neurophysiology, 44,* 514–531.

Poplawsky, A., & Isaacson, R. L. (1987). The GM1 ganglioside hastens the reduction of hyperemotionality after septal lesions. *Behavioral and Neural Biology, 48,* 150–158.

Rainbow, T. C., Parsons, B., & McEwen, B. A. (1982). Sex differences in rat brain oestrogen and progestin receptors. *Nature (London), 300,* 648–649.

Raisman, G., & Field, P. M. (1971). Sexual dimorphism in the preoptic area of the rat. *Science, 173,* 731–733.

Raisman, G., & Field, P. M. (1973). Sexual dimorphism in the neuropil of the preoptic area of the rat and its dependence on neonatal androgen. *Brain Research, 54,* 1–29.

Ranson, S. W., Kabat, H., & Magoun, H. W. (1935). Autonomic responses to electrical stimulation of the hypothalamus, preoptic region and septum, *Archives of Neurology and Psychiatry, 33,* 467–477.

Rausch, R., Serafetinides, E. A., & Crandall, P. H. (1977). Olfactory memory in patients with anterior temporal lobectomy. *Cortex, 13,* 445–452.

Rawlins, J. N. P. (1985). Associations across time: The hippocampus as a temporary memory store. *Behavioral and Brain Sciences, 8,* 479–496.

Redding, F. K. (1967). Modification of sensory cortical evoked potentials by hippocampal stimulation. *Electroencephalography and Clinical Neurophysiology, 22,* 74–83.

Remillard, G. M., *et al.* (1983). Sexual ictal manifestations predominant in women with temporal lobe epilepsy: A finding suggesting sexual dimorphism in the human brain *Neurology New York), 33,* 323–330.

Robinson, B. W. (1967). Vocalizations evoked from forebrain in *Macaca mulatta. Physiology and Behavior, 2,* 345–352.

Robinson, B. W., & Mishkin, M. (1968). Alimentary responses evoked from forebrain structures in *Macaca mulatta. Science, 136,* 260–261.

Rolls, E. T. (1975). *The brain and reward.* Oxford: Pergamon Press.

Rolls, E. T., Burton, M. J., & Mora, F. (1976). Hypothalamic neuronal response associated with the sight of food. *Brain Research, 111,* 53–56.

Rosenzweig, M. R. (1971). Effects of environment on development of brain and behavior. In E. Tolbach, L. R. Aronson, & E. Shaw (Eds.), *The biopsychology of development* (pp. 307–367). New York: Academic Press.

Routtenberg, A. (1968). The two arousal hypothesis: Reticular formation and limbic system. *Psychological Review, 75,* 51–80.

Rosvold, H. E., Mirsky, A. F., & Pribram, K. H. (1954). Influences of amygdalectomy on social behavior in monkeys. *Journal of Comparative and Physiological Psychology, 47,* 173–178.

Rubenstein, E. H., & Delgado, J. M. R. (1963). Inhibition induced by forebrain stimulation in monkey. *American Journal of Physiology, 205,* 941–948.

Ruff, R. L. (1980). Orgasmic epilepsy. *Neurology (New York), 30,* 1252–1253.

Russchen, F. T. (1982). Amygdalopetal projection in the cat. *Journal of Comparative Neurology, 207,* 157–176.

Sarter, M., & Markowitsch, J. J. (1985). The amygdala's role in human mnemonic processing. *Cortex, 21,* 7–24.

Savage, G. E. (1980). The fish telencephalon and its relation to learning. In S. O. E. Ebbesson (Ed.), *Comparative neurology of the telencephalon* (pp. 160–188). New York: Plenum Press.

Sawa, M., & Delgado, J. M. R. (1963). Amygdala unitary activity in the unrestrained cat. *Electroencephalography and Clinical Neurophysiology, 15,* 637–650.

Schaffer, H. R. (1966). The onset of fear of strangers and the incongruity hypothesis. *Journal of Child Psychology and Psychiatry, 7,* 95–106.

Schaffer, H. R., & Emerson, P. E. (1964). The development of social attachment in infancy. *Monographs of the Society for Research in Child Development, 29,* (Whole No. 94).

Schiff, H. B., Sabin, T. D., Geller, A. Alexander, L., & Mark, V. (1982). Lithium in aggressive behavior. *American Journal of Psychiatry, 139,* 1346–1348.

Schreiner, L., & Kling, A. (1953). Behavioral changes following rhinencephalic injury in cat. *Journal of Neurophysiology, 16,* 643–659.

Schreiner, L., & Kling, A. (1956). Rhinencephalon and behavior. *American Journal of Physiology, 184,* 486–490.

Schutze, I., Knuepfer, M. M., Eismann, A., Stumpf, H., & Stock, G. (1987). Sensory input to single neurons in the amygdala of the cat. *Experimental Neurology, 97,* 499–515.

Scoville, W. B., & Milner, B. (1957). Loss of recent memory after bilateral hippocampal lesions. *Journal of Neurology, Neurosurgery and Psychiatry, 20,* 11–21.

Serafetinides, E. A. (1965). The significance of the temporal lobes and of hemisphere dominance in the production of the LSD-25 symptomology in man. *Neuropsychologia, 3,* 69–79.

Sethi, P. K., & Rao, S. T. (1976). Gelastic, quiritarian, and cursive epilepsy. *Journal of Neurology, Neurosurgery and Psychiatry, 39,* 823–828.

Shealy, C., & Peele, J. (1957). Studies on amygdaloid nucleus of cat. *Journal of Neurophysiology, 20,* 125–139.

Sherwin, I. (1981). Psychosis associated with epilepsy. *Journal of Neurology, Neurosurgery and Psychiatry, 44,* 83–85.

Siegel, A., & Edinger, H. (1976). Organization of the hippocampal–septal axis. In J. F. DeFrance (Ed.), *The septal nuclei* (74–114). New York: Plenum Press.

Spencer, S. S., Spencer, D. D., Williamson, P. D., & Mattson, R. H. (1983). Sexual automatisms in complex partial seizures. *Neurology (New York), 33,* 527–533.

Spinelli, D. N. (1970). OCCAM: A computer model for a content of addressable memory in the central nervous system. In K. H. Pribram & D. E. Broadbent (Eds.), *Biology of memory* (pp. 33–60). New York: Academic Press.

Spitz, R. A. (1945). Hospitalism: An inquiry into the genesis of psychiatric conditions in early childhood. *Psychoanalytical Study of the Child, 1,* 53–74.

Spitz, R. A., & Wolf, K. M. (1946). The smiling response: A contribution to the ontogenesis of social relations. *Genetic Psychology Monographs, 34,* 57–125.

Squire, L. R., & Moore, R. Y. (1979). Dorsal thalamic lesion in a noted case of human memory dysfunction. *Annals of Neurology, 6,* 503–506.

Sroufe, L. A., Waters, E., & Matas, L. (1974). Contextual determinants in infant affective response. In M. Lewis and L. Roseblum, (Eds.), *The origins of fear* (pp. 301–350). New York: John Wiley & Sons.

Stein, L., & Ray, O. S. (1959). Self-regulation of brain stimulating current intensity in the rat, *Science, 130,* 570–572.

Steklis, H. D., & Kling, A. (1985). Neurobiology of affiliative behavior in nonhuman primates. In M. Reite &

T. Field (Eds.), *The psychobiology of attachment and separation* (pp. 93–134). Orlando, FL: Academic Press.

Steriade, M. (1964). Development of evoked responses into self-sustained activity within amygdalo–hippocampal circuits. *Electroencephalography and Clinical Neurophysiology, 16,* 221–231.

Steward, O. (1976). Topographic organization of the projections from the entorhinal area to the hippocampal formation of the rat. *Journal of Comparative Neurology, 167,* 285–314.

Stern, K., & Dacey, T. (1942). Glioma of the diencephalon in a manic patient. *American Journal of Psychiatry, 98,* 716.

Strauss, E., Risser, A., & Jones, M. W. (1982). Fear responses in patients with epilepsy. *Archives of Neurology, 39,* 626–630.

Swanson, L. W., & Cowan, W. M. (1979). The connections of the septal region in the rat. *Journal of Comparative Neurology, 186,* 621–656.

Sweet, W. H., Ervin, F., & Mark, V. H. (1969). The relationship of violent behavior in focal cerebral disease. In S. Garattini & E. Sigg (Eds.), *Aggressive behavior.* New York: John Wiley & Sons.

Tanabe, T., Yarita, H., Lino, M., Ooshima, Y., & Takagi, S. F. (1975). An olfactory projection area in orbitofrontal cortex of the monkey. *Journal of Neurophysiology, 38,* 1269–1283.

Tarachow, S. (1941). The clinical value of hallucinations in localizing brain tumors. *American Journal of Psychiatry, 99,* 1434–1443.

Taylor, D. C. (1975). Factors influencing the occurrence of schizophrenia like psychosis in patients with temporal lobe epilepsy. *Psychological Medicine, 5,* 249–254.

Teitelbaum, P. (1961). Disturbances in feeding and drinking behavior after hypothalamic lesions. In M. R. Jones (Ed.), *Nebraska symposium on motivation* (pp. 70–92). Lincoln: University of Nebraska Press.

Teitelbaum, P., & Epstein, A. N. (1962). The lateral hypothalamic syndrome. *Psychological Review, 69,* 74–90.

Terzian, H., & Ore, G. D. (1955). Syndrome of Kluver and Bucy in man by bilateral removal of temporal lobes. *Neurology (New York), 5,* 373–380.

Turner, B. H., Mishkin, M., & Knapp, M. (1980). Organization of the amygdalopetal projections from modality-specific cortical association areas in the monkey. *Journal of Comparative Neurology, 191,* 515–543.

Uhl, R. G., Kuhar, M. J., & Snyder, S. H. (1978). Enkephalin containing pathways: Amygdaloid efferents in the stria terminalis. *Brain Research, 149,* 223–228.

Ursin, H., & Kaada, B. R. (1960). Functional localization within the amygdaloid complex in the cat. *Electroencephalography and Clinical Neurophysiology, 12,* 1–20.

Van Hoesen, G. W., Pandya, D. N., & Butters, N. (1972). Cortical afferents to the entorhinal cortex of the rhesus monkey. *Science, 175,* 1471–1473.

Victor, M., Adams, R. D., & Collins, G. H. (1971). *The Wernicke–Korsakoff syndrome.* Philadelphia: F. A. Davis.

Van Hoesen, G. W. (1981). The differential distribution, diversity and sprouting of cortical projections to the amygdala in the rhesus monkey. In Y. Ben-Ari (Ed.), *The amygdala complex* (pp. 77–90). Amsterdam: Elsevier.

Vochteloo, J. D., & Koolhaas, J. M. (1987). Medial amygdala lesions in male rats reduce aggressive behavior. *Physiology and Behavior, 41,* 99–102.

Vonderache, A. R. (1940). Changes in the hypothalamus on organic disease. *Journal of Nervous and Mental Disease, 20,* 689–712.

Waraczynski, M., & Stellar, J. R. (1978). Reward saturation in medial forebrain bundle self-stimulation. *Physiology and Behavior, 41,* 585–593.

Waters, E., Matas, L., & Stroufe, L. A. (1975). Infant's reactions to an approaching stranger: description, validation and functional significance of wariness. *Child Development, 46,* 348–356.

Wasman, M., & Flynn, J. P. (1962). Directed attack elicited from the hypothalamus. *Archives of Neurology, 6,* 220–227.

Wechsler, A. F. (1973). The effect of organic brain disease on recall of emotionally charged vs. neutral narrative texts. *Neurology (New York), 23,* 130–135.

Weil, A. A. (1956). Ictal depression and anxiety in temporal lobe disorders. *American Journal of Psychiatry, 113,* 149–157.

Weingarten, S. M., Cherlow, D. G., & Holmgren, E. (1977). The relationship of hallucinations to the depth structures of the temporal lobe. *Acta Neurochirurgica, 24,* 199–216.

Weiskrantz, L. (1956). Behavioral changes associated with ablation of the amygdaloid complex in monkeys. *Journal of Comparative and Physiological Psychology, 49,* 381–391.

Wheatley, M. D. (1944). The hypothalamus and affective behavior. *Archives of Neurology and Psychiatry, 52,* 296–316.

Williams, D. (1956). The structure of emotions reflected in epileptic experiences. *Brain, 79,* 29–67.

Wilson, E. O. (1962). Chemical systems. In T. A. Sebeok (Ed.), *Animal communication* (pp. 87–117).

Zybrozyna, A. W. (1963). The anatomical basis of patterns of autonomic and behavior responses effected via the amygdala. In W. Bargmann & J. P. Schade (Eds.), *Progress in brain research* (Vol. 13) (pp. 220–253). Amsterdam: Elsevier.

4

The Frontal Lobes
Neuropsychiatry, Neuropsychology, and Behavioral Neurology

The frontal lobes serve as the "senior executive" of the brain; through the assimilation and fusion of perceptual, volitional, cognitive, and emotional processes, it modulates and shapes character and personality. When damaged, the result can be excessive or diminished cortical and behavioral arousal, disintegration of personality and emotional functioning, difficulty planning or initiating activity, abnormal attention and ability to concentrate, severe apathy or euphoria, disinhibition, and a reduced ability to monitor and control one's thoughts, speech, and actions. Paralysis of the extremities, severe unilateral neglect of visual–auditory space, or, conversely, compulsive utilization of tools or other objects can occur.

The reason for such a wide range of potential disturbance is that rather than a single pair of frontal lobes, there are several frontal regions that differ in regard to embryology, phylogeny, cellular composition, functional specificity, and interconnection and interaction with other brain areas. Each frontal region is concerned with somewhat different functions. Moreover, damage is seldom restricted to one specific frontal area but commonly disrupts adjoining frontal tissues as well. Thus, a host of divergent abnormalities can result, sometimes simultaneously, depending on the extent, site, depth, and laterality of the lesion.

Broadly speaking, the frontal lobes can be subdivided into four major functional–anatomical regions. These include the central motor areas (Brodmann's areas 4, 6, 8, 44, and 45); the lateral convexity (areas 9, 10, 11, 45, 46, and 47); the orbital regions (10, 11, 12, 13, and 14); and the medial inner walls of the hemispheres, which include overlapping tissues from the motor, lateral convexity, and orbital areas, including the anterior cingulate gyrus (area 24). Also of significance is the head of the caudate nucleus, which is buried within the depths of the frontal lobes and is functionally related to the lateral convexity and motor areas, as is the anterior cingulate.

In the ensuing discussion of the neuroanatomy, physiology, functions and symptoms associated with these various regions classifications such as "prefrontal" will not be employed. Rather, the term frontal lobe is reserved for the frontal region of the brain (i.e.,

139

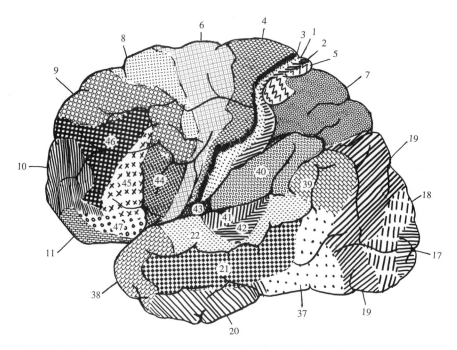

FIGURE 26. The lateral surface of the left cerebral hemisphere with Brodmann's areas indicated.

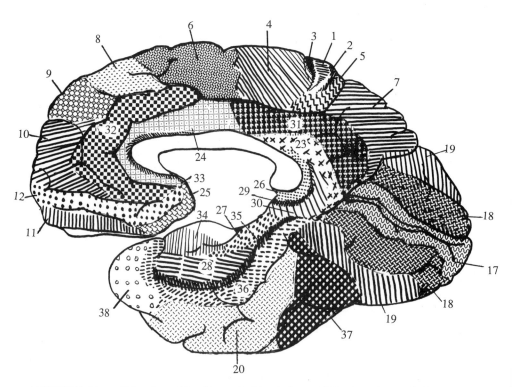

FIGURE 27. The medial surface of the right cerebral hemisphere with Brodmann's areas indicated.

orbital, lateral convexity, portions of the medial walls), whereas the motor areas are simply referred to as the motor regions (Figs. 26 and 27).

MOTOR REGIONS OF THE FRONTAL LOBES

The motor regions consist of three major subdivisions: the primary motor cortex, located along the precental gyrus (area 4); the premotor cortex (area 6); and the supplementary motor cortex, which is located along the medial wall of the hemispheres and includes portions of area 6. The frontal eye fields (area 8 with overlap from areas 9 and 6), Exner's writing area, and Broca's expressive speech area (45, 46) are also related to motor functioning as are the medial frontal lobes.

The Primary Motor Area

Functionally, the primary motor cortex appears to extend well beyond the confines of the precentral gyrus (area 4) and includes portions of area 6 and the somatosensory (1, 2, 3, and 5) regions (Brodal, 1981). These areas are richly interconnected (Jones, Coulter, & Hendry, 1978; Jones & Powell, 1970; Kuypers & Catsman-Berrevoets, 1984), the somatosensory projections providing information important in the sensory guidance of movement. Moreover, axonal projections from the motor and somesthetic regions all give rise to the massive corticospinal (pyramidal) tract, a rope of fibers that descend to the brainstem and spinal cord to make contact with cranial nerve and sensory and spinal motor neurons (Brodal, 1981; Kuypers & Catsman-Berrevoets, 1984). For these reasons, some investigators have referred to the somesthetic and motor regions as the sensorimotor cortex.

The primary motor area is concerned with the coordination and expression of gross and fine motor functioning (Woolsey, 1958) and serves as a final pathway or nodal point, where impulses organized in other brain areas are transferred for expression. Unlike the sensory areas, where information is first received in the primary zones before transmission to the association area, motor impulses begin their organizational journey in the premotor supplementary motor as well other areas before transmission to the primary regions, where they are then acted upon. Because of this, direct electrical stimulation of the primary motor cortex never gives rise to complex, coordinated, or purposeful movements (Penfield & Jasper, 1954; Penfield & Rasmussen, 1950; Rothwell, Thompson, Day, Dick, Kachi, Cowan, & Marsden, 1987), although some gross movement may be elicited.

Rather, electrical stimulation of discrete points within the motor cortex elicit contractions and movements of tiny muscle groups. In fact, an almost one to one correspondence between single motor neurons and particular muscles is evident, such that the entire musculature of the body is neuronally represented in the motor cortex. However, since certain muscle groups play a proportionately greater role in the performance of complex (versus simple) movements a relatively greater number of neurons are involved in their representation. Thus, the fingers have extensive cortical representation, whereas a smaller neuronal field is concerned with the elbow. Indeed, by stimulating the motor cortex, Penfield and colleagues were able to construct a cerebral-motor map of the body (i.e., a motor homunculus) (Fig. 28).

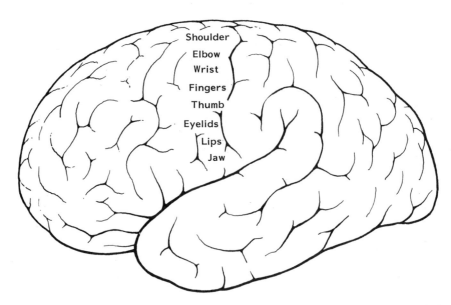

FIGURE 28. The lateral surface of the left cerebral hemisphere with relative location of body parts indicated along the primary motor cortex.

If electrical stimulation is applied when the patient is attempting to move, the result is paralysis (Penfield & Jasper, 1954; Penfield & Rasmussen, 1950). Presumably this is a consequence of blocking the reception of impulses to move, which are initiated and organized elsewhere (i.e., disconnection).

Paralysis

Damage to the motor areas, or to the descending corticospinal tract initially results in a flaccid hemiplegia such that the muscles are completely without tone contralateral to the lesion (Adams & Victor, 1981; Brodal, 1981). If the examiner were to raise and release an effected arm, it would drop in a limp rag-doll fashion.

Over the course of the next several days, the muscles develop increased tone and resistance to passive movements. The reflexes become very brisk and manifest spasticity and hyperreflexia. The leg usually becomes permanently extended and the arm assumes a flexed position (Adams & Victor, 1981; Brodal, 1981). After several weeks or months, a limited capacity to perform gross movements reappears. Fine movements are usually permanently lost (Brodal, 1981).

The Premotor Cortex

The premotor cortex (area 6) is intimately interconnected with the primary motor area, both of which continue on to the medial wall of the hemisphere. Although not containing giant Betz cells (which are found in area 4), the premotor cortex contributes almost one third of the fibers of the corticospinal tract. The premotor cortex sends axons to area 4 and receives projections from this and the supplementary motor area (Jones *et al.*, 1978; Jones & Powell, 1970). It also receives information directly from the primary and secondary somesthetic and visual (areas 17, 18 and 19) cortices (Jones & Powell, 1970; Pandya & Kuypers, 1969) and is heavily involved in the guidance and refinement of movement via the assimilation of sensory information provided by the sensory areas (Godschalk, Lemon, Nijis, & Kuypers, 1981).

Whereas neurons in the primary motor region become active during movement, excitation in the premotor cortex precedes cellular activation of the primary region (Weinrich, Wise, & Mauritz, 1984). Moreover, cells in the premotor cortex become activated before movements are even initiated. These and other findings suggest that the premotor area may be modulating and exerting controlling influences on impulses which are to be transmitted to the primary region for expression. Indeed, the premotor area appears to be highly involved in the programming of various gross and fine motor activities and becomes highly active during the learning of new motor programs (Roland, Skinhoj, Lassen, & Larsen, 1980). Moreover, electrical stimulation elicits complex patterned movement sequences as well as stereotyped and gross motor responses such as head turning or torsion of the body (Fulton, 1934; Passingham, 1981).

Unlike the primary area, damage limited to the premotor cortex does not result in paralysis but disrupts fine motor functioning and dexterity, including simple activities such as finger tapping (Luria, 1980). With extensive damage fine motor skills are completely lost and phenomena such as the grasp reflex are elicited (Brodal, 1981); i.e., if you were to touch the patient's hand it would involantarily clasp shut.

The Supplementary Motor Area and the Medial Frontal Lobes

Will, Apathy, Gegenhalten, Waxy Flexibility, and Catatonia

The supplementary motor area (SMA) is located long the medial walls of the hemispheres but has no clear-cut anatomical boundaries. Its anterior portion abuts the medial overlap of the primary area, and its extends downward along the medial wall where it meets the anterior cingulate gyrus (area 24). The SMA contains a crude neuronal representation of the body (see Goldberg, 1985; for a detailed review).

The SMA receives axonal projections from the primary and association somatosensory areas (Jones & Powell, 1970; Pandya & Vignolo, 1971) and shares rich interconnections with primary motor cortex, the anterior cingulate (Jones *et al.*, 1978), and the basal ganglia (Brodal, 1981). The SMA appears to be concerned with the general problem of guiding and moving the extremities through space. Electrical stimulation has produced complex semipurposeful movements, vocalization (Penfield & Jasper, 1954), and postural synergies involving the trunk and extremities bilaterally (Van Buren & Fedio, 1976). Moreover, single cell recordings (Brinkman & Porter, 1979; Tanji & Kurata, 1982) and blood flow studies (Orgogozo & Larsen, 1979) have indicated increased activity in this area while performing and even imagining complex movements of the fingers and hands. This region becomes highly active during the modification, learning and establishment of new movement programs (Brinkman & Porter, 1979; Roland *et al.*, 1980; Tanji, Tanguchi, & Saga, 1980).

SMA Damage

Paralysis or paresis does not result even with extensive damage, although movements tend to be slow and incoordinated—a condition also seen with mild lesions (Penfield & Jasper, 1954). Difficulties in performing rapid or alternating movements as well as clumsiness, severe agraphia, and impairments of bimanual coordination (Brinkman, 1981; Goldberg, Meyer, & Toglia, 1981; McNabb, Carroll, & Mastaglia, 1988; Penfield & Jasper, 1954; Travis, 1955; Watson, Fleet, Gonzalez-Rothi, & Heilman, 1986), including gegenhalten and waxy flexibility can result. Patients may walk with short steps and suffer disturbances involving posture, balance, and gait. Initially, mutism may be observed (McNabb *et al.,* 1988; Watson *et al.,* 1986).

Gegenhalten and Waxy Flexibility

Rather than paralysis, lesions involving the SMA and surrounding medial tissue are sometimes associated with gengenhalten (counterpull) i.e., involuntary resistance to movement of the extremities (Travis, 1955). If a physician attempts to move an affected arm, it will suddenly stiffen and become increasingly rigid as pressure to move it increases. Although aware, the patient cannot decrease the resistance.

Waxy flexibility has been attributed to deep SMA and medial lesions as well as following surgical destruction of the underlying SMA white matter. If the examiner moves the arm, resistance appears after completion of the movement such that the extremity will remain in whatever position or posture it is placed and then only very slowly return to a normal resting position.

Posturing is also noted. Such patients, for example, might remain in odd and uncomfortable positions for exceedingly long time periods and make no effort to correct the situation (Freeman & Watts, 1942; Rose, 1950). This condition will usually resolve within a few weeks. Nevertheless, in some cases the condition may be mistaken for catatonia.

The Frontal–Medial Walls of the Cerebral Hemispheres

The medial walls of the anterior portion of the hemispheres contain not only the SMA, but the anterior cingulate (area 24), portions of the frontal eye fields (area 8), and areas of overlap from the primary and supplementary motor cortices, lateral convexity (areas 9 and 10) and orbital frontal lobe (areas 11 and 12) (Fig. 29). It maintains massive interconnections with all these regions, as well as with the hippocampus, lateral amygdala, lateral hypothalamus, basal ganglia, and the reticular formation, and receives axonal projections from the sensory cortices (Jones & Powell, 1970, Leichnetz & Astruc, 1976). Through these interconnections, it is involved in the synthesis of motor, sensory, and emotional information. In this manner, ideas and thoughts can become emotionally charged and motivational significance assigned to external perceptions or particular motor activities. Thus, if damaged disturbances of "will" (e.g., apathy) as well as peculiar abnormalities involving motor activity (e.g., gegenhalten, waxy flexibility) are likely. Neglect, indifference, catatonic-like features, or, conversely, compulsive activation of the limbs including, in the extreme, a syndrome referred to as the alien hand may result.

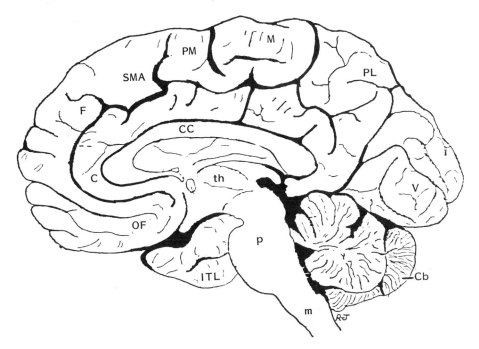

FIGURE 29. The medial surface of the right cerebral hemisphere. The pons (p) and medulla (m) of the brainstem are indicated as well as the thalamus (th), corpus callosum (cc), cingulate (C), orbital frontal lobes (OF), supplementary motor area (SMA), premotor (PM) and the primary motor areas (M), parietal lobule (PL), visual cortex (V), and cerebellum (Cb).

Catatonia

Although a variety of neural pathways and structures have been implicated in the pathogenesis of schizophrenia, there is some evidence that deep medial lesions of the frontal lobe sometimes give rise to emotional blunting, posturing, and what appears to be catatonic-like symptoms. For example, Freeman and Watts (1942) describe one patient who developed waxy flexibility, catatonia, and related symptoms after a gunshot wound (suffered during the war) that passed completely through the frontal lobes.

> The patient layed in a catatonic-like stupor for 2 months, always on one side with slightly flexed arms and legs, never changing his uncomfortable position; if he were rolled into some other position, he would quickly get back into his former one. He did not obey commands, but if food and drink were given to him, he swallowed them naturally. He was incontinent, made no complaints, gazed steadily forward, and showed no interest in anything. He could not be persuaded to talk, and then suddenly he would answer quite correctly about his personal affairs and go back to mutism. From time to time he showed a peculiar explosive laugh, especially when his untidiness was mentioned. Incredibly, the patient "was eventually returned to active duty." (pp. 46–47)

Similarly, Hillbom (1951), reported that among a large sample of individuals who had suffered traumatic missile wounds, those who developed catatonic features (or hebrephrenia) commonly had frontal lobe injuries. In a recent case, a patient with no previous psychiatric history, after having been beat around the head and suffering frontal subdural hematomas (which required drilling burr holes for evacuation) within days developed catatonic behaviors, resisted the efforts of others to move him, and would sit motionless and unresponsive for hours in odd and uncomfortable positions. Interestingly, the patient's symptoms seemed to wax and wane such that he demonstrated some periods of seeming normality.

"Will" and Apathy

Stimulation of the SMA sometimes results in a functional disconnection between this and other areas such that the ability to initiate or complete a voluntary movement is disrupted, and the "Will to move" or speak completely attenuated and abolished (Hassler, 1980; Laplane, Talairach, Meininger, Bancaud, & Orgogozo, 1977; Lur' 1980; Penfield & Jasper, 1954; Penfield & Welch, 1951). Upon partial recovery or with extensive prodding, such patients have complained that thoughts do not enter their head (Luria, 1980); i.e., they are unable to think or generate ideas, and experience a motivational–ideational void (Brutkowski, 1965; Hassler, 1980; Laplane *et al.,* 1977; Luria, 1980; Mishkin, 1964). Subjects may bump into objects, not blink in response to threat, stand about motionless, or, demonstrate waxy flexibility. Thus, it is not surprising that patients, like the soldier described by Freeman and Watts, may initially seem to be in a catononic-like stupor. Similar abnormalities (excluding catatonia) are sometimes seen with convexity lesions bordering on the frontal pole or motor areas, and with anterior cingulate damage.

Forced Grasping, Compulsive Utilization, and the "Alien Hand"

In other instances, semipurposeful uncontrolled motoric responses may become superimposed on the patient's otherwise seemingly apathetic and confused condition. That is, with massive or bilateral destruction of the SMA and portions of the medial walls, there can result semipurposeful, albeit reflexive motoric abnormalities such as forced grasping and "magnetic" groping (Denny-Brown, 1958; McNabb *et al.,* 1988; Travis, 1955). In some cases, patients seem "stimulus bound" and involuntarily respond to or even compulsively use objects or stimuli with which they come in contact (Denny-Brown, 1958; Lhermitte, 1983; Travis, 1955). Presumably, this is caused by a loss of internal motivational controls (i.e., disconnection) and is partially a release phenomenon such that patients appear to be reflexively or magnetically directed solely by external stimuli that trigger involuntary motor reactions.

Forced Grasping and Groping

Forced grasping is the mildest form of this disturbance. If an object touches the palm of the hand, the patient grips it involuntarily and cannot let go. With extensive destruction and/or as the lesion extends mesially, the mere visual presence of an object near the hand triggers groping movements as well as grasping. Denny-Brown (1958) has referred to this as "magnetic apraxia" and "compulsive exploration." He notes that touching the hand will elicit orienting movements to bring the object into the palm. Once it is grasped, the patient cannot release his grip.

This aberration is often accompanied by gegenhalten. Immediately before actually grasping the object, the entire arm will stiffen and one is met with resistance if an attempt is made to move the extremity. When the patient attempts to write, the hand stiffens and becomes seemingly stuck to the paper. When trying to walk, the feet seem to stick to the floor as if glued, and steps are made with great difficulty (Denny-Brown, 1958).

Denny-Brown (1958) believed that magnetic groping was due to a perseveration of contractual reactions (as well as parietal lobe disinhibitory release), for as long a stimulation is applied to the skin, the deficit, including gegenhalten, not only persists but becomes more intense. Magnetic apraxia is also triggered visually. As if stimulus bound, the patient's eyes and head may compulsively follow moving objects. If an object is brought near the face they may compulsively reach out and take it, and/or if near the lips may attempt to mouth or suck it. Such behavior is completely involuntary and will occur even if the patient ''willfully'' attempts to oppose it.

Compulsive Utilization

With extensive mesial damage involving the medial and medial–orbital areas, patients not only magnetically grope but may demonstrate a compulsive involuntary tendency to use whatever objects may be near (Lhermitte, 1983). For example, if an experimenter were to place a hammer and nail close by, the patient might impulsively begin to hammer the nail into the testing table or the wall—even if instructed not to. If the examiner places a pair of spectacles on the table, the patient compulsively puts them on. One such patient put three pair of spectacles on simultaneously (Lhermitte, 1983). If food or water are near, he might eat and drink, even when repeatedly told to refrain and in the absence of hunger or thirst. Damage to this area can cause patients to respond and use whatever objects or tools may be close by, even when they understand that they are not to do so (Lhermitte, 1983).

The ''Alien Hand''

In rare instances, this compulsive groping and utilization behavior can become confined to one limb and involve complex and seemingly purposeful action. This has occurred in cases in which the lesion has predominantly destroyed either the right or left SMA and medial portion of the hemisphere as well as the anterior corpus callosum (McNabb *et al.,* 1988; Goldberg *et al.,* 1981), such that the right and left frontal lobe became partially or fully disconnected.

For example, McNabb *et al.* (1988) describe one woman who had extensive damage involving the medial left frontal lobe and anterior corpus callosum, whose right ''hand showed an uncontrollable tendency to reach out and take hold of objects and then be unable to release them. At times the right hand interfered with tasks being performed by the left hand, and she attempted to restrain it by wedging it between her legs or by holding or slapping it with her left hand. The patient would repeatedly express astonishment at these actions'' (p. 219). A second patient frequently experienced similar difficulties. When ''attempting to write with her left hand the right hand would reach over and attempt to take the pencil. The left hand would respond by grasping the right hand to restrain it'' (p. 221).

Similar problems, however, have also plagued some patients following complete (surgical) destruction of the corpus callosum (Joseph, 1988a,b). In many of these instances, however, the independent alien behaviors demonstrated were often purposeful, intentional, complex, and obviously directed by an awareness maintained by the disconnected right hemisphere. For example, one patient's left hand would not allow him to smoke and would pluck lit cigarettes from his mouth, whereas another patient's left hand (right brain) preferred different foods and even television shows and would interfere with the choices made by the right hand (left hemisphere). One patient was pulled to the television and the left hand changed the channel.

Internal Utilization

As the locus of the lesion becomes even more inferior and posterior, encroaching on the orbital–temporal (amygdaloid) area, external utilization is replaced by attempts at internal (oral) utilization. Instead of using an object by motorically interacting with it, the individual orally interacts and attempts to consume the object. Everything that is seen and touched is placed indiscriminantly in the mouth and orally "explored" (Joseph, 1989).

This latter disturbance, extreme orality, has been referred to as "psychic blindness" and the Kluver–Bucy syndrome, and is a consequence of amygdaloid destruction—a nucleus with massive interconnections with the orbital/inferior medial area (Joseph, 1989).

Implications

Although seemingly disparate, a continuum of related aberrations can result following damage to the medial and motor areas of the frontal lobe. With deep inferior orbital–temporal (amygdaloid) destruction, the patient may engage in internal utilization, e.g., heightened orality and internal utilization behavior. With more medial destruction the patient may instead display external compulsive utilization of objects or in the extreme, complex uncontrollable acts limited to one extremity. With more superior medial damage involving the SMA, the behavioral displays are less complex and may involve involuntary activation of the fingers and extremities, including forced grasping and groping (SMA). However, with damage involving the premotor area there is a loss of fine motor skills, whereas paralysis results from primary motor destruction. Hence, with primary motor damage a patient cannot move although he may want to, whereas with medial and SMA damage the patient may compulsively move although he does not want to. In some instances (such as following partial disconnection of the anterior regions due to corpus callosum involvement), a complex syndrome of motoric responses referred to as the alien hand syndrome may result.

These findings raise the possibility that the motor areas, although guided by sensory impressions, act at the behest of impulses originating in or beyond the medial and orbital–amygdaloid area. When these internal influences are blocked (due to disconnection) but external perceptual activity is preserved, compulsive responding to external stimuli results. The motor areas become released from the internal guidance or from inhibitory influences mediated by the opposing hemisphere. However, with massive medial damage (where internal influences becomes integrated with external sources of input), the patient loses the ability to respond either to internal or to external forces, becoming mute and sometimes seemingly catatonic.

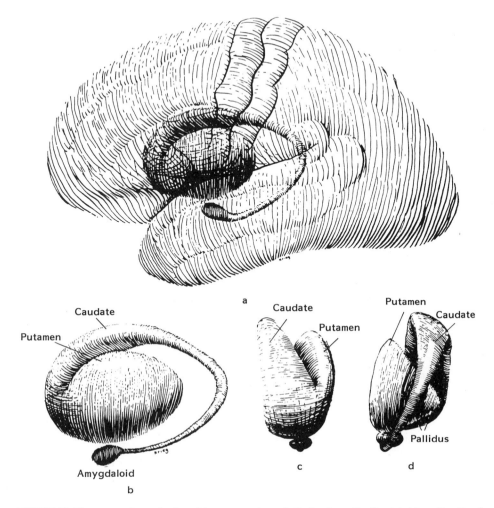

FIGURE 30. The structural organization of the corpus striatum in the basal ganglia. Reprinted from *Functional neuroanatomy* by W. J. S. Krieg, 1966. Brain Books. Chicago.

The Anterior Cingulate

The SMA and portions of the lateral convexity appear to have evolved from the anterior cingulate gyrus (Sanides, 1972). That is, over the course of evolutionary development, the cingulate has grown up and over the medial wall to become, in modified form, part of the SMA and lateral convexity. Indeed, the SMA and portions of the lateral convexity are not only structurally related to the anterior cingulate but maintain massive interconnections with this area (Damasio & Van Hoesen, 1980).

The anterior cingulate (Brodmann's area 24) also maintains extensive interconnections with the lateral amygdala, septum, hippocampus, anterior hypothalamus, caudate and putamen, dorsal–medial nucleus of the thalamus, inferior parietal lobule, as well as the lateral convexity, medial wall, and orbital frontal lobes (Baleydier & Maguiere, 1980; Pandya & Kuypers, 1969; Powell, 1978; Powell, Akagi, & Hatton, 1974). The cingulate appears to maintain an intermediate functional–anatomical position between the limbic system and neurocortex and probably serves as an interface linking volitional, motoric, cognitive, and emotional impulses.

Electrical stimulation of the anterior cingulate gyrus (hereafter referred to simply as the cingulate) in humans has produced primitive motor subroutines, or rather, motor fragments, which if linked together, would constitute an entire movement (see Goldberg, 1985, for review). Thus, the cingulate appears to aid in performing complete movements or movement sequences.

The cingulate may also be involved in setting thresholds for vocalization (Jurgens & Muller-Preuss, 1977), including modulation of some of the prosodic (melodic) features that characterize different speech patterns (e.g., happiness versus sadness). For example, among primates, when this area is electrically stimulated, "limbic" vocalizations indicative of alarm, fear, or "separation anxiety" have been triggered (Robinson 1967). Moreover, all cortical areas which give rise to vocalization maintain direct interconnections with area 24 (Jurgens & Muller-Preuss, 1977).

Among humans and primates, electrical stimulation has also resulted in feelings of anxiety, fear, and pleasure (Meyer *et al.*, 1973). However, these effects may be secondary to indirect involvement of the hypothalamus, amygdala, or even the orbital area (Joseph, 1989).

Similar to damage involving the SMA, lesions of the cingulate trigger a variety of motor abnormalities, including paralysis of will, magnetic apraxia, compulsive utilization, and mutism (Barris & Schuman, 1953; Kennard, 1955; Laplane *et al.*, 1981; Smith, 1944). Damage or surgical removal has also resulted in generalized emotional dampening and unresponsiveness, inability to make active avoidance responses, hypokinetic states, severe social indifference and apathy, and decreased awareness of the environment (Barris & Schuman, 1953; Glees *et al.*, 1950; Kennard, 1955; Laplane *et al.*, 1981; Pechtel, McAvoy, Levitt, Kloing, & Masserman, 1958; Smith, 1944; Tow & Whitty, 1953).

For example, Barris and Schuman (1953) describe one patient who rapidly developed akinetic mutism and indifference following bilateral damage to the anterior cingulate and portions of the SMA. After returning home from work he sat down on the sofa, held up a newspaper as if reading (i.e., utilization behavior), became incontinent of urine (about which he was totally unconcerned), was unresponsive and was unable to reply to questions. The next morning, family members found him sitting on the floor polishing a cigarette lighter, although he was unable in all other respects to respond intelligibly.

Laplane *et al.* (1981) describe a similar patient who, following bilateral infarcts to the cingulate, became indifferent, docile and incontinent and demonstrated both magnetic groping and utilization behavior. However, instead of becoming mute, she developed confabulatory tendencies and distractability.

In addition, initially following surgical anterior cingulotomies patients have complained of difficulties distinguishing between events occurring internally and externally, such that thoughts and waking experience seem dreamlike (Whitty & Lewin, 1957). Confabulation and delusions have been noted, including tangentiality and disinhibited speech (Whitty & Lewin, 1957, 1960). These latter symptoms, however, are probably secondary to damage involving adjacent frontal tissues (Joseph, 1986*a*).

THE POSTERIOR FRONTAL CONVEXITY

The Frontal Eye Fields

The frontal eye fields (FEF) are located along the superior lateral convexity immediately adjacent and anterior to the premotor area and encompass all of area 8 as well as portions of areas 9 and 6. The FEF receives projections from the primary and association visual cortices in the occipital lobe (17, 18, and 19), the auditory association (22), and multimodal visual association areas (20) in the temporal lobe (Barbas & Mesulam, 1981; Jones et al., 1978; Jones & Powell, 1970), and the somatosensory association area (see Crowne, 1983; and Levin, 1984, for review). It also shares interconnections with the caudate, superior colliculus, and oculomotor nucleus (Astruc, 1971; Knuzle & Akert, 1977; Segraves & Goldberg, 1987). Hence, the FEF receives information concerning the auditory, tactual, and visual environment and is multimodally responsive.

The FEF is heavily involved in coordinating and maintaining eye and head movements, and thus orienting and attentional reactions in response to predominantly visual, but also tactile and auditory, stimuli (Barbas & Dubrovsky, 1981; Denny-Brown, 1966; Latto & Cowey, 1971a,b; Pragay, Mirsky, & Nakamura, 1987; Segraves & Goldberg, 1987; Wagman, Krieger, Papetheodorou, & Bender, 1961). It is also involved in focusing attention on certain regions within the visual field, particularly the fovea (Segraves & Goldberg, 1987; Wurtz, Goldberg, & Robinson, 1980).

In addition to supporting focused attention, neurons in the FEF demonstrate anticipatory activity (Pragay, Mirskey, & Nakamura, 1987); i.e., firing before a response is made. In fact, these neurons will continue to fire at a high rate until the moment when behavior is initiated. Yet other cells begin to fire only when the waiting period becomes prolonged (Pragay et al., 1987). In this regard, they probably exert a countering influence, so that attention does not drift.

Electrical stimulation of the FEF results in complete saccades of the eyes (Barbas & Dubrovsky, 1981; Wagman et al., 1981), as well as pupillary dilation. Moreover, cells in the FEF will fire selectively in response to stationary and moving stimuli, to objects which are within arms reach, as well as to tactual stimuli applied to the hands and/or mouth (Rizzolatti, Scandolara, Matelli, & Gentilucci, 1981a,b). In fact, as an object approaches the face and mouth, some of these cells correspondingly increase their rate of activity (Rizzolatti et al., 1981a,b). Hence, cells within the FEF are highly involved in mediating sustained attention and orienting reactions of the head and eyes, maintaining visual fixation and modulating visual scanning, as well as coordinating eye–hand and hand-to-mouth movements.

Visual Scanning Deficits and Neglect

Damage to the FEF can cause abnormalities in fixation, decreased sensitivity to stimuli throughout the visual field, slowed visual scanning and searching (Latto & Cowey, 1971a,b; Teuber, 1964), inattention and neglect, as well as mislocation of sounds (Denny-Brown, 1966; Welch & Stuteville, 1958). With massive lesions, searching and responsiveness become so profoundly reduced that a complete unilateral neglect and failure to attend to any and all stimuli falling to one side of the body results (Heilman &

Valenstein, 1972). Like confabulation, neglect is more frequently seen after right cerebral damage (Joseph, 1986a, 1988a).

Even with less severe destruction performance on tasks involving visual search is disrupted (Teuber, 1964) as is attention to visual detail (Luria, 1980). If shown and asked to describe a complex picture, patients may focus on only one detail, neglecting the remainder of the array, or may look about haphazardly (Luria, 1980). It is probable that patients with certain types of dyslexia suffer from similar abnormalities involving visual search and synthesis.

With large lesions (particularly when involving the right frontal area), they may tend to make leaps of judgment and impulsively guess and describe the meaning of the whole based on the perception of a fragment. For example, focusing only a drummer boy in a battle scene, they may describe the picture as being about musicians or a rock band. Thus, such patients may erroneously extrapolate from an isolated detail around which they construct and confabulate a conclusion (Joseph, 1986a).

In the extreme, instead of a true analysis, they may produce irrelevant associations, as they not only have difficulty analyzing and synthesizing the different components of a visual array (Luria, 1980) but in correcting their impressions through search and feedback as well (Joseph, 1986a, 1988b). In these instances, the lesion typically extends well beyond the confines of the FEF. With extensive damage involving the FEF and convexity, not only confabulation but Capgras syndrome (false identification) and reduplicative paramnesia have been reported—particularly if the damage is bilateral (Alexander, Stuss, & Benson, 1979; Benson, Gardner, & Meadows, 1979; Hecaen, 1964).

Exner's Writing Area

Exner's writing area lies within a small region along the lateral convexity, near the foot of the second frontal convolution of the left hemisphere, occupying the border regions of Brodmann's areas 46, 8, and 6 (see Hecaen & Albert, 1978; Levine & Sweet, 1983). Although some investigators have denied the existence of Exner's area, this region appears to be the final common pathway where linguistic impulses receive their final motoric stamp for the purposes of writing; i.e., the formation of graphemes and their temporal–sequential expression (Fig. 31).

Exner's area, however, is dependent on Broca's expressive speech area with which it maintains extensive interconnections. In fact, Exner's writing center is probably coextensive with Broca's area (Lesser, Lueders, Dinner, Hahn, & Cohen, 1984), which possibly acts to organize and relay impulses received from the posterior language zones to Exner's area in instances where written expression is desired. Exner's area, in turn, transfers this information to the secondary and primary motor areas for final expression. Electrical stimulation of this vicinity in awake moving patients has resulted in the arrest of ongoing motor acts, including the capacity to write or perform rapid alternating movements of the fingers (Lesser et al., 1984). In some instances, writing and speech arrest were noted.

Agraphia

Lesions localized to this vicinity lead to deficiencies involving the elementary motoric aspects of writing, i.e., pure agraphia (Penfield & Roberts, 1959). Grapheme

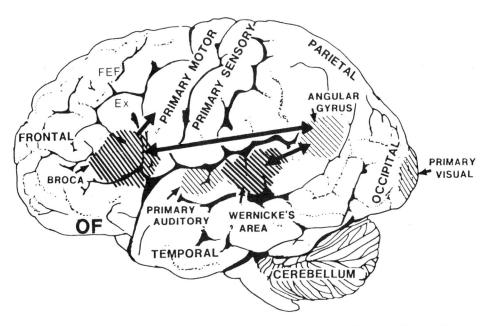

FIGURE 31. The left cerebral hemisphere with the language axis, including the frontal eye fields and Exner's writing area.

formation becomes labored, incoordinated, and takes on a very sloppy appearance. Cursive handwriting is usually more disturbed than printing. Usually there are no gross deficiencies of motor functioning or speech, although mild articulatory disturbances may be observed (e.g., lisping) as well as abnormalities involving fine motor control (cf. Lesser *et al.*, 1984; Levine & Sweet, 1983).

In cases of pure (frontal) agraphia, spelling may or may not be affected, whereas with parietal lesions spelling as well as writing is often abnormal. Rather, with left frontal lesions more frequently there are disturbances of grapheme selection such that the patient may seem to have forgotten how to form certain letters and/or may misplace or even add unnecessary letters when writing (Hecaen & Albert, 1978). When spelling orally or typing, the ability to spell is often better preserved.

Damage localized to this vicinity can be secondary to perinatal trauma, tumors, or vascular abnormalities. Disturbances involving constructional or manipulospatial functioning are not apparent. In fact, one such patient whose damage was secondary to birth injury, although able to write or print only with great difficulty, was able to draw and paint with some professional acumen. However, his ability to copy letters was severely affected. Hence, disturbances secondary to lesions localized to Exner's area are limited to abnormalities involving linguistic–symbolic grapheme motor control.

Broca's Speech Area

Broca's speech area is located in the general vicinity of the posterior-inferior region of the left frontal area (i.e., third frontal convolution), and includes portions of areas 45,

6, and 4 and all of area 44. This region is multimodally responsive and receives projections from the auditory, visual, somesthetic areas (Geschwind, 1965; Jones & Powell, 1970), as well as massive input from the inferior parietal lobule and Wernicke's area via a rope of nerve fibers referred to as the arcuate fasciculus.

Broca's speech area is a final converging destination point through which thought and other impulses come to receive their final sequential (syntactical, grammatical) inprint so as to become organized and expressed as temporally ordered motoric articulations, i.e., speech. Verbal communication, the writing of words (via transmission to Exner's area), and the expression of thought in linguistic form are made possible.

Through this neuronal field, impulses transmitted from the posterior language zones come to be temporally—sequentially prepared for transmission to the adjacent primary and motor neurons which mediate oral–facial muscular activity (i.e., lips, tongue, jaw) and thus the actual expression of speech (Geschwind, 1965, 1979).

Broca's (Expressive) Aphasia

When this region is badly damaged (such as following a massive stroke), the individual loses the capacity to produce fluent speech. Output becomes extremely labored, sparse, and difficult, and they may be unable to say even single words, such as "yes" or "no." Often, immediately following a large stroke patient are almost completely mute and suffer a paralysis of the upper right extremity as well as right facial weakness (since these areas are neuronally represented in the immediately adjacent area 4). Patients are also unable to write, read out loud, or repeat simple words. Interestingly, it has been repeatedly noted that almost immediately following stroke some patients will announce "I can't talk," and then lapse into frustrated partial mutism.

With less severe forms of Broca's (also referred to as expressive, motor, nonfluent, verbal) aphasia, speech remains labored, agrammatical, fragmented, extremely limited to stereotyped phrases ("yes," "no," "shit," "fine") and contaminated with syntactic and paraphasic errors, i.e., "orroble" for auto, "rutton" for button (Goodglass & Kaplan, 1972; Levine & Sweet, 1982, 1983; Tramo, Baynes & Volpe, 1988). Writing remains severely affected, as are oral reading and repetition. Such patients also have mild difficulties with verbal perception and comprehension (Hebben, 1986; Tramo et al., 1988), including the ability to follow three-step commands. Commands to purse or smack the lips, lick, suck, or blow are often, but not always, poorly executed (DeRenzi, Pieczuro, & Vignolo, 1966); a condition referred to as buccal–facial apraxia. Nonspeech oral movements are seldom affected (see Goodglass & Kaplan, 1972; Hecaen & Albert, 1978; Levine & Sweet, 1983, for further discussion).

With mild damage, patients may demonstrate severe confrontive naming and word finding difficulties (anomia), as well as possible right facial, hand, and arm weakness. Speech is often characterized by long pauses, misnaming, paraphasic disturbances and articulatory abnormalities. Stammering and the omission of words may also be apparent. Similarly, electrical stimulation of this region results in speech arrest (Lesser et al., 1984; Ojemann & Whitaker, 1978) and can alter the ability to write and/or perform various oral–facial movements.

Nevertheless, even with anterior lesions or surgical frontal lobectomy sparing Broca's area a considerable impairment of spontaneous speech can result (Luria, 1980; Milner, 1971; Novoa & Ardila, 1987). Disturbances involving grammar and syntax, and reductions in vocabulary and word fluency in both speech and writing are observed (Benson, 1967; Crocket, Bilsker, Hurwitz, & Kozak, 1986; Goodglass & Berko, 1960; Milner, 1964; Novoa & Ardila, 1987; Petrie, 1952; Samuels & Benson, 1979, Tow, 1955). In word fluency tests, however, simple verbal generation (e.g., words starting with the letter L) is usually more severely impaired than semantic naming (e.g., all animals that live in the jungle), presumably a function of semantic processing being more dependent on posterior language areas.

Confabulation and Right Frontal Emotional and Prosodic Speech

Although unable to discourse fluently, persons with severe forms of expressive aphasia may be capable of swearing, making statements of self-pity, praying, singing, and even learning new songs—although in the absence of music, they would be unable to say the very words they had just sung. Presumably the ability to produce nonlinguistic and musical/emotional sounds is due to these functions being mediated by the undamaged right hemisphere and limbic structures (Joseph, 1982, 1988a, 1989).

Emotional and Prosodic Speech

Although language is usually discussed in regard to grammar and vocabulary, it is also emotional, melodic, and prosodic—features that enable a speaker to convey, and a listener to determine, intent, attitude, feeling, and meaning (Joseph, 1988a). A listener comprehends not only what is said, but how it is said—what a speaker *feels*.

Feeling and attitude are conveyed through the melody (musical qualities), inflection, intonation, and prosody of one's voice, and by varying the pitch, inflection, timbre, stress contours, melody, as well as the rate and amplitude of speech—capacities predominantly mediated by the right half of the cerebrum (see Joseph, 1988a). Indeed, just as there is a large region within the left frontal convexity (i.e., Broca's area) which subserves the syntactical, temporal–sequential, motoric, and grammatical aspects of linguistic expression, there appears to be a homologous region within the right frontal area which mediates the expression of emotional/melodic speech (Gorelick & Ross, 1987; Joseph, 1988a; Ross, 1981).

With massive damage involving the right frontal language area, speech may become flat and monotonous, or conversely, the ability to alter or convey melodic/prosodic elements can become exceedingly abnormal and distorted. One such patient, following a bullet wound that damaged part of the right orbital and convexity region, frequently lost control over his voice and at times sounded as if he were crying, wailing, or screeching. He also suffered some paralysis involving the left extremities. Such patents also lose the ability to engage in vocal mimicry or to accurately repeat various statements in an emotional manner (Gorelick & Ross, 1987; Joseph, 1988a; Ross, 1981).

With mild damage, rather than severe distortions or a loss of melody, the intonational qualities of the voice can become mildly abnormal and patients may seem to be speaking with an odd midwestern-like accent, particularly with deep lesions of the right frontal area, perhaps involving the cingulate or basal ganglia. Prosodic distortion in the form of an unusual accent is sometimes seen in seizure disorders involving deep right frontal or frontal–temporal areas.

By contrast, with left frontal lesions, some patients develop what sounds like an unlearned foreign accent, as if they were from Germany, France, etc. (Blumstein, Alexander, Ryalls, Katz, & Dworetzky, 1987; Graff-Radford, Cooper, Colsher, & Damasio, 1986). This is due, in part, to distortions involving the pronunciation of vowels.

When damage is limited to this right frontal emotional–motor speech area, the ability to comprehend and understand prosodic–emotional nuances appears to be somewhat intact (Gorelick & Ross, 1987; Joseph, 1988a; Ross, 1981). Nevertheless, since so few studies have been concerned with these issues, much more research is needed before truly definitive statements can be made.

Confabulation

In contrast to left frontal convexity damage, which can result in speech arrest and/or significant reductions in verbal fluency, right frontal damage has frequently been observed to result in speech release, verbosity (i.e., "motor mouth"), tangentiality, and in the extreme, confabulation (Joseph, 1986a, 1988a). Reductions in fluency, perhaps secondary to motor or frontal pole involvement, can also occur to a mild degree in some cases. That is, spontaneous speech per se may be reduced. However, once speech is initiated confabulatory or tangential tendencies may be observed.

When secondary to right (or deep and/or bilateral) frontal damage, confabulation seem to be due to disinhibition, difficulties monitoring responses, withholding answers, using external or internal cues to make corrections, or suppressing the flow of tangential and circumstantial ideas (Joseph, 1986a, 1988a; Kapur & Coughlan, 1980; Shapiro, Alexander, Gardner, & Mercer, 1981; Stuss, Alexander, Lieberman, & Levine, 1978) such that the Language Axis of the left hemisphere becomes overwhelmed and flooded by irrelevant associations. Frontal lobe confabulators also sometimes demonstrate marked perseveratory tendencies, difficulty shifting response sets, or maintaining a coherent line of reasoning. In some cases, the content of their speech may be bizarre and fantastical, as loosely associated ideas become organized or anchored around fragments of current experience. For example, one 24-year-old patient who received a gunshot wound that resulted in destruction of the right inferior convexity and orbital areas attributed his hospitalization to a plot by the government to steal his ideas. When it was pointed out that he had undergone surgery for removal of bone fragments and the bullet, he pointed to his head and replied, "that's how they are stealing my ideas."

Another patient, formerly a janitor, who suffered a large right frontal subdural hematoma (which required evacuation) soon began claiming to be the owner of the business where he formerly worked. He also alternatively claimed to be a congressman and fabulously wealthy. When asked about his work as a janitor he reported that as a congressman he had been working under cover for the C.I.A. Interestingly, this patient, several months later stated that he realized what he was saying was probably not true. "And yet I feel it and believe it though I know it's not right."

Although diverse forms of cerebral injury may trigger confabulatory responding, this type of disturbance is frequently seen with Korsakoff's psychosis and the accompanying amnesic syndrome. It is thus noteworthy that individuals with Korsakoff's disease and memory loss who were brought to autopsy, were found to have neuronal damage involving predominantly the dorsal–medial nucleus of the thalamus (Victor, Adams, & Collins, 1971)—a nucleus with major interrelaying fiber pathways that project to and from the frontal lobes (Pribram, Chow, & Semmes, 1953; Walker, 1940; Whitlock & Nauta, 1956). Moreover, the dorsal medial nucleus, when damaged, often gives rise to memory disturbances (Squire, 1987, for review) as well as bizarre, delusional and confabulatory speech (Bogousslavsky, Ferrazzini, Regli, Assal, Tanabe, & Delaloye-Bischof, 1988).

Tangentiality and Circumlocutory Speech

With bilateral or right frontal lobe damage, tangentiality is frequently observed in speech (Joseph, 1986a). For example, when a patient with severe right orbital damage was asked if his injury affected his thinking, he replied, "yeah—it's affected the way I think—It's affected my senses—the only thing I can taste are sugar and salt—I can't detect a pungent odor—ha ha—to tell you the truth it's a blessing this way" (Blumer & Benson, 1975, p. 197).

One frontal patient, when asked what he received for Christmas, replied "I got a record player and a sweater. [looking down at his boots] I also like boots, westerns, popcorn, peanuts, and pretzels." Another right frontal patient, when asked in what manner an orange and a banana were alike, replied, "fruit. Fruitcakes—ha ha—tooty fruity." When asked how a lion and a dog were alike he responded, "They both like fruit—ha ha. No. That's not right. They like trees—fruit frees. Lions climb trees and dogs chase cats up trees, and they both have a bark."

Tangentiality is in some manner related to impulsiveness as well as circumlocution. By contrast, patients with circumlocutous speech often have disturbances involving the left cerebral hemisphere and frequently suffer from word-finding difficulty and sometimes receptive or expressive dysphasia. They experience difficulty expressing a particular idea or describing some need, as they have trouble finding the correct words. Thus, they seem to talk around the central point, and only through successive approximations are they able to convey what they mean to say.

Patients with tangential speech lose the point altogether. Instead, words or statements trigger other words or statements that are related only in regard to sound (e.g., like a clang association) or to some obscure and ever-shifting semantic category. Speech may be rushed or pressured, and the patient may seem to be free associating as he jumps from topic to topic.

THE ORBITAL FRONTAL LOBES AND INFERIOR CONVEXITY

The Orbital Frontal Lobes

The orbital frontal lobes receive higher-order sensory information from the sensory association areas throughout the neocortex and maintain rich interconnections with the lateral convexity, anterior cingulate, inferior temporal and inferior parietal lobes, the medial walls, the parahippocampal gyrus (Fuster, 1980; Johnson, Rosvold, & Mishkin, 1968; Jones & Powell, 1970; Pandya & Kuypers, 1969; Van Hoesen, Pandya, & Butters, 1975), and with the hypothalamus and amygdala, all of which are major "limbic" nuclei involved in emotion and autonomic functioning (Joseph, 1989).

The orbital cortices also send fibers directly to the reticularis gigantocellularis of the reticular formation, including the reticular inhibitory regions within the medulla and the excitatory areas throughout the pons (Kuypers, 1958; Rossi & Brodal, 1956; Sauerland *et al.*, 1967). There are also rich interconnections with the medial magnocellular dorsal–medial nucleus of the thalamus (Pribram *et al.*, 1953; Siegel *et al.*, 1977), a major relay nucleus involved in the gating and filtering of information destined for the neocortex (Skinner & Yingling, 1977; Yingling & Skinner, 1977) and limbic system (Joseph, 1989). That is, this portion of the thalamus appears to exert modulating influences on information reception and processing as well as arousal.

Orbital Mediation of Limbic Arousal

The medial portion of the magnocellular dorsal–medial thalamic (MDMT) nucleus (like the orbital region) also receives fibers from the reticular formation and amygdala (Chi, 1970; Krettek & Price, 1974; Siegel, Fukushima, Meibach, Burke, Edinger, & Weiner, 1977). However, this portion of the dorsal–medial thalamus is subject to orbital control. Indeed, the orbital region, through its interconnections with all three regions (i.e., reticular formation, limbic system, MDMT), is able to exert considerable influence on the interactions that take place in these nuclei, including control over various forms of limbic, behavioral, and emotional arousal.

For example, electrical stimulation of the orbital area can cause a hungry animal to stop eating, walk away from its dish, lie down, and even fall into slow-wave synchronized sleep (Lineberry & Siegel, 1971). It can inhibit monosynaptic spinal reflexes (Clemente *et al.*, 1966; Sauerland *et al.*, 1967), as well as reduce and inhibit arousal throughout the neocortex (Lineberry & Siegel, 1971), limbic system (Steriade, 1964), including the reticular formation (Lineberry & Siegel, 1971; Siegel & Wang, 1974). Indeed, the orbital region appears to exert hierarchical control over the MDMT, reticular formation, limbic and autonomic nervous system, thereby mediating generalized arousal throughout the neuroaxis. As pertaining to emotional arousal, it has also been postulated that the orbital area exerts a major influence on the experience of anxiety (Gray, 1987).

Autonomic Influences

Electrical stimulation of the orbital cortex can slow or arrest respiration, alter arterial blood pressure, inhibit pyloric peristalsis, increase salivation, dilate the pupils, decrease gastric motility, and increase skin temperature (Bailey & Sweet, 1940; Chapman, Livingston, & Livingston, 1950; Kaada, 1951, 1972; Livingston, Chapman, & Livingston, 1948; Wall & Davis, 1951). Hence, when the orbital cortex is severely damaged, the autonomic nervous system is liberated from higher order inhibitory control (Rinkel, Greenblatt, Coon, & Solomon, 1950). Blood pressure and skin temperature are lowered, sweating is increased, and widespread disturbances involving gastrointestinal activities, salivation, micturition, diuresis, and sexual arousal can occur (Chapman *et al.*, 1950; Delgado & Livingston, 1948; Langworthy & Richter, 1939; Mettler, Spindler, Mettler, & Combs, 1936; Rinkel, Solomon, Rosen, & Levine, 1950). Urinary bladder control is also diminished resulting in a "disturbance of micturation."

In this regard, as the "senior executive" of the subcortical brain, we can see how activity in this area can effect gastric functioning, including the possible development of ulcers (Freeman & Watts, 1942), and contribute to many of the symptoms that underlie feelings of anxiety.

Emotional Unresponsiveness

Usually immediately following surgical destruction of the orbital frontal lobes, there results severe reductions in activity and emotional/motivational functioning, including apathy, indifference to loud noises or threats, as well as extreme reductions in arousal and motor functioning (Butter *et al.*, 1970; Freeman & Watts, 1942, 1943). With extensive orbital destruction involving portions of the medial wall and anterior tip of the cingulate, reduced responsiveness persists and patients will sit quietly and silently, nearly motionless, making little or no attempt to communicate, as if mute. The ability to respond socially and emotionally seems abolished. Rather, if sufficiently stimulated, humans and animals seem capable of reacting only in an irritable and aversive manner (Butter, Mishkin, & Mirsky, 1968).

In free-ranging monkeys as well as those reared in enclosed settings, global social disintegration is observed following orbital destruction. Animals cease to groom or produce appropriate vocalizations, adults attempt to completely avoid members of their social group, and mothers neglect and rebuff their infants (Myers, Swett, & Miller, 1973; Raleigh, 1976, cited by Kling & Steklis, 1976). Similarly, women with surgical destruction of this vicinity will neglect and/or strike or beat their children without provocation (Broffman, 1950).

In the free-ranging situation, orbital animals in fact ran away from their social groups and remained solitary until their deaths (Myers *et al.*, 1973). By contrast, lateral convexity lesions do not result in changes involving social proximity, grooming, or bonding (Kling & Mass, 1974). Thus complete orbital destruction results in complete abolition of most forms of emotional and social behavior.

Emotional Disinhibition

With less extensive damage, or as swelling and ischemia become reduced so that neighboring structures are not impacted, this initial unresponsiveness phase passes. Rather than a loss of emotion, there is a loss of emotional control, the subject becomes disinhibited, hyperactive, euphoric, extroverted, labile, and overtalkative and develops perseveratory tendencies (Butter, 1969; Butter *et al.*, 1970; Dax, Reitman, & Radley-Smith, 1948; Greenblatt, 1950; Kennard, Spencer, & Fountain, 1941; Kolb, Nonnemann, & Singh, 1974; Reitman, 1946, 1947; Ruch & Shenkin, 1943). Patients are frequently described as markedly irresponsible, antisocial, lacking in tact or concern, having difficulty planning ahead or foreseeing consequences, and suffer from generalized disinhibition. There can result tendencies toward impulsive actions, to laugh inappropriately and make trivial jokes, or to behave in a demanding or transiently aggressive manner. Proneness to criminal behavior, promiscuity, gradiosity, and paranoia have also been observed (Benson & Geschwind, 1971; Blumer & Benson, 1975; Lishman, 1973; Luria, 1980; Stuss & Benson, 1984).

Much of this inappropriate behavior is a consequence of a loss of control over reticular and limbic structures. That is, the orbital region appears as a kind of ''censor,'' or even "conscience," such that when these superego-like influences are removed, heightened levels of generalized and emotional arousal result, and the patient responds in a childish, inappropriate, and unrestrained manner. With less extensive damage, or when the lesions are confined to one hemisphere, the long-term effects are less drastic. However, right orbital damage seems to result in the most severe alterations in mood and emotional functioning (Grafman, Vance, Weingartner, Salazar, & Amin, 1986).

Attention and Differentiation

Among primates and mammals, disturbances involving visual, spatial, auditory, tactile, and olfactory discrimination have consistently been observed with orbital lesions (Fuster, 1980; Oscar-Berman, 1975). That is, due to heightened generalized arousal levels (resulting from orbital release of the reticular formation and other nuclei), competing perceptions do not seem to stand out sufficiently to attract and shift attention; i.e., there is a reduced capacity to deactivate whatever perceptual and behavioral activity is predominant, such that the ability to differentiate and attend to salient versus irrelevant stimuli is reduced.

Moreover, the ability to shift attention is reduced. That is, in a manner analogous to magnetic motor behaviors following medial lesions, orbital destruction may lead to attentional stimulus binding such that the subject appears "stuck in set" and may demonstrate perseverative attentional activity and difficulty shifting responses. However, if the patient or orbitally lesioned animal is purposefully distracted, e.g., through a novel stimulus, this pattern of perseveration is momentarily halted and the ability to shift response and attention is briefly regained (Mishkin, 1964; Pribram et al., 1964). Nevertheless, lesions confined to the orbital area do not result in distractability per se.

Perseveration

Lesions involving the orbital frontal cortex and inferior convexity have consistently resulted in increased activity levels and an abnormal tendency to repeat previous responses in a repetitive perseverative fashion even when the context is no longer appropriate or rewarded, and/or the response is punished and the individual realizes his responses are incorrect (Butter, 1969; Butter et al., 1963; Iverson & Mishkin, 1970; Jones & Mishkin, 1972; Kolb et al., 1974; Luria, 1980; Mishkin, 1964); i.e., the capacity to shift responses is attenuated. Thus, once a behavior is completed, particularly if it is repeatedly performed, the pattern continues to be involuntarily executed such that the ability to change to a different pattern of activity is disrupted. Similar disturbances are seen with inferior medial damage.

Perseverative, repetitive abnormalities can affect motor behavior, intellectual functioning as well as speech. For example, patients may tend to repeat phrases: "Doctor, can I look at this, can I look at this, Doctor, can I look at this," or once a topic seems to have changed they may reintroduce and again repeat certain statements or words. During the administration of the vocabulary subtest from the WAIS-R, for example, an orbitally damaged patient managed to use the word "summer" in five different definitions.

Another patient with damage and suspected subclinical seizures involving the mesial orbital cortex and possibly the basal ganglia, demonstrated a striking perseveration of movement. If asked to draw a star he would dash off four or five. When he attempted to sit, the downward motion continued in repetitive machine-like fashion, and he would slide to the floor.

In severe cases, it is frequently found once a patient has performed a required action, such as drawing a particular figure several times, he continues to draw the first, even when asked to draw a different figure. If asked to draw a star, a cross, and a square, the patient may draw the first or even the second figure correctly but will then impulsively draw the star again. In the less extreme they may simply inappropriately introduce components of a previous response in their next set of actions.

In one instance, a patient with bilateral damage was asked to draw a pair of spectacles and did so correctly. When asked to draw a watch, he again drew the spectacles. When the mistake was pointed out, he again drew a pair of spectacles but this time drew a watch in the center of one of the lens (Luria, 1980).

Conceptually, patients may have difficulty considering or even recognizing alternatives such that they seem to become locked into a particular mode of thinking or activity. For example, Luria (1980) describes "a patient with a wound of the frontal lobes, who, when working in the carpenter's shop of the hospital, inertly went on planing a piece of wood until nothing of its remained. Even then he did not stop but continued to plane the bench" (p. 294).

Although orbital patients may have difficulty inhibiting emotionality, the perseverative abnormality is not the result of disturbances involving impulsivity or the withholding of a behavioral response. For example, across tasks requiring delayed responding, orbital lesions have little or no effect on performance (Brutkowski *et al.*, 1963; see Rosenkilde, 1979, for review). Rather, the problem is in shifting sets and in inhibiting the recurrence of a previous response when the next action is initiated. Once a behavior occurs, it tends to persist and contaminates the performance of unrelated actions (Figs. 32 and 33).

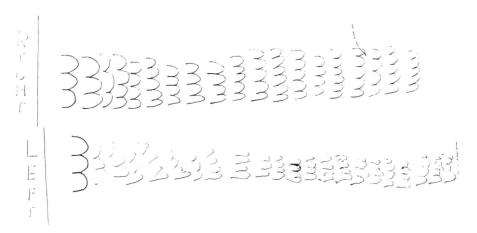

FIGURE 32. Examples of perseveration coupled with micrographia secondary to subcortical bilateral frontal lobe degeneration in a 62-year-old woman. The patient was required to draw a copy of the sample figure and then to draw it repeatedly across the page.

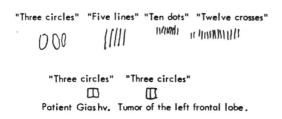

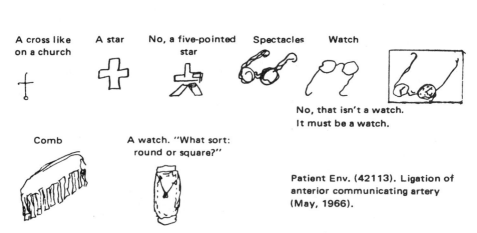

FIGURE 33. Examples of perseveration in a patient following damage to the frontal lobes. From *Higher cortical functions in man* by A. Luria, 1980. New York: Basic Books. Reprinted by permission.

Perseverative reactions, however, may occur with lesions situated well outside the orbital areas. For example, perseveration of speech (of which there are several subtypes), can also occur among individuals with aphasia and with lesions localized to the right or left frontal lobe or damage situated throughout the left hemisphere (Joseph, 1986*a;* Pietro & Rigdrodsky, 1986; Sandson & Albert, 1987). In these instances, as patients grope for words, the same word may be repeated in a number of erroneous contexts in a perseverative fashion.

Inferior Lateral Convexity

Disinhibition and the Withholding of a Response

The inferior lateral convexity appears to be highly involved in the inhibition of behavior and the ability to withhold or delay responses. For example, electrophysiological analysis of cellular activity within the lateral convexity indicates that many neurons alter their discharge rates when a subject is required to wait before responding to a signal. Yet others increase or decrease their activity as the time interval between the onset of the delay and the release of the response increases (Fuster, Bauer, & Jervey, 1982). The majority of these delay neurons are found within the inferior convexity. However, a number of neurons in the superior convexity show similar properties (Pragay *et al.,* 1987).

Similarly, high-frequency electrical stimulation of the lateral and inferior convexity has been shown to disrupt the ability to inhibit, delay, and withhold responses (Goldman,

Rosvold, & Mishkin, 1970; Gross & Weiskrantz, 1964; Stamm & Rosen, 1973), whereas low frequency stimulation actually improves performance on delayed response tasks and enhances behavioral inhibition (Wilcott, 1974, 1977). Interestingly, electrical stimulation of the right frontal region, as compared to the left, more greatly disrupts delayed response performance.

Conversely, when the lateral and inferior convexity are damaged there results a consistent disturbance across tasks requiring the withholding and delay of a response (Brutkowski, Mishkin, & Rosvold, 1963; Gross & Weiskrantz, 1964; Mishkin & Pribram, 1956; Stepien & Stamm, 1970). That is, subjects become disinhibited and impulsive—disturbances that in turn affect all aspects of behavior. Patients may spontaneously speak or make comments without thinking and act on sudden impulses without regard for consequences. Depending on the extent of the lesion, both emotion and cognitive activity can be affected.

In addition, humans and animals tend to become hyperreactive and may demonstrate increased activity levels (Bradford, 1950; French, 1959; Latto & Cowey, 1971a; Rose, 1950). For example, noise, threat, or novel stimuli result in significantly heightened activity in frontal animals coupled with distractability (French, 1959). Among humans, a perpetual shifting of attention may result, as they are inordinately distracted by noises in the hall or even specks on the testing table. However, if potential distractors are removed or the subject is placed in a darkened room, activity and hyperresponsiveness declines (French, 1964; French & Harlow, 1955).

With more restricted or lateralized lesions, long term effects are more mild. For example, right-sided damage being more frequently associated with motor decontrol, such as edginess (Grafman et al., 1986) and even mania.

Summary

Lesions of the supplementary, secondary, and primary motor areas give rise respectively to compulsive utilization and magnetic groping and grasping, diminished fine motor functioning and paralysis. Damage to the posterior (particularly the left) lateral convexity involving Broca's speech area, Exner's writing area, or the frontal eye fields reduces motor responsiveness and behavioral expression, i.e., aphasia, agraphia, apraxia, and deficiencies involving visual search and orienting. With inferior convexity and right frontal lesions, there is increased responsiveness and impulsivity. Perseverative aberrations are found with orbital, inferior medial and inferior convexity lesions, whereas deep medial–orbital damage can also result in compulsive utilization behavior. With medial lesions involving the corpus callosum, complex involuntary behavior acts may be performed, i.e., the alien hand. Hence, regardless of where a frontal lesion occurs, motor functioning is in some manner affected.

Damage to the medial wall produces symptoms that in some respects parallel those associated with convexity damage. For example, lesions to the primary motor strip cause paralysis of movement, whereas damage to the medial wall and cingulate can result in paralysis of will. Damage involving the inferior convexity is associated with disinhibition and impulsiveness, whereas destruction of the inferior medial wall is associated with compulsive utilization. When the orbital area is also compromised, disinhibition, manic-excitement, and internal utilization behaviors (increased sexuality, orality) may occur.

Disturbances involving emotion can result with medial–cingulate or convexity damage. With complete destruction of the orbital area, emotional and social functioning is abolished, but with less extensive damage, rather than a loss of emotion there is a loss of emotional control. These findings suggest that the orbital region acts as the "senior executive" of the social–emotional brain and exerts tremendous inhibitory as well as expressive influences on emotion and generalized arousal through its massive interconnections with various limbic nuclei, the dorsal–medial nucleus of the thalamus, and the reticular formation.

The orbital region also seems to coordinate and integrate emotional and perceptual activity. For example, fibers from the sensory association areas, including the inferior parietal lobule, project into the orbital frontal cortex. Thus, the orbital region is continually informed as to the perceptual processing being performed in the neocortex and can thus integrate and assign emotional–motivational significance to cognitive impressions; the association of emotion to ideas and thoughts. It is in this manner that thoughts can come to be upsetting or emotionally arousing. It is also in this manner that disturbances such as anxiety can result (Gray, 1987). The medial frontal cortex and cingulate are also involved in these processes. Thus, with complete destruction of these areas, emotion can no longer be assigned to external events, thoughts, or ideas, and the patient seems apathetic and blunted. The lateral convexity is much less concerned with emotional and motivational functioning. Rather, the domain of the convexity appears to involve the integration and coordination of perceptual and cognitive processes with volitional-expressive activities.

LATERAL–FRONTAL CORTICAL MONITORING

With the exception of olfactory information, which projects to the limbic system and is relayed to the orbital region via the olfactory tracts (Cavada, 1984; Joseph, 1989), all sensory impulses are first transferred to the thalamus before being transmitted to the primary auditory, visual, and somesthetic receiving areas. From the primary zones this information is sent to three separate major locations: to the immediately adjacent sensory association area, back to the thalamus, and to the motor cortex of the frontal lobes (Joseph, 1989b).

The motor area then relays this information to the lateral convexity which simultaneously receives fiber projections from the sensory association areas (Cavada, 1984; Jones, Coulter, & Hendry, 1978; Jones & Powell, 1970; Pandya & Kuypers, 1969) and the inferior parietal lobule. Hence, the frontal cortex is interlocked with the posterior sensory areas through converging and reciprocal connections with the first, second, and third level of modality specific analysis, including the multimodal associational integration performed by the inferior parietal lobule. It is therefore able to sample activity within all cortical sensory/association regions at all levels of information analysis (Fig. 34).

Frontal–Thalamic Control of Cortical Activity

The role of the lateral convexity is not limited to sampling but also involves regulation of information flow to and within the neocortex. This is accomplished, in part, through projections linking the frontal lobes with the dorsal–medial thalamic nucleus.

Reticular Thalamus

Fibers passing to and from the thalamus and to the cortical sensory receiving areas give off collaterals to the reticular thalamic nucleus, which also sends fibers that envelop and innervate most of the other thalamic nuclei (Scheibel & Scheibel, 1966; Updyke, 1975) (Figs. 35–36). The reticular thalamus acts to selectively gate transmission from the thalamus to the neocortex and continually samples thalamic–cortical activity (Skinner & Yingling, 1977; Yingling & Skinner, 1977).

Lateral Frontal–Thalamic System

The reticular thalamus is controlled by the lateral convexity of the frontal lobes, the recticular formation and the lateral portion of the dorsal–medial thalamus with which it maintains dense interconnections (Skinner & Yingling, 1977; Yingling & Skinner, 1977). The convexity and lateral dorsal–medial nucleus (LDM) are also richly interconnected and together exert significant steering influences on the reticular thalamus. That is, the lateral–frontal convexity appears to exert specific influences on the LDM so as to promote or diminish the flow of information to the cortex and thus modulate specific perceptual and cognitive activities occurring within the neocortex—activity that it is simultaneously

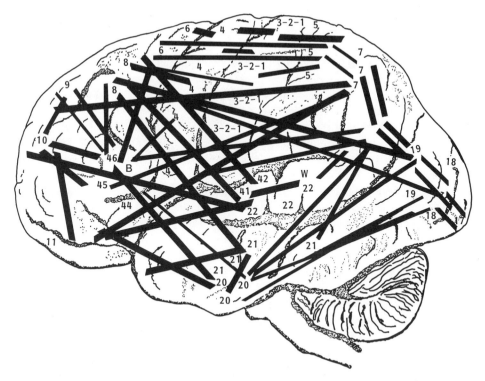

FIGURE 34. Schematic depiction of pathways interlinking the various regions of the brain. Numbers refer to Brodmann's areas.

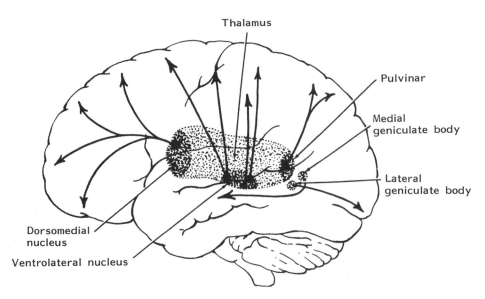

FIGURE 35. Diagram of principle thalamocortical projections. Reproduced, with permission, from *Correlative neuroanatomy,* 20th Ed., by J. DeGroot & J. G. Chusid, copyright Appleton & Lange, E. Norwalk, CT, 1988.

sampling. This is in contrast to the orbital region with its connections to the reticular formation and the medial magnocellular segment of the dorsal–medial thalamus and its influences on generalized arousal and limbic activation/inhibition.

To recapitulate, the lateral–frontal system is able to influence cognitive/perceptual cortical functioning by sampling activity occurring throughout the neocortex at all levels of informational analysis and by its modulating influences on the lateral portion of the dorsal–medial and reticular thalamic nuclei. The lateral frontal region is thus able to act at any stage of processing, from initial reception to motor expression so as to facilitate or inhibit further analysis, selectively acting to determine what type of processing occurs throughout the neocortex.

Through integration and inhibitory action and its neocortical and thalamic links, the lateral convexity is able to coordinate interactions between various regions of the neuroaxis so as to organize, mobilize, and direct overall cortical and behavioral activity and to minimize conflicting demands, impulses, distractions and/or the processing of irrelevant information.

When damaged, depending on the site (e.g., inferior versus posterior convexity) or laterality of the lesion, there can result behavioral disinhibition, flooding of the sensory association areas with irrelevant information, hyperreactively, distractability, impulsiveness, and/or apathy, reduced motor-expressive activities (e.g., speech arrest), and sensory neglect. Similar disturbances can result when the dorsal medial nucleus or the bidirectional pathways linking the thalamus and frontal lobe are severed (cf. Skinner & Yingling, 1977). In summary, the orbital region exerts modulating influences on subcortical and generalized limbic arousal, whereas the lateral regions are more concerned with the control of information processing as well as arousal at the neocortical level.

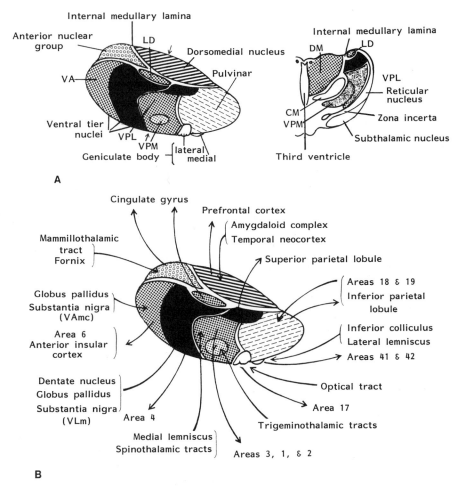

FIGURE 36. Schematic diagram of (A) the major thalamic nuclei and (B) their principal efferent and afferent projections. From *Human neuroanatomy* by R. C. Truex & M. R. Carpenter, 1969. Courtesy of The Williams & Wilkins Co., Baltimore, MD.

PERSONALITY AND BEHAVIORAL ALTERATIONS SECONDARY TO FRONTAL INJURY

The Frontal Lobe Personality

Lesions involving the nonmotor frontal regions are usually not accompanied by gross disturbances of visual, auditory, and tactile sensation. However, with severe and massive lesions, attentional functioning may become grossly compromised, behavior may become fragmented, and initiative and the general attitude toward the future may be lost. The patient's range of interests may shrink, they may be unable to adapt to new situations; carry out complex, purposive, and goal-directed activities; or evaluate their attempts

(Freeman & Watts, 1942; Girgis, 1971; Hecaen, 1964; Joseph, 1986a; Luria, 1980; Petrie, 1952; Rylander, 1939; Tow, 1955).

With trauma, stroke, neoplasm or surgical destruction, patients may show a reduction in activity and take very long to achieve very little. They may be unconcerned about their appearance, their disabilities, and demonstrate little or no interest in self-care or the manner in which they dress or even if their clothes are soiled or inappropriate (Bradford, 1950; Broffman, 1950; Freeman & Watts, 1942; Petrie, 1952; Strom-Olsen, 1946; Tow, 1955). Although often demonstrating restlessness, they may tire easily and show careless work habits and a desire to get things over and done with quickly. They may in fact immediately develop a tendency just to lie in bed unless forcibly removed (Broffman, 1950; Freeman & Watts, 1942, 1943; Rylander, 1948; Tow, 1955), a condition that may pass with recovery.

Patients with mild and subtle damage may seem to take hours to get dressed, to finish their business in the bathroom, and even to stop and purchase simple items. A curious mixture of obsessive compulsiveness and passive aggressiveness may be suggested by their behavior. In severe cases, compulsive utilization may occur, as well as distractability and perseveration. As described by Freeman and Watts (1943) regarding their lobotomy cases, patients may pick up and play with various objects for long periods of time or spend hours in the bathtub playing with the bubbles. "Sometimes a pencil and a piece of paper will be enough to start an endless letter that may end up with the mechanical repitition of a phrase, line after line and even page after page" (Freeman and Watts, 1943, p. 801). Not all patients behave in this manner, however.

Even with mild injuries to the frontal lobes patients may demonstrate periods of tangentiality, grandiosity, irresponsibility, laziness, hyperexcitability, lability, personal untidiness and dirtiness, poor judgment, irritability, fatuous jocularity, and tendencies to spend funds extravagantly. Failure to be concerned about consequences, tactlessness, and changes in sex drive and even hunger and appetite (usually accompanied by weight gain) may occur. Disturbances of attention, perseverative tendencies, and a reduction in the ability to produce original or imaginative thinking, as well as fantasy, seem to be associated with mild or severe cases, at least initially following injury (Figs. 37–40).

Urinary Incontinence

Urinary and (in rare instances) fecal incontinence are associated with frontal lobe damage, as well as excessive eating, drinking, and smoking (Bianchi, 1922; Fulton, Jacobsen, & Kennard, 1932; Freeman & Watts, 1942; Greenblatt, 1950; Langworthy & Richter, 1939; Rose, 1950; Watts & Fulton, 1934). Patients may freely urinate upon themselves while lying in bed, sitting in front of the T.V., or while at the dinner table and seem totally unconcerned about their condition. One patient, standing at her front door, was observed to empty her bladder while waving goodbye to a friend. She stopped on request but completed the act as she walked to the toilet (Rose, 1950). Apparently, urinary bladder capacity is significantly reduced after frontal damage, and with severe destruction (such as following lobotomy) the bladder may become spastic and hypertonic (Rinkel, Soloman, Rosen, & Levine, 1950). This is caused by loss of frontal inhibitory control. However, even in mild cases patients may report occasional instances of involuntary urination.

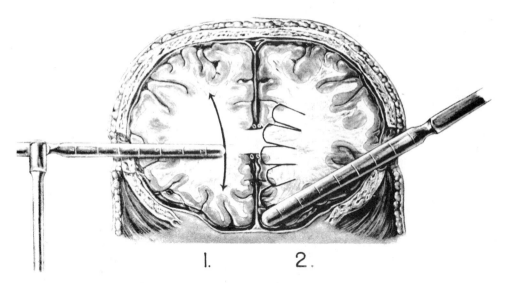

FIGURE 37. Frontal lobotomy. Destruction of the lateral fibers via a lateral approach. From *Psychosurgery in the treatment of mental disorders and intractable pain* by W. Freeman & J. W. Watts, 1950. Courtesy of Charles C. Thomas, Springfield, IL.

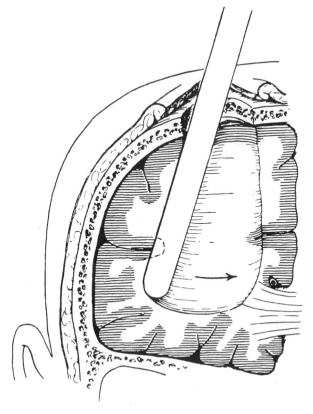

FIGURE 38. Frontal lobotomy. Destruction of the medial fibers via a superior approach. From "Technic of Prefrontal Lobotomy" by J. L. Poppen, 1948, *Journal of Neurosurgery, 5*, p. 514. Reprinted by permission.

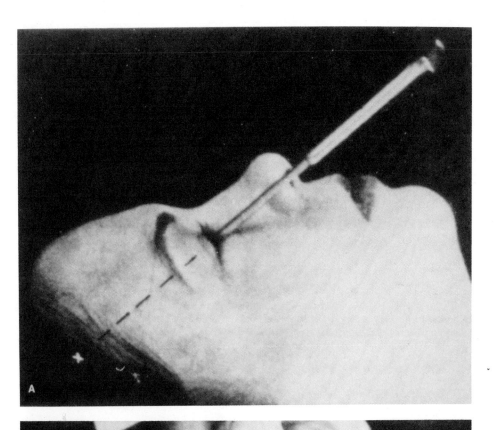

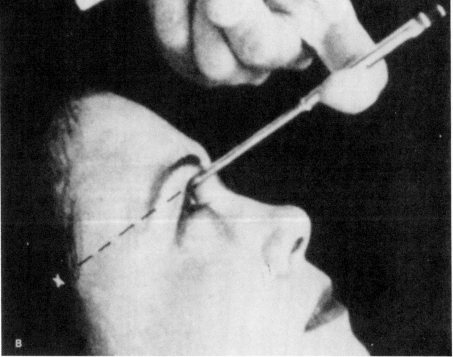

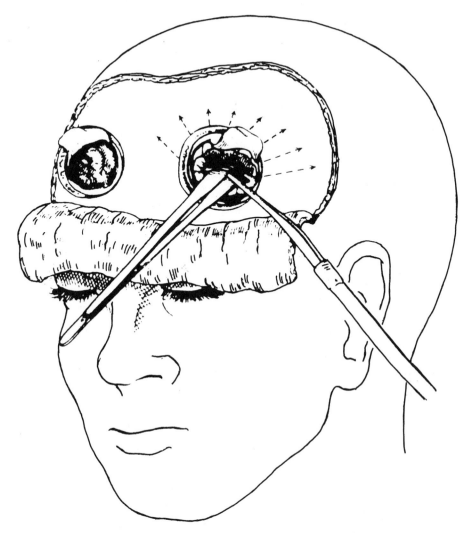

FIGURE 40. Orbital undercutting. The frontal lobes were lifted upward via a spatula, and an incision was made so as to cut the medial orbital fibers. From *Neurosurgical techniques* by A. Asenjo, 1963. Courtesy of Charles C. Thomas, Springfield, IL.

←

FIGURE 39. Transorbital lobotomy. Freeman often coupled this type of lobotomy with electroconvulsive shock. According to Freeman, the "shock treatment disorganizes the cortical patterns that underlie the psychotic behavior, and by severing the connections between the thalamus and frontal pole the pattern is prevented from reforming." From "Transorbital leucotomy" by W. Freeman, 1949, *Proceedings of the Royal Society of Medicine, 42*, p. 8. Reprinted with permission.

Alterations in Appetite

With bilateral or anterior orbital damage, appetite may become exceedingly excessive, and patients (or animals) may eat two or three times their normal amount (Anand, Dua, & China, 1958; Bianchi, 1922; Fulton *et al.,* 1932; Langworthy & Richter, 1939). One patient I examined who suffered a series of small bilateral strokes gained more than 150 pounds within 8 months. A second patient with a degenerative disturbance involving the inferior medial and orbital areas, in addition to perseveration and compulsive utilization, gained over 200 pounds within 1½ years. Indeed, it has been reported that in some patients the craving for food became so intense they repeatedly crammed their mouths with food, became cyanotic, and died with their mouth still full (Greenblatt, 1950).

In other instances patients might eat non-nutritive objects such as cigarette butts or drink enormous amounts of fluid. Hence, hyperphagia, extreme orality, even coprophagia may occur (Butter & Snyder, 1972; Butter, Snyder, & McDonald, 1970). Similar disturbances result from hypothalamic/limbic damage (Joseph, 1989).

Disinhibition and Impulsiveness

Following massive frontal injuries, patients may become emotionally labile, irritable, euphoric, aggressive, and quick to anger, and yet be unable to maintain a grudge or sustain other emotions mood states (Bradford, 1950; Greenblatt, 1950; Rylander, 1939; Strom-Olsen, 1946). They may become unrestrained, overtalkative, and tactless, saying whatever "pops into their head", with little or no concern as to the effect their behavior may have on others or what personal consequences may result (Bogousslavsky, Ferrazzini, Regli, Assal, Tanabe, & Delaloye-Bischof, 1988; Broffman, 1950; Freeman & Watts, 1943; Joseph, 1986a; Luria, 1980; Miller *et al.,* 1986; Partridge, 1950; Rylander, 1939, 1948; Strom-Olsen, 1946).

Patients may seem inordinately disinhibited and influenced by the immediacy of a situation, buying things they cannot afford, lending money when they themselves are in need, and acting and speaking "without thinking." Seeing someone who is obese, they may call out in a friendly manner, "Hey, fatty," and comment on their presumed eating habits. If they enter a room and detect a faint odor, it's: "Hey, what stinks?" or "Who farted?"

In many instances following severe injuries, there may be periods of gross disinhibition, which may consist of loud, boisterous, and grandiose speech; singing, yelling, beating on trays; or even destruction of furniture and tearing of clothes. Some patients may impulsively strike doctors, nurses, or relatives and behave in a thoroughly callous and irresponsible manner (Benson & Geschwind, 1971; Freeman & Watts, 1942, 1943; Strom-Olsen, 1946). One patient, with a tumor involving the right frontal area, following resection, attempted to throw a fellow patient's radio through the window because he did not like the music. He also loudly sang opera in the halls. Indeed, during the course of his examination, he would frequently sing his answers to various questions.

Disturbances involving impulsiveness can also be quite subtle. Luria (1980, p. 294), describes one patient with a slow-growing frontal tumor "whose first manifestation of illness occurred when, on going to the train station, got into the train which happened to arrive first, although it was going in the opposite direction."

Uncontrolled Laughter and Mirth

Frontal lobe patients can act in a very childish and puerile manner, laughing at the most trivial of things, making inappropriate jokes, teasing, and attempting to engage total strangers in hilarious conversation (Ackerley, 1935; Freeman & Watts, 1942, 1943; Kramer, 1954; Luria, 1980; Petrie, 1952; Rylander, 1939, 1948). Some may initially appear almost completely emotionally unrestrained. Pathological laughter, joking, and punning may occur superimposed on a labile effect, and many of the patients seem vastly amused by their own jokes (Ironside, 1956; Kramer, 1954; Martin, 1950). Indeed, such patients can be quite funny, but often they are not. In part, this humor is a function of tangentiality and disinhibition such that loosely connected ideas or events come to be strung together in an unusual fashion. The tendency to exaggerate and to comment impulsively on whatever happens to draw their attention is also contributory.

Nevertheless, rather than funny, many seem crude and inappropriate. In other instances, they may laugh without reason and with no accompanying feelings of mirth. Kramer (1954) for example, describes four cases of uncontrollable laughter after lobotomy and noted that these patients were unable to stop their laughter on command or upon their own volition. The laughter would come on like spells, occurring up to a dozen times a day, and/or continue into the night, requiring sedation in some cases. In these instances, however, the laughter had no contagious aspects but seemed shrill and "frozen." When questioned about the laughter, the patients either confabulated a reason or seemed completely perplexed as to the cause. Similar disturbances have been noted with damage to the hypothalamus, a nucleus having major interconnections with the orbital regions (Joseph, 1989).

Focal tumors of the orbital regions have also been reported to give rise to gelastic seizures (Chen & Foster, 1973; Daly & Moulder, 1957; Loiseau, Cohandon, & Cohandon, 1971); that is, seizures which induce uncontrollable laughter. Often the damage appears more extensive on the right. In addition to laughter, punning and *Witzelsucht* (puerility) language might become excessively and inappropriately profane, and the patient may seem inordinately inconsiderate, outspoken, and obstinate (Broffman, 1950; Partridge, 1950; Strom-Olsen, 1946).

Disinhibited Sexuality

In some cases, there is a loss of control over sexual behavior, and patients may engage in inappropriate sexual activity (Benson & Geschwind, 1971; Brutkowski, 1965; Freeman & Watts, 1942, 1943; Girgis, 1971; Lishman, 1973; Miller *et al.,* 1986; Strom-Olsen, 1946). One patient, after a right frontal injury, began patronizing up to four prostitutes a day, whereas his premorbid sexual activity had been limited to Tuesday evenings with his wife of 20 years (Joseph, 1988*a*).

Another patient I examined, with a right frontal stroke began propositioning nurses and on one occasion when a particularly large breasted woman chanced to be near he reached out and fondled her. It is thus not unusual for hypersexual disinhibited frontal lobe-injured patients to become forceful and indiscriminant in their activity. One patient, who was described as quite gentle, concerned, caring, and loving before his injury, became exceedingly forceful afterward and raped several women. This type of behavior, however, occurs only in a few cases.

Similar behavior has been described regarding certain individuals following lobotomy (Freeman & Watts, 1943). "Sometimes the wife has to put up with some exaggerated attention on the part of her husband, even at inconvenient times and under circumstances which she may find embarrassing. Refusal, however, has led to one savage beating that we know of, and to an additional separation or two" (p. 805). Curiously, in these situations Freeman and Watts (1943, p. 805) have suggested that "spirited physical self-defense is probably the best strategy of the woman. Her husband may have regressed to the cave-man level, and she owes it to him to be responsive at the cave-woman level. It may not be agreeable at first, but she will soon find it exhilarating if unconventional."

Seizure activity arising from the deep frontal regions have also been associated with increased sexual behavior, including sexual automatisms, exhibitionism, genital manipulation, and masturbation (Spencer, Spencer, Williamson, & Mattson, 1983). In most instances, "sexual" seizures are associated with right frontal or right temporal seizure foci (Joseph, 1988a). Nevertheless, in many cases, patients may become hyposexual (Greenblatt, 1950; Miller *et al.*, 1986).

Apathy and Pseudodepressive Features

In many instances, however, patients may appear severely apathetic, indifferent, and lethargic and may develop bradykinesia, inertia, and mutism (Blumer & Benson, 1975; Freeman & Watts, 1942, 1943; Girgis, 1971; Hacaen, 1964; Luria, 1980; Strom-Olsen, 1946). Periods of impulsiveness, tangentiality, perseveration, and irritability may also be evident, although pseudodepressive features predominate. There is a loss of drive and initiative, inactivity, a narrowing of interests, untidiness, excessive sleep, confusion, and defects of memory and attention. Indeed, even among those who initially behave in a floridly disinhibited fashion tend over time to behave in a generalized apathetic manner.

For example, one patient who "prior to his accident requiring amputation of the left frontal pole, had been garrulous, enjoyed people, had many friends, was active in community affairs" (and was described as having) "true charisma," following his head injury became quiet and remote, spent most of his time sitting alone smoking, and was frequently incontinent of urine, and occasionally of stool. He remained unconcerned and was frequently found soaking wet, calmly sitting and smoking. When asked, he would deny illness (Blumer & Benson, 1975, p. 196).

Bilateral frontal damage in monkeys has also been reported to result in a severe generalized apathetic and disinterested/indifferent state. As described by Kennard (1939), these monkeys would sit with their head sunk between their shoulders, neither blinking nor turning their heads in response to noise, threats, or the presence of intruders, but would stare absently straight ahead with no facial expression. In a similar study, following massive frontal destruction a monkey who was formerly quite active and the dominant leader of his group became inactive, indifferently watched others, failed to respond emotionally, and seemed to have lost all interest and ability to engage in complex social behavior (Batuyev, 1969).

According to Freeman and Watts (1943), inertia and apathy usually immediately follow surgical destruction of the frontal lobes. "This is characterized by more or less complete blankness. Whoever has charge of the patient will have to pull him out of bed, otherwise he may stay there all day. It is especially necessary since he won't get up voluntarily even to go to the toilet.''

In some this initial state of inertia disappears, whereas in others it becomes a lasting or even progressively severe disturbance. "The previously busy housewife who has always been a dirt chaser, and who has kept her fingers perpetually busy with darning, crocheting, knitting, and so on, sits with her hands in her lap watching the 'snails whiz by.' Like a child she must be told to wipe the dishes, to dust the sideboard, to sweep the porch'' and even then the patient completes only half the task as there is no longer any interest or initiative (Freeman & Watts, 1943, p. 803).

In his summary of two large-scale frontal tumor studies, Hecaen (1964) noted that most patients seemed confused, disorganized, apathetic, hypoactive, and to be suffering from inertia and feelings of indifference. However, puerility was also common among these patients, and many demonstrated decreased judgment with either total or partial unawareness of the environment.

Summary

Overall, there appear to be two extremes in the qualitative features of abnormal personality and emotion which may result from frontal injury. One group of patients may tend to display disinhibition, hyperactivity, impulsivity, including tangentiality and con-fabulatory tendencies, whereas a second group may demonstrate apathy, hypoactivity, confusion, lethargy, and depression. Many patients, however, demonstrate both extremes coupled with periods of intensification, amelioration, and islands of seeming normality. In part, the type and pattern of abnormality depend on whether the lesion involves the orbital, medial, inferior, or lateral convexity, or the frontal pole, as well as the laterality of the destruction.

THE RIGHT AND LEFT FRONTAL LOBES

Neuropsychiatric Disorders

In general, symptoms associated with frontal lobe lesions, particularly those involv-ing the convexity, are often differentially expressed depending on the laterality of the lesion. For example, in one study of 670 patients with missile wounds, "a specific association" between emotional–psychiatric disability and right frontal wounds was noted (Lishman, 1968). In particular, the so-called "frontal lobe personality" (e.g., euphoria, childishness, egoism, irritability) was almost exclusively associated with right but not left front wounds. Similarly, confabulation, hypersexuality, tangentiality, and manic like behaviors seem to be more frequently associated with right frontal dysfunction (Joseph, 1986a; 1988a). In contrast, reduced responsiveness is more frequently linked to lesions of the left convexity.

Depression

Patients with severe forms of Broca's expressive aphasia often become frustrated, tearful, sad and depressed (Robinson & Benson, 1981). This is because comprehension is usually relatively intact, and they are painfully aware of their deficit (Gainotti, 1972). In other words, depression in these cases appears to be a normal reaction and as such is mediated by normal tissue, i.e., the undamaged right hemisphere (Joseph, 1982, 1988a).

Depressive-like features, however, also seem to result with left anterior damage sparing Broca's area such as when the frontal pole of either hemisphere is compromised (Robinson, Kubos, Starr, Rao, & Price, 1984; Robinson & Szetela, 1981; Sinyour, Jacques, Kaloupek, Becker, Goldenberg, & Coopersmith, 1986). In part, this is probably due to its close proximity and interconnections with the medial region, an area which when damaged induces hypokinetic and apathetic states. Hence, although these patients look depressed, often they are severely apathetic, indifferent, hypoactive, and poorly motivated. When questioned, instead of being worried or truly concerned about their condition, the overall picture is one of confusion, disinterest, and blunted emotionality (Kleist, 1934, cited in Freeman & Watts, 1942; Hecaen, 1964) i.e., there is a lack of worrisome thoughts or depressive ideation.

By contrast, it has been reported that psychiatric patients classified as depressed (who presumably show no obvious signs of neurological impairment), demonstrate a significant lower integrated amplitude of the EEG-evoked response over the left versus right frontal lobe (d'Elia & Perris, 1974; Perris, 1974); i.e., the left frontal region is insufficiently activated. On the basis of EEG and clinical observation, d'Elia and Perris have argued that the involvement of the left hemisphere is proportional to the degree of depression. They have also noted that with recovery from depression the amplitude of the evoked response increases to normal right and left hemisphere levels. Reduced bioelectric arousal over the left frontal region has also been reported following depressive mood induction (Tucker, Stenslie, & Roth, & Shearer, 1981).

In part, apathetic and depressive features may result from left frontal convexity and frontal pole damage due to a severance of fibers which link emotional impulses (such as those being transmitted via the orbital and medial region) with external sources of input or cognitive activity which are transmitted to the convexity (i.e., disconnection). For example, areas 9 and 10 of the frontal lobe receive converging sensory fibers from the auditory, visual, and somesthetic cortices (Jones & Powell, 1970; Pandya & Kuypers, 1969); the inferior parietal lobule; as well as the anterior cingulate and medial wall. Areas 9 and 10 then project into, as well as receive fibers from, the orbital regions, which share projections with the hypothalamus, amygdala, septal nuclei—limbic nuclei that govern and mediate almost all forms of emotionality (Joseph, 1989). Indeed, it was the recognition that the frontal lobes acted as a bridge between emotion and idea that led to the wide-scale use of frontal lobotomy, i.e., surgical destruction of interlinking fibers, a technique that, when used during the 1940s and 1950s, often involved little more than blindly swishing a surgical ice pick inside somebody's brain.

Moreover, convexity lesions, like medial damage, may result in a disconnection not only between cognitive—perceptual and emotional activity, but would prevent limbic system output from reaching the motor areas such that emotional—motivational impulses are unable to become integrated with motor activities. The patient is thus motorically hypoemotionally aroused (i.e., depressed), and appears to be demonstrating psychomotor retardation.

Just as left frontal convexity motor damage can result in left-sided apraxia (due to right hemisphere disconnection from left parietal temporal–sequential output), the reverse can also occur. That is, with left frontal damage, linguistic impulses not only fail to become expressed, but emotional output from the right hemisphere and limbic system fails to become integrated with linguistic ideation (i.e., thought). Ideas no longer come to be assigned emotional significance. In the extreme, the motivational impetus to even engage in thought production is cut off.

As pertaining to laterality, left frontal (versus right) lesions are associated with reductions in intellectual and conceptual capability (to be explained), often leading to confusion and reduced ability to appreciate and appropriately respond to the external or internal environment. In these instances, one possible consequence is apathy, indifference, hyporesponsiveness, and depressive-like symptoms. However, it is possible that among psychiatric patients and otherwise normal, albeit depressed, patients that the left frontal region appears relatively inactive because the right frontal area is preoccupied with being depressed; the right frontal region is excessively aroused. That is, excessive right frontal arousal leads to massive left frontal inhibition, i.e., the bilateral arousal system of the right hemisphere inhibiting the left (to be explained). Depressive and apathetic disturbances, however, also occur with right hemisphere lesions, particularly those involving the parietal regions and the frontal pole (Joseph, 1988a).

Obsessive-Compulsive Disorders

There is strong, albeit, inconclusive evidence that frontal lobe dysfunction may give rise to obsessive-compulsive (Ob-C) disorders, particularly when the left frontal region is compromised (Flor-Henry, Yeudall, Koles, & Howarth, 1979; Miller, in press). It is noteworthy that Ob-C disturbances are also frequently accompanied by strong feelings of depression and anxiety (Goodwin & Guze, 1979)—affective states linked to alterations in the functional integrity of the anterior and left frontal regions of the brain.

Compulsions involving simple as well as complex motor acts are associated with frontal injuries. Moreover, abnormal activation of the frontal lobes have been reported to elicit recurrent and intrusive ideational activity ("forced thinking"), as well as compulsive urges to perform aberrant actions, e.g., shouting (Penfield & Jasper, 1954; Ward, 1988). A more frequent complication, however, are perseverations of speech and motor functioning.

The mixture of perseveration and compulsions, when subtle, may take on the appearance of obsessions. Of course, perseveration is not due to an obsessive disorder. Nevertheless, obsessions are perseverative in nature, often involving intrusive recurring thoughts, feelings, or impulses to perform certain actions (Goodwin & Guze, 1979). This disinhibition of verbal representation, i.e., forced, repetitive, and intrusive thinking, as pointed out by Miller (in press), strongly reinforces the impression of an Ob-C frontal lobe association. Motorically obsessive compulsions may involve repetitive stereotyped acts, including the perseverative manipulation and touching of objects (Goodwin & Guze, 1979)—abnormalities that are also associated with certain forms of frontal lobe damage.

Thus, in many ways, there appears to be a convergence of symptoms, suggesting that some patients suffering from certain subtypes of severe obsessive-compulsive irregularities may be victims of abnormalities involving the frontal lobes.

Schizophrenia

It has also been reported that some individuals classified as schizophrenic demonstrate EEG and other abnormalities suggestive of bilateral or left frontal dysfunction or hypoarousal (Ariel, Golden, Berg, Quaiffe, Dirksen, Forsell, Wilson, & Graber, 1983; Ingvar & Franzen, 1974; Kolb & Whishaw, 1983; Levin, 1984). It is likely, however, that only certain subpopulations of schizophrenics actually suffer from frontal lobe dysfunction, such as those with catatonia, posturing, mannerisms, and emotional blunting.

For example, patients displaying unusual mannerisms, catatonia, "emotional blunting," apathy, and/or "Hebephrenia" (blunting associated with puerile, silly childishness as well as obsessive-compulsiveness; cf. Hamilton, 1976), are certainly "frontal lobe" candidates. Indeed, Hillbom (1951), notes exactly this association among individuals with head trauma and missle wounds who later developed schizophrenic-like symptoms, including catatonia and hebrephrenia; i.e., left frontal patients are more likely to develop these symptoms. However, it is also likely that lesions involving the left temporal lobe or dysfunctional nuclei buried deep within the frontal lobe, i.e., the caudate and other portions of the basal ganglia, may in fact be the causative agents in some instances.

For example, Richfield, Twyman and Berent (1987) report a 25-year-old female honor student (soon to be married) who, after complaining of headaches and nausea, disappeared for 3 days. "When found, she had undergone a dramatic personality change manifested by alterations in affect, motivation, cognition, and self-care." These changes were largely permanent. "Her abnormal behaviors included vulgarity, impulsiveness, violent outbursts, enuresis, indifference, hypersexuality, shoplifting and exposing herself. She was inattentive and uninterested in her surroundings but could be encouraged to concentrate for short periods of time. She would frequently lie down to sleep. Her affect was flat" (p. 768). Computed tomography (CT) scan indicated bilateral damage to the head of the caudate nuclei. Thus, in some respects this patient's behavior suggested the acute onset of a schizoaffective disorder. However, repeated psychiatric hospitalizations and treatment with major tranquilizers over the course of the next 2 years were of no assistance. And no wonder—Her problem was neurologic, not psychiatric (as illustrated by Richfield *et al.*, 1987). And yet, the wards of many psychiatric hospitals are probably filled with such unfortunates, with their neurological abnormalities unrecognized.

As pertaining to schizophrenia, the caudate and basal ganglia are also implicated as they are major sites of dopamine concentration (i.e., the dopamine theory of schizophrenia), and many of the major antipsychotic drugs act on dopamine receptors within these nuclei.

Mania

When the orbital and portions of the inferior lateral convexity are damaged, behavior often becomes inappropriate, labile, and disinhibited. Individuals may become hyperactive, distractable, hypersexual, tangential, and confabulatory. However, although laughing and joking one moment, these same patients can quickly become irritated, angered, enraged, destructive, or conversely tearful with slight provocation. This pattern is one of mania and/or hypomanic excitement.

Mania and manic-like features have been reported in many patients with injuries, tumors, and even seizures involving predominantly the frontal lobe and/or the right hemisphere (Bogousslavsky *et al.*, 1988; Clark & Davison, 1987; Cohen & Niska, 1980; Cummings & Mendez, 1984; Forrest, 1982; Girgis, 1971; Jack, Rivers-Bulkley, & Rabin, 1983; Jamieson & Wells, 1979; Joseph, 1986a, 1988a; Lishman, 1973; Miller *et al.*, 1986; Oppler, 1950; Rosenbaum & Berry, 1975; Starkstein, Pearlson, Boston, & Robinson, 1987; Stern & Dancey, 1942). For example, one patient described as a very stable, happily married family man became very talkative, restless, grossly disinhibited, and sexually preoccupied; he spent money extravagantly and recklessly purchased a business that soon went bankrupt (Lishman, 1973). Frontal lobe destruction was indicated.

In another case, a 46-year-old woman was admitted to the hospital and observed to be careless about her person and room, incontinent of urine and feces, to sleep very little and to act in a hypersexual manner. Her symptoms had developed several months earlier, when she began accusing a neighbor of taking things she had misplaced and on other occasions stripping in front of him. She began going about in just her nightdress, informing people she was descended from queens, was very rich, and that many men wanted to divorce their wives and marry her. During her hospitalization, she was frequently quite loud, disoriented to time and place, and extremely tangential, jumping from subject to subject. After several years she died, and a meningioma involving the orbital surface of her frontal lobes was discovered (Girgis, 1971).

Oppler (1950) reported one patient who developed flight of ideas, increased activity, emotional lability, including elation, extreme fearfulness, distractability, puerility, and argumentative behavior. Subsequently a tumor was discovered and removed from the right frontal–parietal area.

Over the course of the last several years, I have had eight male patients referred to me for differential diagnosis involving mania versus cerebral dysfunction. All but one had good premorbid histories and had worked at their respective jobs for at least 6 years until the time of their injuries. Seven had suffered trauma to the right cranium, and one was discovered to have a small tumor developing in the right frontal area. Following their injuries, all developed delusions of grandeur, pressured speech, flight of ideas, decreased need for sleep, indiscriminant financial activity, extreme emotional lability, and increased libido. In four of the seven head-injured patients CT-scan indicated damage involving the right frontal area and all 7 demonstrated right hemisphere and frontal deficits on neuropsychological testing. In several cases contra coup injuries were also apparent (Joseph, 1988a).

Intellectual and Conceptual Alterations

It has frequently been claimed that intelligence is not affected even with massive injuries to the frontal lobes. However, this view is completely erroneous. Even in mild cases, although intelligence per se may not seem to be reduced, the ability to employ one's intelligence effectively is almost always compromised to some extent. Frontal lobe damage reduces one's ability to profit from experience, to anticipate consequences, or to learn from errors (Bianchi, 1922; Drewe, 1974; Goldstein, 1936–37, 1944; Halstead, 1947; Milner, 1964, 1971; Nichols & Hunt, 1940; Joseph, 1986a; Petrie, 1952, Porteus & Peters, 1947; Rylander, 1939; Tow, 1955). There is a reduction in creativity, fantasy, dreaming, abstract reasoning, the capacity to synthesize ideas into concepts or to grasp situations in their entirety. Interests of an intellectual nature seem to be diminished or, with severe damage, abolished (Bianchi, 1922; Freeman & Watts, 1942, 1943; Goldstein, 1936–37, 1944; Partridge, 1950; Tow, 1955). For example, Freeman and Watts (1943, p. 803) noted that "patients who formerly were great readers of good literature will be interested only in comic books or movie magazines. Men of considerable intellectual achievement will read avidly the sports page, and when discussion turns on the great events of the day will pass off some cliches as their own opinions."

In mild or severe cases, thinking may be contaminated by perseverative intrusions of irrelevant and tangential ideas, randomly formed associations, and illogical intellectual activity. These patients are also often affected by the immediacy of their environment and have difficulty making plans or adequately meeting long-term goals in an appropriate manner. For example, one patient, formerly an executive at a local electronics firm, arrived at my office with a toothbrush, toothpaste, hairbrush, and wash rag sticking out of his shirt pocket. When I asked, pointing at his pocket, "What's all that for?" he replied with a laugh, "Just in case I want to wash my face and brush my teeth," and in so saying he quickly drew the toothbrush from his pocket and began to demonstrate. During the course of the examination, he laughingly wanted to show me how the hole in his head (from the craniotomy and bullet wound) could bulge in or out when he held his breath or held his head upside down. He climbed up on my desk so that I could better see his head when held upside down. Although this patient had suffered a bullet wound damaging the orbital area and mesial convexity of the right frontal lobe (he had shot himself in the mouth), his overall WAIS-R IQ was above 130 (98% rank: "Very Superior"). Nevertheless, throughout the examination, he behaved in a silly, puerile manner, often joking and laughing inappropriately.

Frontal lobe patients also may have difficulty thinking up or considering alternative problem-solving strategies and thus developing alternative lines of reasoning. For example, Nichols and Hunt (1940) dealt a patient five cards down, including the ace of spades, which always fell to the right on two successive deals and then to the left for two trials. The patient's task was to learn this pattern and turn up the ace. The patient failed to master this after 200 trials.

Some frontal lobe patients may also have extreme difficulty sorting even common everyday objects according to category (Rylander, 1939; Tow, 1955), for example, sorting and grouping drinking containers (glasses) with other drinking containers (mugs) and tools with tools. Similarly, they may have difficulty performing the Wisconsin Card Sorting Task (Crockett et al., 1986; Drewe, 1974; Milner, 1964, 1971), which involves sorting geometric figures according to similarity in color, shape, or number. However, the manner in which a patient fails on this task is dependent on the locus and laterality of the damage.

For example, patients with orbital damage seem to have relatively little difficulty performing this category of sorting task (Drewe, 1974; Milner, 1971). Similarly, patients with right frontal damage, although they show a tendency to make perseverative type errors (i.e., persisting in a choice pattern that is clearly indicated as incorrect), perform significantly better than those with left frontal damage (Drewe, 1974; Milner, 1964, 1971). Thus overall, patients with left medial and convexity lesions perform most poorly, and have the greatest degree of difficulty thinking in a flexible manner or developing alternative response strategies.

IQ. In a number of studies of conceptual functioning in which either the Raven's Progressive Matrices or Porteus Mazes were administered both before and after surgical destruction of the frontal lobes it has been consistently found that significant declines result (Petrie, 1952; Porteus & Peters, 1947; Tow, 1955). As with most tests, the usual pattern is to improve with practice. Hence, these results (and those mentioned above) indicate that frontal lobe damage disrupts abstract reasoning skills, verbal–nonverbal pattern analysis, learning and intellectual ability, as well as the capacity to anticipate the consequences of one's actions or to profit from experience.

Significant disturbances and reductions in intellectual ability have also been reported with administration of the Wechsler Intelligence Scales (Petrie, 1952; Smith, 1966). In one study where patients undergoing frontal leucotomy for intractable pain were administered the Wechsler both pre- and post surgery, a 20 point drop in the IQ was reported (Koskoff, 1948, cited by Tow, 1955). Again, however, the effects of frontal damage on IQ is dependent on the locus of the damage.

For example, left frontal patients show lower Wechsler IQs than did those with right frontal lesions (Petrie, 1952; Smith, 1966). In fact, 17 of 18 patients with left frontal damage reported by Smith (1966) scored lower across all subtests as compared with those with right frontal lesions. Indeed, patients with left-sided destruction perform as poorly as those with bilateral damage (Petrie, 1952).

In analyzing subtest performance, Smith (1966) notes that left frontal patients scored particularly poorly on Picture Completion (which requires identification of missing details). This is presumably because the left cerebral hemisphere is more concerned with the perception of details (or parts, segments) versus wholes (Joseph, 1982, 1988a). Petrie (1952), however, reports that performance on the Comprehension subtests (i.e., judgment, common sense) was most significantly impaired among left frontal patients. By contrast, patients with severe right frontal damage have difficulty performing Picture Arrangement—often leaving the cards in the same order in which they are laid (McFie & Thompson, 1972). This may be a consequence of deficiencies in the capacity to discern social–emotional nuances, a function in which the right hemisphere excels (Joseph, 1988a).

Nevertheless, since so few studies have been conducted, it is probably not reasonable to assume that lesions lateralized to the right or left frontal lobe will always effect performance on certain subtests, particularly if there is a mild injury. It is also important to consider in what manner lateralized effects on IQ may be contributing to or secondary to reduced motivation and apathy since bilateral and left frontal damage often give rise to this constellation of symptoms. If the patient is apathetic they are not going to be motivated to perform at the best of their ability.

Attention

There is a tremendous amount of evidence indicating the frontal lobes are highly involved in attentional functioning (see also Crowne, 1983; Fuster, 1980; Luria, 1980; Knight, Hillyard, Woods, & Neville, 1981; Pragay *et al.*, 1987). Hence, attentional disturbances are frequently associated with frontal lobe lesions. Some patients, although fully alert and oriented, are easily distracted and show wandering or a perpetual shifting of attention (Bianchi, 1922; Stuss & Benson, 1984). They may seem distracted by noises in the hall, specks on the testing table, or extraneous objects around the room.

Others may seem easily overwhelmed by complexity or behave as if their sensory–perceptual capacities were significantly narrowed (Yarcorzynski & Davis, 1942). In severe cases attention may be focused for only short time periods. For example, if asked to count, they may stop after reaching 10 or 15 (Rose, 1950) and then must be prodded to continue.

On the other hand, some patients seem remarkably able to maintain directed attention, at least when performing simple tasks. I have frequently observed, and it has been reported, that frontal patients can perform tasks such as digit span without difficulty (Benson, Gardner, & Meadows, 1976; Partridge, 1950; Petrie, 1952; Stuss, Alexander, Lieberman, & Levine, 1978). Indeed, patients may seem to be locked into this as if all potentially interfering stimuli were completely blocked out (perseverative attention?). Nevertheless, although repetition of digits may be normal, or even well above average, when required to recite digits backwards, performance often is abnormal (Partridge, 1950; Petrie, 1952). Hence, although able to attend (or at least echo what has been said), the ability to maintain sustained concentration is often disturbed.

As might be expected, a secondary consequence of attentional abnormalities are disturbances of memory. If a patient is not paying attention, he is not going to remember (see Squire, 1987, regarding memory and the frontal lobes). Memory is not always affected, however (e.g., Delaney, Rosen, Mattson, & Novelly, 1980). Nevertheless, the type of attentional disturbance depends in part on the laterality of the lesion as well as on the extent to which it involves the convexity or orbital zones. For example, some right frontal patients are impaired on sustained attention tasks when stimuli are presented at the rate of 1 stimulus per second. However, if presented with 7 stimuli per second, performance is improved (Wilkins, Shallice, & McCarthy, 1987). This suggests that right frontal patients may be understimulated and show wandering attention if not fully engaged.

The left frontal lobe appears to be more concerned with verbal attentional functioning and with the monitoring of temporal—sequential and detailed events (Milner, 1971; Petrides & Milner, 1982), whereas the right is more attentive to nonverbal auditory, visual, tactual, and social–emotional stimuli (Joseph, 1988a). For example, damage involving either the right or left frontal lobe may impair performance on the Picture Completion subtest of the WAIS-R (i.e., detecting a missing detail such as a dog leaving no footprints), but for different reasons. Left frontal patients may do poorly because of inattention to detail (e.g., "There's nothing wrong with this picture"). Right frontal patients may perform deficiently due to impulsive tendencies to say the first thing that comes to mind ("The dog doesn't have a leash"). Higher false-positive rates also occur when the frontal lobes are damaged.

Right Frontal Dominance for Arousal

The right cerebral hemisphere is clearly dominant in regard to the mediation and control over most aspects of social–emotional functioning (Joseph, 1988a). There are also a variety of findings that strongly suggest that the right frontal lobe is dominant in the control and mediation of emotion and various aspects of attention and that it exerts bilateral influences on arousal (DeRenzi & Faglioni, 1965; Heilman & Van Den Abell, 1979, 1980; Joseph, 1982, 1986a, 1988a; Tucker, 1981). For example, the intact, normal right hemisphere is quicker to react to external stimuli, and has a greater attentional capacity compared to the left (Dimond, 1976, 1979; Heilman & Van Den Abell, 1979; Jeeves & Dixon, 1970; Joseph, 1988a,b). In split-brain studies, the isolated left hemisphere occasionally tends to become unresponsive, suffers lapses of attention, and is more limited in attentional capacity (Dimond, 1976, 1979; Joseph, 1988*a,b*). The right frontal lobe is also larger than the left, suggesting a greater degree of interconnections with other brain tissue.

Moreover, it has been demonstrated that visual and somesthetic stimuli, or active touch exploration with either the right or left hand, elicits evoked EEG responses preferentially and of greater magnitude over the right hemisphere (Desmedt, 1977). The right hemisphere also becomes desynchronized (aroused) following left- or right-sided stimulation (indicating it is bilaterally responsive), whereas the left brain is activated only by unilateral (right side) stimulation (Heilman & Van Den Abell, 1980).

It is also possible that the right and left frontal lobes may exert different influences on arousal (Tucker, 1981). The right frontal lobe may exert predominantly bilateral inhibitory influences. The left frontal region may be more involved in unilateral excitatory (expressive) activation. Thus when the left frontal region is damaged, the right acts unopposed and there is excessive inhibition, for example, as manifested by speech arrest, depression, and/or apathy. However, with lesions involving the right frontal lobe, not only is there a loss of inhibitory control, but the left may act unopposed such that there is excessive excitement, as manifested by speech release, confabulation, and disinhibited behavior.

Nevertheless, because left cerebral excitatory influences are predominantly unilateral, with massive right cerebral damage, although the left hemisphere is aroused, the left is unable to activate the right half of the brain. This results in unilateral inattention and neglect of the left half of the body and space (Damasio, Damasio, & Chui, 1980; Heilman & Valenstein, 1972; Joseph, 1986*a,* 1988*a,b*). That is, the patient's (undamaged) left hemisphere may ignore his or her left arm or leg, and if their neglected extremities are shown to them, may claim they belong to the doctor or a person in the next room.

That such disturbances occur only rarely with left frontal or left hemisphere damage further suggests that the right brain is able to continue to monitor events occurring on either side of the body. Thus although the damaged left brain is hypoaroused (or inhibited by the right), there is no neglect.

In contrast, with partial right frontal damage, rather than a loss of arousal, there results a loss of inhibitory restraint, and the patient demonstrates confabulatory tendencies (speech release), heightened sexuality, manic-like excitement, and a host of other disinhibitory disturbances. Nevertheless, more research is needed to clarify these and other issues; notions regarding lateralized inhibitory versus excitatory influences should be considered highly speculative.

SUMMARY

The frontal lobes serve as the "senior executive" of the brain and, together with the motor area, make up almost half the cerebrum. They act to mediate information processing throughout the neuroaxis via cortical sampling, thalamic gating, and inhibitory control over various nuclei, including the limbic system and reticular formation. For example, the orbital regions appear to exert controlling influences over limbic arousal whereas the convexity seems more concerned with influencing information processing throughout the neocortex. Through these and other interactions, the frontal lobes act to maintain and shift attention; exert organizational control over all aspects of expression (e.g., thought, speech, motor); anticipate consequences; consider alternatives; plan and formulate goals; shape, direct, and modulate personality and emotional functioning; and integrate ideas, emotions, and perceptions.

Although bearing in mind the large expanse of tissue that comprises the frontal lobes, as well as the considerable overlap in functional representation and interconnections between the different quadrants of the anterior half of the brain, it certainly appears that certain regions are more closely associated with specific functions and characteristic patterns of deficit. But it also appears that such capacities as motor, emotion, and personality functioning may become compromised to some extent, regardless of where within the frontal lobe a lesion may occur.

Massive damage to the medial walls of the frontal lobes (including the supplementary motor area and cingulate gyrus) often initially results in reduced speech output, mutism, variable motor abnormalities and mannerisms, including agraphia, forced groping, compulsive utilization, gegenhalten, and waxy flexibility, as well as, in the extreme, catatonia. Patients may seem apathetic, indifferent, and/or severely depressed.

There is some speculation that, over the course of evolutionary development, the anterior cingulate has grown up and over the medial wall to become part of the lateral convexity and motor areas. Hence, with convexity lesions, and particularly left frontal lesions, symptoms qualitatively similar (at least in part) to those following medial damage may arise. These include reduced expressive abilities and motor output (Broca's aphasia, agraphia, apraxia), and apathy and depressive-like personality features. Left convexity lesions are also associated with reduced intellectual functioning and possibly with some forms of schizophrenic and obsessive-compulsive abnormalities.

Regardless of laterality, lesions involving the orbital frontal lobes, if partial, can give rise to a loss of emotional control and social–emotional restraint, coupled with disinhibition and irresponsible behavior. However, if massive, instead of a loss of emotional control, there is a loss of emotion. Moreover, orbital lesions (as well as inferior medial and inferior convexity) are often associated with perseverative abnormalities. In part, the above is a function of orbital mediation of limbic arousal and emotional–social ideational association. By contrast, the convexity is more involved in controlling neocortical arousal and integrating perceptual with motor and ideational activities. Thus, convexity lesions may result in hyper- (or hypo-) reactivity to external stimuli and difficulty in delaying and withholding responses.

Inferior convexity lesions also often result in a loss of restraint, including hyperexcitability, and perseveration. Similarly, right frontal convexity lesions may initially give rise to disinhibitory states and, in the extreme, patients may seem delusional and maniclike.

In many respects, whereas the left convexity seems to resemble the medial-frontal lobes, the right frontal region seems more closely associated with the orbital areas. In part this may be attributable to the greater right frontal involvement with emotional functioning as well as its more intimate connections with and control over the limbic system, of which the orbital region is part.

It must be emphasized, however, that not only is there considerable overlap in functional representation, lesions are seldom confined to one particular region of the frontal lobe. On the basis of symptoms alone, one cannot with complete assurance localize damage to a particular quadrant of the anterior half of the cerebrum. Moreover, as a result of uterine or birth trauma, brain damage experienced during childhood, or even early rearing experiences, considerable functional reorganization can occur (Goldman, 1971; Joseph, 1982, 1986b, 1988b). Not all brains are alike. Moreover, long-term effects are often quite different from what is seen initially or during the first year following injury. In general, the frontal patients I have followed over several years' time have tended to become more sluggish and apathetic in their behavior—even those who were floridly manic when first examined. Similarly, if the damage is mild, the disturbances may be quite subtle. Given these caveats, and the fact that more research is needed, it is best to consider this discussion and review as a general outline of the functions and symptoms of the frontal lobes.

REFERENCES

Ackerly, S. S. (1935). Instinctive emotional and mental changes following pre-frontal lobe extirpation. *American Journal of Psychiatry, 92,* 717–727.

Adams, R. D., & Victor, M. (1981). *Principles of neurology.* New York: McGraw-Hill.

Alexander, M. P., Stuss, D. T., & Benson, D. F. (1979). Capgras syndrome: A reduplicative phenomenon. *Neurology (New York), 29,* 334–339.

Anand, B. K., Dua, S., & China, G. S. (1958). Higher nervous control over food intake. *Indian Journal of Medical Research, 46,* 277–287.

Ariel, R. N., Golden, C. J., Berg, R. A., Quaife, M. A., Dirksen, J. W., Forsell, T., Wilson, J., & Graber, B. (1983). Regional blood flow in schizophrenia. *Archives of General Psychiatry, 40,* 258–263.

Astruc, J. (1971). Corticofugal connections of area 8 (frontal eye field) in *Macaca mulatta. Brain Research, 33,* 241–256.

Bailey, P., & Sweet, W. H. (1940). Effects on respiration, blood pressure and gastric motility of stimulation of orbital surface of frontal lobes. *Journal of Neurophysiology, 3,* 276–281.

Baleydier, C., & Maguiere, F. (1980). The duality of the cingulate gyrus of the monkey. *Brain 103,* 525–554.

Barbas, H., & Dubrovsky, B. (1981). Excitatory and inhibitory interactions of extraocular and dorsal neck muscle afferents in the cat frontal cortex. *Experimental Neurology, 74,* 51–66.

Barbas, H., & Mesulam, M. M. (1981). Organization of afferent input to subdivision of area 8 in the rhesus monkey. *Journal of Comparative Neurology, 200,* 407–431.

Barris, R. W., & Schuman, H. R. (1953). Bilateral anterior cingulate gyrus lesions: Syndrome of the anterior cingulate gyri. *Neurology (New York), 3,* 44–52.

Batuyev, A. S. (1969). The frontal lobes and the processes of synthesis in the brain. *Brain Behavior and Evolution, 2,* 202–212.

Benson, D. F. (1967). Fluency in aphasis correlation with radioactive scan localization. *Cortex, 3,* 373–394.

Benson, D. F., Gardner, H., & Meadows, J. C. (1976). Reduplicative paramnesia. *Neurology (New York), 26,* 147–151.

Benson, D. F., & Geschwind, N. (1971). Psychiatric conditions associated with focal lesions of the central nervous system. In S. Arieti & M. Reiser (Eds.), *American handbook of psychiatry* (Vol. 4, pp. 208–243). New York: Basic Books.

Bianchi, L. (1922). *The mechanism of the brain and the function of the frontal lobes.* Edinburgh: Livingstone.

Blumer, D., & Benson, D. F. (1975). Personality changes with frontal and temporal lesions. In D. F. Benson & D. Blumer (Eds.), *Psychiatric aspects of neurologic disease*. Orlando, FL: Grune & Stratton.

Blumstein, S. E., Alexander, M. P., Ryalls, J. H., Katz, W., & Dworetzky, B. (1987). On the nature of the foreign accent syndrome: A case study. *Brain and Language, 31,* 215–244.

Bogousslavsky, J., Ferrazzini, M., Regli, F., Assal, G., Tanabe, H., & Delaloye-Bischof, A. (1988). Manic delirium and frontal-like syndrome with paramedian infarction of the right thalamus. *Journal of Neurology, Neurosurgery and Psychiatry, 51,* 116–119.

Bradford, R. (1950). Nursing procedures and problems. In M. Greenblatt, R. Arnot, & H. C. Solomon (Eds.), *Studies in lobotomy*. Orlando, FL: Grune & Stratton.

Brinkman, C. (1981). Lesions in supplementary motor area interfere with a monkey's performance on a bimanual coordination task. *Neuroscience Letters, 27,* 267–270.

Brinkman, C., & Porter, R. (1979). Supplementary motor area in the monkey: Activity of neurons during performance of a learned motor task. *Journal of Neurophysiology, 42,* 681–709.

Brodal, A. (1981). *Neurological anatomy*. New York: Oxford University Press.

Broffman, M. (1950). The lobotomized patient during the first year at home. In M. Greenblatt, R. Arnot, & H. C. Solomon (Eds.), *Studies in lobotomy*. Orlando, FL: Grune & Stratton.

Brutkowski, S. (1965). Functions of prefrontal cortex in animals. *Physiological Review, 45,* 721–746.

Brutkowski, S., Mishkin, M., & Rosvold, H. E. (1963). Positive and inhibitory motor CRs in monkeys after ablation of orbital or dorsolateral surface of the frontal cortex. In E. Guttman & P. Hnik (Eds.), *Central and peripheral mechanisms of motor functions*. (pp. 133–141). Prague: Czechoslovak Academy of Science.

Butter, C. M. (1969). Perseveration in extinction and in discrimination reversal tasks following selective frontal ablations in Macaca mulatta. *Physiology and Behavior, 4,* 163–171.

Butter, C. M., Mishkin, M., & Mirsky, A. F. (1968). Emotional response toward humans in monkeys with selective frontal lesions. *Physiology and Behavior, 3,* 213–215.

Butter, C. M., Mishkin, M., & Rosvold, H. L. (1963). Conditioning and extinction of food rewarded responses after selective ablations of frontal cortex in the rhesus monkey. *Experimental Neurology, 7,* 65–75.

Butter, C. M., & Snyder, D. R. (1972). Alterations in aversive and aggressive behaviors following orbital frontal lesions in rhesus monkeys. *Acta Neurobiologica Experimentalis, 32,* 525–566.

Butter, C. M., Snyder, D. R., & McDonald, J. A. (1970). Effects of orbital frontal lesions on aversive and aggressive behaviors in rhesus monkeys. *Journal of Comparative and Physiological Psychology, 72,* 132–144.

Cavada, C. (1984). Transcortical sensory pathways to the prefrontal cortex with special attention to the olfactory and visual modalities. In F. Reinoso-Suarez & Ajmone-Marsan (Eds.), *Cortical integration* (pp. 317–328). New York: Raven Press.

Chapman, W. P., Livingston, R., & Livingston, K. E. (1950). The effects of lobotomy and of electrical stimulation of the orbital surface of the frontal lobe upon respiration and blood pressure in man. In M. Greenblatt, R. Arnot, & H. C. Solomon (Eds.), *Studies in lobotomy*. Orlando, FL: Grune & Stratton.

Chen, R., & Foster, F. N. (1973). Cursive and gelastic epilepsy. *Neurology (New York), 23,* 1019–1029.

Chi, C. C. (1970). An experimental silver study of the ascending projections of the central gray substance and adjacent tegmentum in the rat with observation in the cat. *Journal of Comparative Neurology, 139,* 259–273.

Clark, A. F., & Davison, K. (1987). Mania following head injury. *British Journal of Psychiatry, 150,* 841–844.

Clemente, C. D., Chase, M. H., Knauss, T. K., Sauerland, E. K., & Sterman, M. B. (1964). Inhibition of a monosynaptic reflex by electrical stimulation of the basal forebrain or the orbital gyrus in the cat. *Experientia, 22,* 844–845.

Cohen, M. R., & Niska, R. W. (1980). Localized right cerebral hemisphere dysfunction and recurrent mania. *American Journal of Psychiatry, 137,* 847–848.

Crocket, D., Bilsker, D., Hurwitz, T., & Kozak, J. (1986). Clinical utility of three measures of frontal lobe dysfunction in neuropsychiatric samples. *Internal Journal of Neuroscience, 30,* 241–248.

Crowne, D. P. (1983). The frontal eye field and attention. *Psychological Bulletin, 93,* 232–260.

Cummings, J. L., & Mendez, M. F. (1984). Secondary mania with focal cerebrovascular lesions. *American Journal of Psychiatry, 41,* 1084–1087.

Daly, D., & Moulder, D. (1957). Gelastic epilepsy. *Neurology (New York), 7,* 26–36.

Damasio, A. R., Damasio, H., & Chui, H. C. (1980). Neglect following damage to frontal lobe or basal ganglia. *Neuropsychologia, 18,* 123–132.

Damasio, A. R., & Van Hoesen, G. W. (1980). Structure and function of the supplementary motor area. *Neurology (New York), 30,* 359.

Dax, E. D., Reitman, F., & Radley-Smith, E. (1948). Prefrontal leucotomy. *Digest of Neurology and Psychiatry, 16,* 533–534.

Delaney, R. C., Rosen, A. J., Mattson, R. H., & Novelly, R. A. (1980). Memory function in focal epilepsy: A comparison of non-surgical unilateral temporal lobe and frontal lobe samples. *Cortex, 16,* 103–117.

d'Elia, G., & Perris, C. (1974). Cerebral functional dominance and memory functioning. *Acta Psychiatrica Scandinavica, 155,* 143–157.

Delgado, J. M. R., & Livingston, R. B. (1948). Some respiratory, vascular, and thermal responses from stimulation of the orbital surface of frontal lobe. *Journal of Neurophysiology, 11,* 39–55.

Denny-Brown, D. (1958). The anture of apraxia. *Journal of Nervous and Mental Disease, 126,* 15–56.

Denny-Brown, D. (1966). *The cerebral control of movement.* Liverpool: Liverpool University Press.

DeRenzi, E., & Faglioni, P. (1965). The comparative efficiency of intelligence and vigilance tests detecting hemisphereic damage. *Cortex, 1,* 410–433.

DeRenzi, E., Pieczuro, A., & Vignolo, L. A. (1966). Oral apraxia and aphasia. *Cortex, 2,* 56–73.

Desmedt, J. E. (1977). Active touch exploration of extrapersonal space elicits specific electrogenesis in the right cerebral hemisphere of intact right-handed man. *Proceedings of the National Academy of Science U.S.A. 74,* 4037–4040.

Dimond, S. J. (1976). Depletion of attentional capacity after total commissurotomy in man. *Brain, 99,* 347–356.

Dimond, S. J. (1979). Tactual and auditory vigilance in split-brain man. *Journal of Neurology, Neurosurgery and Psychiatry, 42,* 70–74.

Drewe, E. A. (1974). The effect of type and area of brain lesion on Wisconsin Card Sorting Task performance. *Cortex, 10,* 159–170.

Flor-Henry, P., Yeudall, L. T., Koles, J., & Howarth, B. G. (1979). Neuropsychological and power spectral EEG investigations of the obsessive-compulsive syndrome. *Biological Psychiatry, 14,* 119–129.

Forrest, D. V. (1982). Bipolar illness after right hemispherectomy. *Archives of General Psychiatry, 39,* 817–819.

Freeman, W., & Watts, J. W. (1942). *Psychosurgery.* Springfield: Charles C Thomas.

Freeman, W., & Watts, J. W. (1943). Prefrontal lobotomy. *American Journal of Psychiatry, 99,* 798–806.

French, G. M. (1959). A deficit associated with hypermotility in monkeys with lesions of the dorsolateral frontal granular cortex. *Journal of Comparative and Physiological Psychology, 52,* 25–28.

French, J. D. (1964). The frontal lobes and association. In J. M. Warren & K. Akert (Eds.), *The frontal granular cortex and behavior* (pp. 56–74). New York: McGraw-Hill.

French, G. M., & Harlow, H. F. (1955). Locomotor reaction decrement in normal and brain-damaged monkeys. *Journal of Comparative and Physiological Psychology, 48,* 496–501.

Fulton, J. F. (1934). Grasping and groping in relation to the syndrome of the premotor area. *Archives of Neurology and Psychiatry, 31,* 221–235.

Fulton, J. F., Jacobson, C. F., & Kennard, M. A. (1932). A note concerning the relation of the frontal lobes to posture and forced grasping in monkeys. *Brain, 55,* 524–536.

Fuster, J. M. (1980). *The prefrontal cortex. Anatomy, physiology, and neuropsychology of the frontal lobes.* New York: Raven Press.

Fuster, J. M., Bauer, R. H., & Jervey, J. P. (1982). Cellular discharge in the dorsolateral prefrontal cortex of the monkey in cognitive tasks. *Experimental Neurology, 77,* 679–694.

Gainotti, G. (1972). Emotional behavior and hemispheric side of lesion. *Cortex, 8,* 41–55.

Geschwind, N. (1965). Disconnection syndromes in animals and man. *Brain, 88,* 237–294, 585–644.

Geschwind, N. (1979). Specialization of the human brain. *Scientific American, 241,* 180–201.

Girgis, M. (1971). The orbital surface of the frontal lobe of the brain. *Acta Psychiatrics Scandinavica (Supplement), 22,* 1–58.

Glees, P., Cole, J., Whitty, C. W. M., & Cairns, H. (1950). The effects of lesions in the cingulate gyrus and adjacent areas in monkeys. *Journal of Neurology, Neurosurgery and Psychiatry, 13,* 178–190.

Godschalk, M., Lemon, R. N., Nijis, H. G. T., & Kuypers, H. G. J. M. (1981). Behavior of neurons in monkeys peri-arcuate and precentral cortex before and during visually guided arm and hand movements. *Experimental Brain Research, 44,* 113–116.

Goldberg, G. (1985). Supplementary motor area structure and function: Review and hypothesis. *The Behavioral and Brain Sciences, 8,* 567–616.

Goldberg, G., Meyer, N. H., & Toglia, J. U. (1981). Medial frontal cortex infarction and the alien hand sign. *Archives of Neurology, 38,* 683–686.

Goldman, P. S. (1971). Functional development of the prefrontal cortex in early life and the problem of neuronal plasticity. *Experimental Neurology, 32,* 366–387.

Goldman, P. S., Rosvold, H. W., & Mishkin, M. (1970). Evidence for behavioral impairment following prefrontal lobectomy in the infant monkey. *Journal of Comparative and Physiological Psychology, 70,* 454–463.

Goldstein, K. (1936–37). The significance of the frontal lobes for mental performance. *Journal of Neurology and Psychopothology, 17,* 27–40.

Goldstein, K. (1944). The mental changes due to frontal lobe damage. *Journal of Psychology, 17,* 187–208.

Goodglass, H., & Berko, J. (1960). Agrammatism and inflectional morphology in English. *Journal of Speech and Hearing Research, 3,* 257–267.

Goodglass, J., & Kaplan, E. (1972). *The assessment of aphasia and related disorders.* Philadelphia: Lea & Febiger.

Goodwin, D. W., & Guze, S. B. (1979). *Psychiatric diagnosis.* New York: Oxford University Press.

Gorelick, P. B., & Ross, E. D. (1987). The aprosodias: Further functional–anatomical evidence for the organization of affective language in the right hemisphere. *Journal of Neurology, Neurosurgery and Psychiatry, 50,* 553–560.

Graff-Radford, N. R., Cooper, W. E., Colsher, P. L., & Damasio, A. R. (1986). An unlearned foreign ''accent'' in a patient with aphasia. *Brain and Language, 28,* 86–94.

Grafman, J., Vance, S., Weingartner, H., Salazar, A. M., & Amin, D. (1986). The effects of lateralized frontal lesions on mood regulation. *Brain, 109,* 1127–1148.

Gray, J. A. (1987). *The psychology of fear and stress.* New York: Oxford University Press.

Greenblatt, M. (1950). *Studies in lobotomy.* Orlando, FL: Grune & Stratton.

Gross, C. G., & Weiskrantz, L. (1964). Some changes in behavior produced by lateral frontal lesions in the macaque. In J. M. Warren & K. Akert (Eds.), *The frontal granular cortex and behavior* (pp. 74–101). New York: McGraw-Hill.

Halstead, W. C. (1947). *Brain and intelligence.* Chicago: University of Chicago Press.

Hamilton, M. (1976). *Fish's schizophrenia.* Bristrol: John Wright & Sons.

Hassler, R. (1980). Brain mechanisms of intention and attention with introductory remarks on other volitional processes. *Progress in Brain Research, 54,* 585–614.

Hebben, N. (1986). The role of the frontal and temporal lobes in the phonetic organizations of speech stimuli: A multidimensional scaling analysis. *Brain and Language, 19,* 342–357.

Hecaen, H. (1964). Mental changes associated with tumors of the frontal lobes. In J. M. Warren & K. Akert (Eds.), *The frontal cortex and behavior* (pp. 335–352). New York: McGraw-Hill.

Hecaen, J., & Albert, M. L. (1978). *Human neuropsychology.* New York: John Wiley & Sons.

Heilman, K. M., & Valenstein, E. (1972). Frontal lobe neglect in man. *Neurology (New York), 22,* 660–664.

Heilman, K. M., & Van Den Abell, T. (1979). Right hemispheric dominance for mediating cerebral activation. *Neuropsychologia, 17,* 315–321.

Heilman, K. M., & Van Den Abell, T. (1980). Right hemisphere dominance for attention. The mechanism underlying hemispheric asymmetries of inattention (neglect). *Neurology (New York), 30,* 327–330.

Ingvar, D. H., & Franzen, G. (1974). Abnormalities of cerebral blood-flow distribution in patients with chronic schizophrenia. *Acta Psychiatrica Scandinavica, 50,* 425–462.

Ironside, R. (1956). Disorders of laughter due to brain lesions. *Brain, 79,* 589–609.

Iversen, S. D., & Mishkin, M. (1970). Perseverative interference in monkeys following selective lesions of the inferior prefrontal convexity. *Experimental Brain Research, 11,* 476–486.

Jack, R. A., Rivers-Bulkley, N. T., & Rabin, P. L. (1983). Seconday mania as a presentation of progressive dialysis encephalopathy. *Journal of Nervous and Mental Disease, 171,* 193–195.

Jamieson, R. C., & Wells, C. E. (1979). Manic psychosis in a patient with multiple metastic brain tumors. *Journal of Clinical Psychiatry, 40,* 280–282.

Jeeves, M. A., & Dixon, N. F. (1970). Hemispheric differences in response rates to visual stimuli. *Psychonomic Science, 20*, 249–251.

Johnson, T. N., Rosvold, H. E., & Mishkin, M. (1968). Projections of behaviorally defined sectors of the prefrontal cortex to the basal ganglia, septum, and diencephalon of the monkey. *Experimental Neurology, 21*, 20–34.

Jones, B., & Mishkin, M. (1972). Limbic lesions and the problem of stimulus-reinforcement associations. *Experimental Neurology, 36*, 362–377.

Jones, E. G., Coulter, J. D., & Hendry, S. H. C. (1978). Intracortical connectivity of architectonic fields in the somatic sensory, motor, and parietal cortex of monkeys. *Journal of Comparative Neurology, 181*, 291–348.

Jones, E. G., & Powell, T. P. S. (1970). An anatomical study of converging sensory pathways within the cerebral cortex of the monkey. *Brain, 93*, 793–820.

Joseph, R. (1982). The neuropsychology of development: Hemispheric laterality, limbic language, and the origin of thought. *Journal of Clinical Psychology, 44*, 3–33.

Joseph, R. (1986a). Confabulation and delusional denial: Frontal lobe and lateralized influences. *Journal of Clinical Psychology, 42*, 845–860.

Joseph, R. (1988b). Reversal of dominance for language and emotion in a corpus callosotomy patient. *Journal of Neurology, Neurosurgery and Psychiatry, 49*, 628–634.

Joseph, R. (1988a). The right cerebral hemisphere: Emotion, music, visual–spatial skills, body-image, dreams and awareness. *Journal of Clinical Psychology, 44*, 630–673.

Joseph, R. (1988b). Dual mental functioning in a "split-brain" patient. *Journal of Clinical Psychology, 44*, 770–779.

Joseph, R. (1989). The limbic system. Emotion, laterality, unconscious mind. *The Psychoanalytic Review,*

Jurgens, U., & Muller-Preuss, P. (1977). Convergent projections of different limbic vocalization areas in the squirrel monkey. *Experimental Brain Research, 29*, 75–83.

Kaada, B. R. (1951). Somato-motor, autonomic and electrocorticographic responses to electrical stimulation of "rhinencephalon" and other structures in primates, cat, and dog. *Acta Physiologica Scandinavica, 83*, 1–285.

Kaada, B. R. (1972). Cingulate, posterior orbital, anterior insular and temporal pole cortex. In J. Field, H. W. Magoun, & V. A. Hall (Eds.), *Handbook of Physiology* (Vol. II, pp. 1345–1372). Washington, D.C.: American Physiological Society.

Kapur, N., & Coughlan, A. K. (1980). Confabulation and frontal lobe dysfunction. *Journal of Neurology, Neurosurgery and Psychiatry, 43*, 461–463.

Kennard, M. A. (1939). Alterations in response to visual stimuli following lesions of frontal lobes in monkeys. *Archives of Neurology and Psychiatry, 41*, 1153–1165.

Kennard, M. A. (1955). Effects of bilateral ablation of cingulate area on behavior in cats. *Journal of Neurophysiology, 18*, 159–169.

Kennard, M. A., Spencer, S., & Fountain, G. (1941). Hyperactivity in monkeys following lesions of the frontal lobes. *Journal of Neurophysiology, 4*, 512–522.

Kling, A., & Mass, R. (1974). Alterations of social behavior with neural lesions in nonhuman primates. In B. Holloway (Ed.), *Primate aggression, territoriality, and zenophobia* (pp. 361–386). Orlando, FL: Academic Press.

Kling, A., & Steklis, H. D. (1976). A neural substrate for affiliative behavior in nonhuman primates. *Brain Behavior and Evolution, 13*, 216–238.

Knight, R. T., Hillyard, S. A., Woods, D. L., & Neville, H. J. (1981). The effects of frontal cortex lesions on event-related potentials during auditory selective attention. *Electroencephalography and Clinical Neurophysiology, 52*, 571–582.

Knuzle, H., & Akert, K. (1977). Efferent connections of cortical area 8 (frontal eye field). *Journal of Comparative Neurology, 173*, 147–164.

Kolb, B., Nonneman, A. J., & Singh, R. J. (1974). Double dissociation of spatial impairments and perseveration following selective prefrontal lesions in rats. *Journal of Comparative and Physiological Psychology, 87*, 772–780.

Kolb, B., & Whishaw, I. Q. (1983). Performance of schizophrenic patients on tests sensitive to left or right frontal, temporal, or parietal function in neurological patients. *Journal of Nervous and Mental Disease, 171*, 435–443.

Kramer, H. C. (1954). Laughing spells in patients after lobotomy. *Journal of Nervous and Mental Disease, 140*, 517–522.

Krettek, J. E., & Price, J. L. (1974). A direct input from the amygdala to the thalamus and the cerebral cortex. *Brain Research, 67*, 169–174.

Kuypers, H. G. J. M. (1958). Corticobulbar connexions to the pons and lower brain stem in man. *Brain, 81*, 364–388.

Kuypers, H. G. J. M., & Catsman-Berrevoets, C. E. (1984). Frontal corticosubcortical projections and their cells of origin. In F. Reinoso-Suarez & C. Ajmone-Marsan (Eds.), *Cortical integration* (pp. 171–194). New York: Raven Press.

Langworthy, O. R., & Richter, C. P. (1939). Increased activity produced by frontal lobe lesions in cats. *American Journal of Physiology, 126*, 158–161.

Laplane, D., Degos, J. D., Baulac, M., & Gray, F. (1981). Bilateral infarction of the anterior cingulate gyri and of the fornices. *Journal of Neurological Sciences, 51*, 289–300.

Laplane, D., Talairach, J., Meininger, V., Bancaud, J., & Orgogozo, J. M. (1977). Clinical consequences of cortisectomies involving the supplementary motor area in man. *Journal of the Neurological Sciences, 34*, 301–314.

Latto, R., & Cowey, A. (1971a). Fixation changes after frontal eye-field lesions in monkeys. *Brain Research, 30*, 25–36.

Latto, R., & Cowey, A. (1971b). Visual field defect after frontal eye field lesions in monkeys. *Brain Research, 30*, 1–24.

Leichnetz, G. R., & Astruc, J. (1976). The different projections of the medical prefrontal cortex in the squirrel monkey *(Saimiri sciureus)*. *Brain Research, 109*, 455–472.

Lesser, R. P., Lueders, H., Dinner, D. S., Hahn, J., & Cohen, L. (1984). The location of speech and writing function in the frontal language area. *Brain, 107*, 275–291.

Levin, S. (1984). Frontal lobe dysfunction in schizophrenia. I and II. *Journal of Psychiatric Research, 18*, 27–55, 57–72.

Levine, D. N., & Sweet, E. (1982). The neuropathologic basis of Broca's aphasia and its implications for the cerebral control of speech. In M. Arbib, D. Caplan, & J. Marshall (Eds.), *Neural models of language processes*. Orlando, FL: Academic Press.

Levine, D. N., & Sweet, E. (1983). Localization of lesions in Broca's motor aphasia. In A. Kertesz (Ed.), *Localization in neuropsychology*. Orlando, FL: Academic Press.

Lhermitte, F. (1983). "Utilization behaviour" and its relation to lesions of the frontal lobes. *Brain, 106*, 237–255.

Lineberry, C. G., & Siegel, J. (1971). EEG synchronization, behavioral inhibition, and mesencephalic unit effect produced by stimulation or orbital cortex, basal forebrain and caudate nucleus. *Brain Research, 34*, 143–161.

Lishman, W. A. (1968). Brain damage in relation to psychiatric disability after head injury. *British Journal of Psychiatry, 114*, 373–410.

Lishman, W. A. (1973). The psychiatric sequelae of head injury: A review. *Psychological Medicine, 3*, 304–318.

Livingston, R., Chapman, W., & Livingston, K. (1948). Stimulation of orbital surface of man prior to lobotomy. *Research publication: The frontal lobes* (pp. 421–433). Washington, D.C.: U.S. Government Printing Office.

Loiseau, P., Cohandon, F., & Cohandon, S. (1971). Gelastic epilepsy, a review and report of 5 cases. *Epilipsia, 12*, 313–320.

Luria, A. R. (1980). *Higher cortical function in man*. New York: Basic Books.

McFie, J. & Thompson, J. A. (1972). Picture arrangement: A measure of frontal lobe function? *British Journal of Psychiatry, 121*, 547–552.

McNabb, A. W., Carroll, W. M., & Mastaglia, F. L. (1988). "Alien hand" and loss of bimanual coordination after dominant anterior cerebral artery territory infarction. *Journal of Neurology, Neurosurgery and Psychiatry, 51*, 218–222.

Meyer, C., MacElhaney, M., Martin, W., & MacGraw, C. P. (1973). Stereotaxic cingulotomy with results of acute stimulation and serial psychological testing. In L. V. Laitinen, & K. E. Livingston (Eds.), *Surgical approaches to psychiatry* (pp. 38–57). Lancaster: Medical Publishing Co.

Mettler, F. A., Spindler, J., Mettler, C. C., & Combs, J. D. (1936). Disturbances in gastrointestinal function after localized ablations of cerebral cortex. *Archives of Surgery, 32*, 618–620.

Miller, B. L., Cummings, J. L., McIntyre, H., Ebers, G., & Grode, M. (1986). Hypersexuality or altered sexual preferences following brain injury. *Journal of Neurology, Neurosurgery and Psychiatry, 49,* 867–873.

Miller, L. (in press). Neuropsychology, personality and cognitive style. Toward a general theory. *Psychoanalytic Review.*

Milner, B. (1964). Some effects of frontal lobectomy in man. In J. M. Warren & K. Akert (Eds.), *The frontal granular cortex and behavior* (pp. 313–334). New York: McGraw-Hill.

Milner, B. (1971). Interhemispheric differences in the localization of psychological process in man. *British Medical Bulletin, 27,* 272–277.

Mishkin, M. (1964). Perseveration of central sets after frontal lesions in monkeys. In J. M. Warren & K. Akert (Eds.), *The frontal granular cortex and behavior* (pp. 219–241). New York: McGraw-Hill.

Mishkin, M., & Pribram, K. H. (1956). Analysis of the effects of frontal lesion in monkeys. II. Variation of delayed response. *Journal of Comparative and Physiological Psychology, 49,* 36–40.

Myers, R. E., Swett, C., & Miller, M. (1973). Loss of social group affinity following prefrontal lesions in free-ranging macaques. *Brain Research, 64,* 257–269.

Nichols, I., & Hunt, J. McV. (1940). A case of partial bilateral frontal lobectomy. *American Journal of Psychiatry, 96,* 1063–1087.

Novoa, O. P., & Ardila, A. (1987). Linguistic abilities in patients with prefrontal damage. *Brain and Language, 30,* 206–225.

Ojemann, G. A., & Whitaker, H. A. (1978). Linaguage localization and variability. *Brain and Language, 6,* 239–260.

Oppler, W. (1950). Manic psychosis in a case of parasagital meningioma. *Archives of Neurology and Psychiatry, 47,* 417–430.

Orgogozo, J. M., & Larsen, B. (1979). Activation of the supplementary motor area during voluntary movement in man suggest it works as a supramodal motor area. *Science, 206,* 847–850.

Oscar-Berman, M. (1975). The effects of dorsolateral–frontal and ventrolateral orbitofrontal lesions on spatial-discrimination learning and delayed response in two modalities. *Neuropsychologia, 13,* 237–246.

Pandya, D. N., & Kuypers, H. G. J. M. (1969). Corticocortial connections in the rhesus monkey. *Brain Research, 13,* 13–16.

Pandya, D. N., & Vignolo, L. A. (1971). Intra and interhemispheric projections of the precentral premotor and arcuate areas in the rhesus monkey. *Brain Research, 26,* 217–233.

Partridge, M. (1950). *Pre-frontal leucotomy. A survey of 300 cases personally followed over 1 and ½–3 years.* Oxford: Blackwell.

Passingham, R. E. (1981). Broca's area and the origins of human vocal skills. *Philosophical Transactions of the Royal Society of London (Biology), 292,* 167–175.

Pechtel, C., McAvoy, T., Levitt, M., Kloing, A., & Masserman, J. H. (1958). The cingulate and behavior. *Journal of Nervous and Mental Disease, 126,* 148–152.

Penfield, W., & Jasper, H. (1954). *Epilepsy and the functional anatomy of the human brain.* Boston: Little-Brown.

Penfield, W., & Rasmussen, T. (1950). *The cerebral cortex of man: A clinical study of localization of function.* New York: Macmillan.

Penfield, W., & Roberts, L. (1959). *Speech and brain mechanisms.* Princeton: Princeton University Press.

Penfield, W., & Welch, K. (1951). Supplementary motor area of cerebral cortex. Clinical and experimental study. *Archives of Neurology and Psychiatry, 66,* 289–317.

Perris, C. (1974). Averaged evoked responses (AER) in patients with affective disorders. *Acta Psychiatrica Scandinavica, 225,* 1–107.

Petrides, M., & Milner, N. (1982). Deficits on subject-ordered tasks after frontal temporal lobe lesions in man. *Neuropsychologia, 20,* 249–262.

Petrie, A. (1952). *Personality and the frontal lobes.* New York: Blakiston.

Pietro, M. J. S., & Rigdrodsky, M. S. (1986). Patterns of oral-verbal perseveration in adult aphasics. *Brain and Language, 29,* 1–17.

Porteus, S. D., & Peters, H. N. (1947). Psychosurgery and test validity. *Journal of Abnormal (Social) Psychology, 42,* 473–488.

Powell, E. W. (1978). The cingulate bridge between allocortex, isocortex, and thalamus. *Anatomical Records, 190,* 783–794.

Powell, E. W., Akagi, K., & Hatton, J. B. (1974). Subcortical projections of the cingulate gyrus in the cat. *Journal de Hirnforsch, 15*, 269–278.

Pragay, E. B., Mirskey, A. F., & Nakamura, R. K. (1987). Attention-related activity in the frontal association cortex during a go/no-go discrimination task. *Experimental Neurology, 96*, 841–500.

Pribram, K. H., Ahumada, A., Hartog, J., & Ross, L. A. (1964). A progress report on the neurological processes disturbed by frontal lesions in primates. In J. M. Warrent & K. Akert (Eds.), *The frontal granular cortex and behavior* (pp. 28–55). New York: McGraw-Hill.

Pribram, K. H., Chow, K. L., & Semmes, J. (1953). Limit and organization of the cortical projections from the medial thalamic nucleus in the monkey.*Journal of Comparative Neurology, 98*, 433–448.

Reitman, F. (1946). Orbital cortex syndrome following leucotomy. *American Journal of Psychiatry, 103*, 238–241.

Reitman, F. (1947). Observations of personality changes after leucotomy. *Journal of Nervous and Mental Disease, 105*, 582–589.

Richfield, E. K., Twyman, T., & Berent, S. (1987). Neurological syndrome following bilateral damage to the head of the caudate nuclei. *Annals of Neurology, 22*, 768–771.

Rinkel, M., Greenblatt, M., Coon, G. P., & Solomon, H. C. (1950). Relations of the frontal lobe to autonomic nervous system in man. In M. Greenblatt, M. Arnot, & H. C. Solomon (Eds.), *Studies in lobotomy*. Orlando, FL: Grune & Stratton.

Rinkel, M., Solomon, H. C., Rosen, D., & Levine, J. (1950). Lobotomy and urinary bladder. In M. Greenblatt, M. Arnot, & H. C. Solomon (Eds.), *Studies in lobotomy*. Orlando, FL: Grune & Stratton.

Rizzolatti, G., Scandolara, C., Matelli, M., & Gentillucci, M. (1981*a*). Afferent properties of periacuate neurons in macaque monkeys. 1, 2. *Behavioral Brain Research, 2*, 125–146, 147–163.

Rizzolatti, G., Scandolara, C., Gentillucci, M., & Camarda, R., (1981*b*). Response properties and behavioral modulation of "mouth" neurons on the post-arcuate cortex (area 6) in macaque monkeys. *Brain Research, 225*, 421–424.

Robinson, B. W. (1967). Vocalization evoked from forebrain in macaca mulatta. *Physiology and Behavior, 2*, 345–352.

Robinson, R. G., & Benson, D. F. (1981). Depression in aphasic patients: Frequency severity and clinical-pathological correlations *Brain and Language, 14*, 282–291.

Robinson, R. G., Kubos, K. L., Starr, L. B., Rao, K., & Price, T. R. (1984). Mood disorders in stroke patients. *Brain, 107*, 81–93.

Robinson, R. R., & Szetela, B. (1981). Mood change following left hemisphere brain injury. *Annals of Neurology, 9*, 447–453.

Roland, P. E., Skinhoj, E., Lassen, N. A., & Larsen, B. (1980). Different cortical areas in man in organization of voluntary movements in extrapersonal space. *Journal of Neurophysiology, 43*, 137–150.

Rose, A. S. (1950). Postoperative behavior. In M. Greenblatt, M. Arnot, & H. C. Solomon (Eds.), *Studies in lobotomy*. Orlando, FL: Grune & Stratton.

Rosenbaum, A. H., & Berry, M. J. (1975). Positive therapeutic response to lithium in hypomania secondary to organic brain syndrome. *American Journal of Psychiatry, 132*,1072–1073.

Rosenkilde, C. E. (1979). Functional heterogeneity of the prefrontal cortex in the monkey: A review. *Behavioral and Neural Biology, 25*, 301–345.

Ross, E. D. (1981). The aprosodias. Functional–anatomic organization of the affective components of language in the right hemisphere. *Archives of Neurology, 38*, 561–569.

Ross, E. D., & Mesulam, M. M. (1979). Dominant language functions of the right hemisphere? Prosody and emotional gesturing. *Archives of Neurology, 36*, 144–148.

Rossi, G. F., & Brodal, A. (1956). Corticofugal fibers to the brain stem reticular formation. *Journal of Anatomy, 90*,42–62.

Rothwell, J. C., Thompson, P. D., Day, B. L., Dick, J. P. R., Kachi, T., Cowan, J. M. A., & Marsden, C. D. (1987). Motor cortex stimulation in intact man. *Brain, 110*, 1173–1190.

Ruch, T. C., & Shenkin, H. A. (1943). The relationship of area 13 on the orbital surface of the frontal lobes to hyperactivity and hyperphagia. *Journal of Neurophysiology, 6*, 349–360.

Rylander, G. (1939). Personality changes after operation on the frontal lobes. A clinical study of 32 cases. *Acta Psychiatrica et Neurologica, 20* (Suppl. XX), 3–327.

Rylander, G. (1948). Personality analysis before and after frontal lobotomy. *Research Publication of the Association of Nervous and Mental Disease, 27*, 691–700.

Samuels, J. A., & Benson, D. F. (1979). Some aspects of language comprehension in anterior aphasia. *Brain and Language, 8,* 275–286.

Sandson, J., & Albert, M. L. (1987). Perseveration in behavioral neurology. *Neurology, (New York), 37,* 1736–1741.

Sanides, F. (1972). Representation in cerebral cortex. In G. H. Bourne (Ed.), *The structure and function of nervous tissue* (Vol. 5, pp. 329–453). Orlando: FL: Academic Press.

Sauerland, E. K., Nakamura, Y., & Clemente, C. D. (1967). The role of the lower brain stem in cortically induced inhibition of somatic reflexes in the cat. *Brain Research, 6,* 164–180.

Scheibel, M. E., & Scheibel, A. B. (1966). Patterns of organization in specific and nonspecific thalamic fields. In D. P. Papura & M. D. Yahr (Eds.), *The thalamus* (pp. 13–46). New York: Columbia University Press.

Segraves, M. A., & Goldberg, M. E. (1987). Functional properties of corticotectal neurons in the monkey's frontal eye field. *Journal of Neurophysiology, 58,* 1387–1418.

Shapiro, B. E., Alexander, M. P., Gardner, H., & Mercer, S. (1981). Mechanisms of confabulations. *Neurology, (New York), 31,* 1070–1076.

Siegel, A., Fukushima, T., Meibach, R., Burke, L., Edinger, H., & Weiner, S. (1977). The origin of the afferent supply to the mediodorsal thalamic nucleus: Enhanced HRP transport by selective lesions. *Brain Research, 135,* 11–23.

Siegel, J., & Wang, R. Y. (1974). Electroencephalographic, behavioral, and single unit activity produced by stimulation of forebrain inhibitory structures in cats. *Experimental Neurology, 42,* 28–50.

Sinyour, D., Jacques, P., Kaloupek, D. G., Becker, R., Goldenberg, M., & Coopersmith, H. (1986). Poststroke depression and lesion location. *Brain, 109,* 537–546.

Skinner, J. E., & Yingling, C. D. (1977). Central gating mechanisms that regulate event related potentials and behavior. In J. Desmedt (Ed.), *Attention, voluntary contraction, and event related cerebral potentials* (pp. 30–69). Basel, S. Karger.

Smith, A. (1966). Intellectual functions in patients with lateralized frontal tumors. *Journal of Neurology, Neurosurgery and Psychiatry, 29,* 52–59.

Smith, W. K. (1944). The results of ablation of the cingular region of the cerebral cortex. *Federal Proceedings, 3,* 42–55.

Spencer, S. S., Spencer, D. D., Williamson, P. D., & Mattson, R. H. (1983). Sexual automatisms in complex partial seizures. *Neurology (New York), 33,* 527–533.

Squire, L. (1987). *Memory and brain.* New York: Oxford University Press.

Stamm, J. S., & Rosen, S. C. (1973). The locus and crucial time of implication of prefrontal cortex in the delayed response task. In K. H. Pribram & A. R. Luria (Eds.), *Psychophysiology of the frontal lobes* (pp. 139-153). Orlando, FL: Academic Press.

Starkstein, S. E., Pearlson, G. E., Boston, J., & Robinson, R. G. (1987). Mania after brain injury. *Archives of Neurology, 44,* 1069–1073.

Stepien, I., & Stamm, J. S. (1970). Impairments on locomotor tasks involving spatial opposition between cue and reward frontally ablated monkeys. *Acta Neurobiologica Experimentalis, 30,* 1–12.

Steriade, M. (1964). Development of evoked responses and self-sustained activity within amygdalo-hippocampal circuits. *Electroencephalography and Clinical Neurophysiology, 16,* 221–231.

Stern, K., & Dancey, T. (1942). Glioma of the diencephalon in a manic patient. *American Journal of Psychiatry, 98,* 716.

Strom-Olsen, J. (1946). Discussion on prefrontal leucotomy with reference to indication and results. *Proceedings of the Royal Society of Medicine, 39,* 443–444.

Stuss, D. T., Alexander, M. P., Lieberman, A., & Levine, H. (1978). An extraordinary form of confabulation. *Neurology (New York), 28,* 1166–1172.

Stuss, D. T., & Benson, F. (1984). Neuropsychological studies of the frontal lobes. *Psychological Bulletin, 95,* 3–28.

Tanji, J., & Kurata, K. (1982). Comparison of movement-related neurons in two cortical motor areas of primates. *Journal of Neurophysiology, 40,* 644–653.

Tanji, J., Tanguchi, K., & Saga, T. (1980). Supplementary motor area: Neuronal response to motor instructions. *Journal of Neurophysiology, 43,* 60–68.

Teuber, H. L. (1964). The riddle of frontal lobe function in man. In J. M. Warren & Akert (Eds.), *The frontal granular cortex and behavior* (pp. 410–477). New York: McGraw-Hill.

Tow, P. M. (1955). *Personality changes following frontal leucotomy.* New York: Oxford University Press.

Tow, P. M., & Whitty, C. W. M. (1953). Personality changes after operations of the cingulate gyrus in man. *Journal of Neurology, Neurosurgery and Psychiatry, 16,* 186–193.

Tramo, M. J., Baynes, K., & Volpe, B. T. (1988). Impaired syntactic comprehension and production in Broca's aphasia: CT lesion localization and recovery patterns. *Neurology (New York), 38,* 95–98.

Travis, A. M. (1955). Neurological deficiencies following supplementary motor area lesions in macaca mulatta. *Brain, 78,* 174–198.

Tucker, D. M. (1981). Lateral brain, function, emotion, and conceptualization. *Psychological Bulletin, 89,* 19–46.

Tucker, D. M., Stenslie, C. E., Roth, R. S., & Shearer, S. L. (1981). Right frontal lobe activation and right hemisphere performance: decrement during a depressed mood. *Archives of General Psychiatry, 38,* 169–174.

Updyke, B. V. (1975). The patterns of projection of cortical areas 17, 18, 19, onto the laminae of the dorsal lateral geniculate nucleus of the cat. *Journal of Comparative Neurology, 163,* 377–396.

Van Buren, J. M., & Fedio, P. (1976). Functional representation on the medial aspect of the frontal lobes in man. *Journal of Neurosurgery, 44,* 275–289.

Van Hoessen, G. E., Pandya, D. N., & Butters, N. (1975). Some connections of the entorhinal (area 28) and perirhinal (area 35) cortices of the rhesus monkey. *Brain Research, 95,* 25–38.

Victor, M., Adams, R. E., & Collins, G. H. (1971). *The Wernicke-Korasakoff syndrome.* Philadelphia: F. A. Davis.

Wagman, I. H., Krieger, H. P., Papetheodorou, C. A., & Bender, M. B. (1961). Eye movements elicited by surface and depth electrode stimulation of the frontal lobe of Macaca mulatta. *Journal of Comparative Neurology, 117,* 179–188.

Wall, P. D., & Davis, G. D. (1951). Three cerebral cortical systems affecting autonomic function. *Journal of Neurophysiology, 14,* 507–517.

Walker, A. E. (1940). The medial thalamic nucleus: A comparative anatomical, physiological, and clinical study. *Journal of Comparative Neurology, 73,* 87–115.

Ward, C. D. (1988). Transient feelings of compulsion caused by hemispheric lesions: Three cases. *Journal of Neurology, Neurosurgery, and Psychiatry, 51,* 266–268.

Watson, R. T., Fleet, S., Gonzalez-Rothi, L., & Heilman, K. M. (1986). Apraxia and the supplementary motor area. *Archives of Neurology, 43,* 787–792.

Watts, J. W., & Fulton, J. F. (1934). Intussuseption—The relation of the cerebral cortex to intestinal motility in the monkey. *New England Journal of Medicine, 210,* 883–890.

Weinrich, M., Wise, S. P., & Mauritz, K. H. (1984). A neurophysiological study of the premotor cortex in rhesus monkey. *Brain, 107,* 385–414.

Welch, K., & Stuteville, P. (1958). Experimental production of unilateral neglect in monkeys. *Brain, 81,* 341–347.

Whitlock, D. G., & Nauta, W. J. H. (1956). Subcortical projections from the temporal neurocortex in *Macaca mulatta. Journal of Comparative Neurology, 106,* 183–212.

Whitty, C. W., & Lewin, W. (1957). Vivid day dreaming—An unusual form of confusion following anterior cingulectomy. *Brain, 80,* 72–76.

Whitty, C. W., & Lewin, W. (1960). A Korsakoff syndrome in the post cingulectomy confusional state. *Brain, 83,* 648–653.

Wilcott, R. C. (1974). Skeletal and autonomic inhibition from low frequency electrical stimulation of the cat's brain. *Neuropsychologia, 12,* 487–495.

Wilcott, R. C. (1977). Electrical stimulation in the prefrontal cortex and delayed response in the cat. *Neuropsychologia, 15,* 115–121.

Wilkins, A. J., Shallice, T., & McCarthy, R. (1987). Frontal lesions and sustained attention. *Neuropsychologia, 25,* 359–365.

Woolsey, C. N. (1958). Organization of somatic sensory and motor area of the cerebral cortex. In H. F. Harlow & C. N. Woolsey (Eds.), *Biological and biochemical bases of behavior* (pp. 63–81). Madison WI: University of Wisconsin Press.

Wurtz, R. H. Goldberg, M. E., & Robinson, D. L. (1980). Behavioral modulation of visual response in the monkey. In J. M. Sprague & A. N. Epstein (Eds.), *Progress in psychobiology and physiological psychology.* Orlando, FL: Academic Press.

Yarcorzynski, G. K., & Davis, L. (1942). Modifications of perceptual responses with unilateral lesions of the frontal lobes. *Transactions of the American Neurological Association, 68,* 122–130.

Yingling, C. D., & Skinner, J. E. (1977). Gating of thalamic input to cerebral cortex by nucleus reticular is thalami. In J. Desmedt (Ed.), *Attention, voluntary contraction and event related cerebral potentials* (pp. 70–96). Basel: S. Karger.

The Parietal Lobes

The parietal lobe is commonly thought to be concerned predominantly with processing of somesthetic, kinesthetic, and proprioceptive information. Like the large expanse of tissue in the frontal portion of the brain, however, the parietal lobes are not homologous tissue but consist of cells that are responsive to a variety of divergent stimuli, including movement, hand position, objects within grasping distance, audition, eye movement, as well as complex and motivationally significant visual stimuli. Damage to the parietal lobe can therefore result in a variety of disturbances, which include abnormalities involving somesthetic sensation, the body image, visual–spatial relations, temporal–sequential motor activity, language, grammar, numerical calculation, emotion, and attention, depending on which area has been lesioned, as well as the laterality of the damage.

PARIETAL TOPOGRAPHY

The parietal lobe may be subdivided into a primary receiving area (involving Brodmann's areas 3,1,2) within the postcentral gyrus, an immediately adjacent somesthetic association area (Brodmann's area 5), a polymodal (visual, motor, somesthetic) receiving area located in the superior–posterior parietal lobule (area 7), and a multimodal–assimilation area within the inferior parietal lobule (areas 7, 39, and 40) that encompasses the angular and supramarginal gyrus.

The primary somesthetic, as well as portions of the association area, contribute almost one third of the fibers, which make up the corticospinal (pyramidal) tract. Thus, this region is clearly involved in motor functioning. Moreover, the primary motor and somesthetic regions are richly interconnected (Jones & Powell, 1970). This is because, in order to make motoric responses with some precision, there must be tremendous sensory feedback concerning proprioception, the positions of the various joints and tendons, and other information provided by the somesthetic cortices. Together, the motor and somesthetic areas comprise a single functional unit that some have referred to as the sensorimotor cortex (Luria, 1980).

THE PRIMARY SOMESTHETIC RECEIVING AREAS

There are two main pathways through which somesthetic information reach the parietal lobule. These are the lemniscal and spinothalamic projections systems, both of which terminate in the thalamus, where the information is then relayed to the somatosensory primary receiving area (Broadmann's area 3). Via these pathways, the entire body surface comes to be spatially represented in the cortex. However, body parts are represented in terms of their sensory importance, i.e., how richly the skin is innervated. For example, more cortical space is devoted to the representation of the fingers and the hand than to the elbow. Because of this, the cortical body map is very distorted. Almost all the cells in area 3 receive input only from the contralateral half of the body; thus, only half the body is represented.

The primary receiving areas for somesthesis continues up and over the top of the hemisphere and runs along the medial wall where the lower half of the body is represented. Specifically, the rectum, genitals, foot, and calf are located along the medial wall, the leg along the superior surface of the hemisphere, and the shoulder, arm, hand, and then face along the lateral convexity (Penfield & Jasper, 1954; Penfield & Rasmussen, 1950). The hand, however, is particularly well represented (Warren, Hamalainen, & Gardner, 1986).

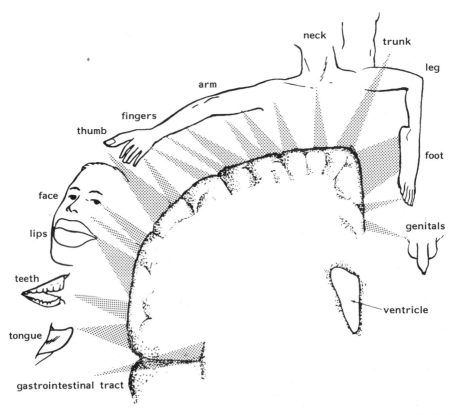

FIGURE 41. The sensory homunculus of the somesthetic cortex. From *Physiological psychology* by P. M. Milner, 1970. Courtesy of Holt, Rinehart & Winston, Inc., New York.

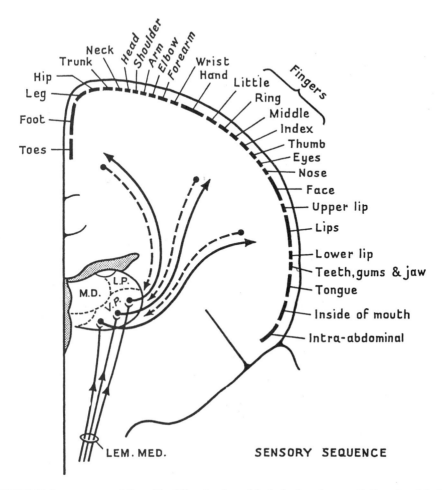

FIGURE 42. Sensory representation of the different regions of the body along the somesthetic cortex of the left hemisphere. The afferent pathways for discriminative somatic sensation are indicated by the unbroken lines. From *Brain's clinical neurology* by R. Bannister, 1975. Courtesy of Oxford University Press, New York.

Nevertheless, it is predominantly elementary and simple contralateral somesthetic information that is processed in this region (Figs. 41–43). Electrical stimulation of the primary somesthetic area gives rise to simple, albeit well localized sensations on the opposite half of the body (Penfield & Jasper, 1954; Penfield & Rasmussen, 1950) such as numbness, pressure, tingling, itching, tickling and warmth.

Information received and processed in area 3 is relayed to the immediately adjacent areas 2 and 1, each of which also contains a specialized spatial map of the body (Kaas, Nelson, Sur, & Merzenich, 1981; Sur, Nelson, & Kaas, 1982). Specifically, area 3 appears to maintain a cutaneous map and can also signal muscle length (e.g., flexion or extension), whereas area 2 maintains a map of the joint receptors and can signal the position and posture of the limbs based on input from the muscle spindles. Area 1 appears to maintain an overlapping cutaneous joint-body map (Evarts, 1969; Mountcastle & Powell, 1959; Schwartz, Deecke, & Fredrickson, 1973). Thus a considerable amount of processing occurs here.

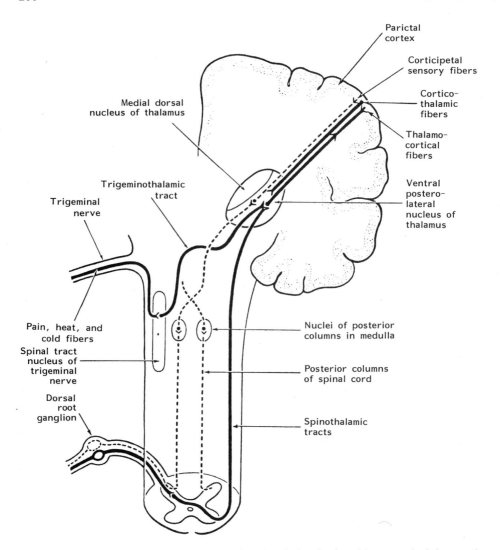

FIGURE 43. The principal sensory pathways leading from the spinal cord and cranial nerves to the thalamus and somesthetic cortex. From *Brain's clinical neurology* by R. Bannister, 1975. Courtesy of Oxford University Press, New York.

Moreover, within this tiny expanse of tissue, there is a sequential hierarchical convergence of input from areas 3 to 1, onto area 2. That is, information is analyzed and then passed from area 3 to 1 and from 3 and 1 onto area 2. Indeed, a single neuron in area 2 receiving multiple input from several cells in area 3, as well as vestibular input. Together these three strips of tissue comprise an interactional functional unit.

Cells in these three distinct, albeit primary receiving areas are responsive to touch, texture, shape, motion, and the direction of stimulus movement, including temporal–sequential patterning, and can directly monitor the position and movement of the extremities (Levitt & Levitt, 1968; Mountcastle, 1957; Warren, Hamalainen, & Gardner, 1986*a,b;* Whitsel, Roppolo, & Werner, 1972). In this manner, we can detect an insect crawling up or down our leg and the direction in which it is moving, as well as determine the position of our arms and legs without looking at them. Many cells are also responsive to changes in temperature as well as the presence of noxious stimuli applied to the skin.

Because most of these neurons receive input concerning pressure, light touch, the movement of joints, and muscular activity (Levitt & Levitt, 1968; Mountcastle, 1957), they can signal and determine whatever posture or position the body is in as well as the amount of force or pressure being exerted by the limbs (Jennings, Lamour, Solis, & Fromm, 1983), i.e., if carrying or lifting some object.

In summary, the primary receiving area receives very precise information regarding events occurring anywhere along the internal/external body and responds to converging inputs from muscle spindles, cutaneous and joint receptors, as well as proprioceptive and vestibular stimuli. In this manner, not only the body but the global properties of objects held in the hand can be determined (Iwamura & Tanaka, 1978), i.e., stereognosis.

Laterality

There is clear evidence that the right parietal areas is dominant in regard to most aspects of somesthetic information processing (as discussed in detail in Chapter 1). Thus, neurons in this half of the brain appear to be more sensitive and more responsive and to more greatly monitor events occurring on either half of the body, but particularly the left. In fact, this relationship was noted more than 150 years ago by Weber.

According to Weber (1834/1977), the left half of the body exceeds the right in regard to most forms of tactual sensitivity. The left hand and the soles of the left foot, as well as the left shoulder are more accurate in judging weight, have a more delicate sense of touch and temperature, such that "a greater sense of cold or of heat is aroused in the left hand" (p. 322). That is, the left hand judges warm substances to be hotter and cold material to be colder, as compared with the right hand, even when both hands are stimulated simultaneously.

Lesions

Surgical or other forms of destruction involving the primary somesthetic receiving areas results in a complete, albeit temporary loss of sensation from the entire half of the body (Russell, 1945). Longer-term effects include elevation of detection thresholds, loss of position and pressure sense, including two-point discrimination, and a greatly reduced ability to detect movement of the fingers. In addition, the capacity to determine texture, shape, temporal–sequential patterning, or to recognize objects by touch or to discriminate among different forms or their properties (e.g., size, texture, length, shape, and stereognosis) is significantly attenuated (Corkin, Milner, & Rasmussen, 1970; Curtis, Jacobsen, & Marcus, 1972; LaMotte & Mountcastle, 1979; Randolf & Semmes, 1974). Passive (nonmovement) sensation is less impaired. In some instances, however, over time a remarkable recovery of somesthetic discrimination sense may be observed (Semmes, 1973).

Nevertheless, even with complete removal of the postcentral gyrus, stimuli applied to the face are much better perceived as compared with the same stimuli applied to the hand. Conversely, lesions that spare the hand area of the postcentral gyrus, but that destroy the remaining tissue, will result in mild or no permanent sensory deficits when the hands are tested, with the exception of stereognosis (Semmes, 1965). However, sensation across other body parts will be impaired. Therefore, when testing for parietal lobe dysfunction, not only the face and hands, but other body parts should be examined.

This region is also highly concerned with motor functioning, as it is extensively interconnected with the primary motor area and gives rise to almost one third of the corticospinal tract. Damage to this region can give rise to motor disturbances, such as paresis accompanied by hypotonia, and/or produce inaccuracy and reduced speed of movement (Cole & Glees, 1954; Luria, 1980). The ability (or will) to initiate movement may also be reduced.

THE SOMESTHETIC ASSOCIATION AREA

In addition to receiving information already analyzed in the immediately adjacent primary somesthetic cortices, some cells in the association area (Brodmann's area 5) also receive input from the contralateral primary zone (via the corpus callosum) as well as from the motor association areas (area 6) in the frontal lobes (Jones & Powell, 1970); thus, both halves of the body, the trunkal area in particular (Robinson, 1973) come to be represented in this region. Indeed, the two halves of the body appear to be superimposed such that the body is bilaterally represented (Whitsel, Petrucelli, & Werner, 1969). However, as based on behavioral and electrophysiological data from intact and brain-damaged patients, bilateral representation is predominantly maintained within the right half of the brain.

Hand-Manipulation Cells

A small percentage of cells in the somesthetic association area also appear to be concerned with more complex activities such as the movement of the hand and arm and the manipulation of objects (Mountcastle et al., 1975). Indeed, a detailed representation of the cutaneous surface of the body, and in particular, the hand, is maintained in this area (Burton, Mitchell, & Brent, 1982). These are referred to as hand-manipulation cells. In fact, electrical stimulation of area 5 can result in limb movements (Hyvariene, 1982). Others are especially responsive to particular temporal–sequential patterns of sensation (LaMotte & Mountcastel, 1979) and can determine direction and rhythm of movement. It is presumably through the activity of these cells that one can "hear" by the detection of vibrations (such as reported by the deaf).

The Body in Space

Signals from joint and cutaneous receptors are transmitted to association neurons (Skata & Iwanura 1978). Many association cells also receive converging input from primary neurons concerned with different body parts (Sakata, Shibutani, & Kawano, 1973) and are thus able to determine positional interrelationships. For example, a single association neuron may receive information regarding the elbow and the shoulder and may become activated only when these two body parts are simultaneously stimulated or in motion. A considerable number of cells are especially sensitive to the posture and position of the trunk and extremities during movement (Hyvarienen, 1982). By associating this convergent input, these cells are able to monitor, coordinate, and guide limb movement as well as determine the position of the body in space.

Through the integrative and associative activities of the cell assemblies within area 5, an interactional image of the body is maintained. In this manner, an individual is able to ascertain the position of the body and the limbs at rest and in motion (Gross *et al.*, 1974). In part, this may be accomplished through comparisons with a more stable image of the body which is possibly maintained via the combined interactions of neurons in areas 3, 1, and 2. Thus, when the body has moved, this new information (received and processed in area 5) can be compared with the more stable trace (maintained in the primary regions), so that the new position of the limbs and body can be ascertained.

Nevertheless, to determine position, sensation per se is not sufficient. Rather, sensation must be combined with input regarding movement or positional change. It is for this reason that in the absence of movement (and in the absence of visual cues, such as when we wake up in the middle of the night) we sometimes cannot tell where or in what position our arms or legs may be in. However, with a slight movement, we can immediately determine position.

Lesions

Destruction of the somesthetic association area results in many of the same disturbances that occur following lesions of the primary region. This includes abnormalities involving two-point discrimination, position sense, and pressure sensitivity. However, the detection threshold is not altered (LaMotte & Mountcastle, 1979). For example, a patient may recognize touch but be unable to localize what part of the body has been stimulated. For example, one patient I examined who had had a right parietal stroke consistently made errors of localization, naming his elbow when I touched his leg and his shoulder when his wrist was touched; in fact he expressed considerable astonishment when I allowed him to open his eyes after each test so as to see where the stimulation was actually being applied.

In addition, although a patient may be able to recognize that he is holding something in his hand he may be unable to determine what it might be (astereognosis). In these later instances, however, the cortical area representing the hand must be compromised.

With small lesions involving only a particular part of the somesthetic cortex (e.g., the area representing the arm and shoulder), the deficit will be only manifested when the part of the body represented is examined. For example, the patient may be able to localize touch and determine the direction of a moving stimulus when it is applied to the hand, face, or leg but be unable to do so along the shoulder or arm if this area of the cortex has been compromised.

The laterality of the lesion is also important, right sided damage having more drastic effects on somesthesis and stereognostic functioning than left parietal lesions. In addition, although lesions to either parietal lobe can give rise to astereognosis (an inability to recognize objects tactually explored), lesions to the right parietal lobes are likely to give rise to bilateral abnormalities, whereas left parietal injuries generally effect only the right hand (Hom & Reitan, 1982). Nevertheless, astereognostic deficits require that the somesthetic area representing the hand (see below) be comprised (Roland, 1976).

Large lesions, however (extending into the posterior parietal lobe, area 7), also decrease the ability to perform size, roughness, weight and shape discriminations (Blum, Chow & Pribram, 1950; Denny-Brown & Chambers, 1958; Garcha, Ettlinger, & Mac-Cabel, 1982; Ridley & Ettlinger, 1975; Semmes & Turner, 1977).

Pain

In some instances, such as when the more inferior portion of area 5, or the supramarginal gyrus (Brodmann's area 40) has been destroyed, patients may demonstrate a lack of emotional responsiveness to painful stimuli, seem behaviorally indifferent, develop an increased pain threshold, tolerate pain for an unusually lengthy time period and fail to respond even to painful threat (Berkley & Parmer, 1974; Biemond, 1956; Geschwind, 1965; Hyvarinen, 1982; Schilder, 1935) particularly with right parietal destruction (Cubelli, Caselli, & Neri, 1984). However, this has been noted to occur when lesions to either hemisphere (Hecaen & Albert, 1978). Frequently, elementary sensation is intact, and the ability to differentiate, for example, between dull and sharp is retained. The deficit is usually bilateral.

Some researchers have claimed that the lesions sometimes involves the frontal-parietal cortex (Hecaen & Albert, 1978). However, the supramarginal gyrus of the inferior parietal lobule (Geschwind, 1965; Hyvarinen, 1982; Schilder, 1935) is the most likely candidate for this condition, particularly in that a second somesthetic area is located in this region as well as yet another image of the human body (Penfield & Rasmussen, 1950). In this regard, Schilder (1935), argued that the loss of reaction to pain is caused by disturbances in perception of body image. That is, the experience or threat of pain is no longer related to the body image. Geschwind, (1965), however, raises the possibility that this condition might be caused by disconnection from the limbic system. If this were the case, somesthetic (painful) sensation would no longer be assigned emotional significance. Loss of sensation or an inability to react to pain may also occur from subcortical lesions, especially within the thalamus.

AREA 7 AND THE SUPERIOR–POSTERIOR PARIETAL LOBULE

Polymodal Information Processing

Information processed and analyzed in the primary and association somesthetic areas is then transmitted to area 7 where polymodal analyses take place. Jones & Powell (1970) considered area 7 to be concerned with the highest levels of somesthetic integration. However, the posterior parietal region is concerned with much more that somesthesis, as it receives massive input from the visual receiving areas in the occipital and middle temporal lobe, motor and nonmotor areas in the lateral frontal convexity, as well as the inferior parietal lobule (Jones & Powell, 1970; Wall, Symonds, & Kaas, 1982). Cells in area 7 also have auditory receptive capacities, including the ability to determine sound location (Hyvarinen, 1982). Thus, area 7 is heavily involved in the analysis and integration of higher-order visual, auditory, and somesthetic information; single neurons often have quite divergent capabilities.

Three-Dimensional Analysis of Body–Spatial Interaction

A single neuron in this area, through the reception of converging input from the primary and association somesthetic regions, can monitor activities occurring in many different body parts simultaneously, such as the position and movement of the arms, trunk, and legs (Leinonen, Hyvarinen, Nyman, & Linnakoski, 1979). Through the reception of auditory and visual input, area 7 is thus also able to create a three-dimensional image of the body in space (Lynch, 1980).

Moreover, cells in this area not only receive information about body part interrelationships (such as is maintained by area 5), but the interaction of the body with external objects and events. Indeed, many cells in this vicinity become highly active when the hand is moved toward or while reaching for and/or manipulating objects (Mountcastle, Lynch, Georgopoulos, Sakata, & Acuna, 1975; Robinson, Goldberg & Stanton, 1978; Yin & Mountcastel, 1977). They also act to coordinate and guide whole-body positional movement through visual and auditory space.

As stated by Mountcastle, Motter, and Andersen, (1980), "the parietal lobe, together with the distributed system of which it is a central node, generates an internal neural construction of the immediately surrounding space, of the location and movements of objects within it in relationship to body position, and of the position and movements of the body in relation to that immediately surrounding space. The region appears in general to be concerned with continually updating information regarding the relationship between internal and external coordinant systems" (p. 522).

Visual–Spatial Properties

Cells in area 7 accomplish these interactions through the convergence of somesthetic information from area 5, visual input from the visual association areas, as well as the reception of vestibular signals (Hyvarinene, 1982; Kawano & Sasaki, 1984). Indeed, a considerable number of these neurons have quite large visual receptive fields, sometimes occupying a whole quadrant or hemifield or the entire visual (Robinson et al., 1978). However, the receptive visual fields of these neurons do not usually include the fovea and are more sensitive to objects in the periphery (Motter & Mountcastle, 1981). In this regard, these cells are not concerned with the identification of form, but rather with place and distance.

Because many of the neurons in area 7 receive highly processed visual (as well as limbic) input, including information regarding ocular movement and direction of gaze, they are responsive to, and can determine a variety of, visual-object qualities and interrelationships, such as motivational significance, direction of movement, distance, spatial location, figure-ground relationships, and depth, including the discrimination and determination of an object's three-dimensional position in space, (Andersen, Essick, & Siegel, 1985; Kawano, Sasaki, & Yamashita, 1984; Lynch, 1980; Sakata, Shibutani, & Kawano, 1978, 1980). They are largely insensitive to velocity or speed of movement. In addition, many cells respond most to stimuli within grasping distance, whereas others respond most to stimuli just beyond arms reach.

Neurons in this supramodal region are able to accomplish this by responding to somesthetic positional information provided by area 5, visual input from areas 18 and 19, and the midtemporal lobe, as well as from extraretinal signals regarding convergence and accommodation of the eyes, and the position and movement of the eyes while tracking. Indeed, electrical stimulation of this area elicits eye movements as well as convergence, accommodation, and pupil dilation (Jampel, 1960). By integrating these signals these cells are able to monitor and mediate eye movement and visual fixation, map out the three-dimensional positions of various objects in visual space, and determine the relationship of these objects to the body and to other objects.

Thus, the visual analysis performed by many of these cells is largely concerned with visual–spatial functions (Robinson *et al.,* 1978; Sakata *et al.,* 1980). In this regard, it is noteworthy that this area maintains extensive interconnections with two other regions highly concerned with visual functions and eye movements: the frontal eye fields and the superior colliculus (Jones & Powell, 1970; Kawamura, Sprague & Nimi, 1974; Knuenzle & Akert, 1977; Pandya & Kuypers, 1969) as well as areas 18 and 19 in the visual cortex (Jones & Powell, 1970).

Conversely, when this area is damaged, depth perception, figure-ground analysis, and the ability to tract objects or to manipulate objects correctly in space (e.g., constructional and manipulospatial skills) are compromised.

Visual Attention

Many neurons in area 7 can act so as to increase or decrease visual fixation, direct attention to objects of motivational significance, and promote the maintenance of visual grasp such that a moving object continues to be visually scanned and followed (Lynch *et al.,* 1977). Indeed, electrical stimulation of this area induces lateral eye movements.

By contrast, lesions to this area often disrupt attentional functioning, such that in the extreme (e.g., following a right parietal lesion), patients fail to attend to the left half not only of visual space, but to the left half of the body.

Motivational and Grasping Functions

A number of cells in area 7 have been described as exerting "Command" functions (Mountcastle, 1976; Mountcastle *et al.,* 1980), especially those located along the inferior lateral convexity. These cells are motivationally responsive, can direct visual attention, become excited when certain objects are within grasping distance and can motivate and guide hand movements, including the grasping and manipulation of specific objects (Hyvarinen & Poranene, 1974; Lynch *et al.,* 1977; Mountcastle, 1976). Most of these latter cells cease to fire when the object fixated upon is actually grasped, suggesting that they may be exerting some type of driving force or at least an alerting function so that objects of desire or of general (versus specific) interest will be attended to (Rolls, Perret, & Thorpe *et al.,* 1979).

It has been argued that many neurons in area 7 actually execute a matching function between the internal drive state of the subject and the object being attended. That is, by responding to signals transmitted from the limbic system, i.e. the cingulate gyrus (Mesulam, Van Hoesen, Pandya, & Geschwind, 1977), as well as the middle and inferior temporal lobe, these cells in turn direct visual attention to objects of potential interest and, when detected, act so as to maintain visual grasp (cf. Lynch *et al.*, 1977).

In other words, when an object is recognized as being of motivational significance (determined by the limbic system and visual form recognition neurons in the temporal lobe), this information is relayed to neurons in area 7. Although not concerned with form recognition, these cells will guide as well as monitor eye movement, so that the object of interest is fixated upon. These cells then exert motor command functions so that the hand is guided toward the object until it is grasped.

LESIONS AND LATERALITY

Attention and Visual Space

Lesions involving the superior, as well as the inferior parietal lobule (of which area 7 is part) and the parietal–occipital junction can greatly disturb the ability to make eye movements, maintain or shift visual attention, visually follow moving objects, and in the extreme result in oculomotor paralysis (Hecaen & De Ajuriaguerra, 1954). Right parietal lesions are associated with deficiencies involving depth perception and stereopsis, including the ability to determine location, distance, spatial orientation, and object size (Benton & Hecaen, 1970; Ratcliff & Davies-Jones, 1972). Visual-constructional abilities may also be compromised (see Cowey, 1981; Critchley, 1953), and many patients suffer from visual–spatial disorientation, appearing clumsy.

Patients with right parietal lesions show defective performance on line-orientation tasks (Warrington & Rabin, 1970; Benton, Hannay, & Varney, 1975), maze learning (Newcombe & Russell, 1969), the ability to discriminate between unfamiliar faces (Milner, 1968) or to select from the visual environment stimuli that are of importance (Critchley, 1953), whereas those with right parietal–occipital damage are deficient on tasks requiring detection of embedded figures (Russo & Vignolo, 1967).

Others may also have severe problems with dressing (e.g., dressing apraxia) and may become easily lost or disoriented even in their own homes. One patient I examined, who had sustained a gunshot wound involving predominantly the right superior posterior parietal area, was unable to find his way to and from his hospital room (although he had been an inpatient for more than 3 months) and on several occasions had difficulty finding his way out of the bathroom. Indeed, in one instance he was discovered feeling his way along the walls in an attempt to find the door.

Localization of Objects in Space

Patients with right parietal lesions perform defectively on visual localization tasks (Hannay, Varney, & Benson, 1976). However, Ratcliff and Davies-Jones (1976) found that the localization of stimuli within grasping distance is disrupted equally by lesions to the posterior region of either hemisphere. Hence, the right parietal lobe appears to play an important role in generalized localization, whereas the left exerts influences in regard to objects that may be directly grasped and manipulated.

Apraxia

Owing to the involvement of the parietal region in mediating hand, arm, and body movements in space (Lynch, Mountcastle, Talbot, & Yin, 1977), as well as temporal sequencing, damage to this vicinity can also result in apraxia such that patients have difficulty controlling or temporally sequencing the extremities. This is especially evident with left rather than right parietal injuries. Gross inaccuracies as well as clumsiness can also result when making reaching movements or in attempting to pick up small objects in visual space (see Lynch, 1980, for review). Tendon reflexes may be slowed, and hypotonia coupled with either a paucity of, or a slowness in, movement initiation, or both, may result with parietal lesions (Denny-Brown & Chambers, 1958; LaMotte & Acunam, 1978; Lynch, 1980). With left parietal damage there may result difficulty visually recognizing objects (agnosia), and left–right orientation may be grossly deficient.

Emotion

Some of the effects of lesions in this region also include altered emotional–motivational functioning, body and visual–spacial neglect, as well as clumsiness and visual–spatial disorganization. With massive right parietal lesions involving area 7, many patients are often initially hypokinetic and seem very passive, inattentive, unresponsive and take very little interest in their environment (Critchley, 1953; Heilman & Watson, 1977). Moreover, when their disabilities are pointed out (e.g., paresis, paralysis), they may seem indifferent or conversely euphoric (Critchley, 1953).

Area 7, as well as area 5 (and the inferior parietal lobule) receive auditory information (Hyvarinen, 1982; Roland *et al.,* 1977) and are capable of discerning the emotional–motivational significance of this input as well as differentiating between different vocal–emotional characteristics—especially right parietal neurons. When the right parietal region is damaged, patients not only seem unconcerned about their disability, but they may have difficulty perceiving and differentiating between different forms of emotional speech (Tucker, Watson, & Heilman, 1977).

THE INFERIOR PARIETAL LOBULE

Developmentally, of all cortical regions, the inferior parietal lobule is one of the last to mature functionally and anatomically (Blinkov & Glezer, 1968; Joseph & Gallagher, 1985; Joseph *et al.,* 1984). Thus many capacities mediated by this area (e.g., reading, calculation, the performance of reversible operations in space) are late to develop, appearing between the ages of 5 and 8.

Sitting at the junction of the temporal, parietal, and occipital lobes, the inferior region (which includes the angular and supramarginal gyri) has no strict anatomical boundaries, is partly coextensive with the posterior–superior temporal gyrus, and includes part of area 7. It maintains rich interconnections with the visual, auditory, and somesthetic associations areas, the superior colliculus through the pulvinar, the lateral geniculate nucleus of the thalamus, and massive interconnections with the frontal lobes, inferior temporal region, and other higher order assimilation areas throughout the neocortex (Bruce, Desimone, & Gross, 1986; Burton & Jones, 1976; Geschwind, 1965; Jones & Powell, 1970; Seltzer & Pandya, 1978; Zeki, 1974).

The Multimodal Assimilation Area

The inferior parietal lobule contains cells that are multimodally responsive, a single neuron simultaneously receiving highly processed somesthetic, visual, auditory, and movement-related input from the various association areas. Hence, many of the neurons in this area are multispecialized for simultaneously analyzing auditory, somesthetic, and spatial–visual associations, have visual receptive properties which encompass almost the entire visual field, and respond to visual stimuli of almost any size, shape, or form (Bruce, Desimone, & Gross, 1982, 1986; Hyvarinen & Shelepin, 1979).

Inferior parietal neurons are involved in the assimilation and creation of cross modal associations and act to increase the capacity for the organization, labeling and multiple categorization of sensorimotor and conceptual events (Geschwind, 1965). One can thus create visual, somesthetic, or auditory equivalents of objects, actions, feelings, and ideas, simultaneously, such as conceptualizing a chair as a word, visual object, or in regard to sensation, usage, and even price.

Language Capabilities

Because of it's involvement in functions such as those described above, one side effect of damage to the left angular gyrus, is a condition called anomia, i.e., severe word finding and confrontive naming difficulty. These patients have difficulty naming objects, describing, pictures, and so forth. Moreover, lesions involving the angular gyrus, or when damage occurs among the fiber pathways linking the left inferior parietal lobule with the visual cortex, pure-word blindness can also result. This is because of an inability to receive visual input from the left and right visual cortex and to transmit this information to Wernicke's area so that auditory equivalents may be called up. Such patients are thus unable to read and suffer from alexia.

Because the inferior parietal lobule also acts as a relay center, where information from Wernicke's region can be transmitted, through the arcuate fasciculus, to Broca's area (for expression) destructive lesions, particularly to the supramarginal gyrus of the left cerebral hemisphere can result in conduction aphasia (Benson, Sheremata, Bouchard, Segarram, Price, & Geschwind, 1973). Although comprehension would be intact and a patient would know what she wanted to say, she would be unable to say it. Nor would she be able to repeat simple statements, read out loud, or write to dictation. This is because Broca's area is disconnected from the posterior language zones.

Agraphia

It has been argued that the sensorimotor engrams necessary for the production and perception of written language are stored within the parietal lobule of the left hemisphere

(Strub & Geschwind, 1983). When lesioned, patients sometimes have difficulty writing and forming letters because of an inability to access these engrams (Strub & Geschwind, 1983; Vignolo, 1983), i.e., they suffer from agraphia, an inability to write. (This is discussed in detail in Chapter 2, The Left Cerebral Hemisphere.) Writing samples may be characterized by mispellings, letter omissions, distortions, temporal–sequential misplacements, and inversions (Kinsbourn & Warrington, 1964). Sometimes agraphia is accompanied by alexia, an inability to read (Benson & Geschwind, 1969; Hecaen & Kremin, 1977).

Lateralized Temporal–Sequential Functions

Because it is a recipient of so much information and aids the rest of the brain in various forms of analysis, one function of the inferior parietal lobe is to maintain track of input/output so that information may be organized appropriately in either a sequential (i.e., first, middle, last), or spatial framework. Thus, another side effect of lesions localized to the inferior parietal lobule is a disruption of visual–spatial functioning, temporal–sequencing ability (e.g., apraxia), as well as logic, grammar, and the capacity to perform calculations, depending on which hemisphere is compromised.

Patients with lesions involving the inferior–parietal–occipital border of either hemisphere may have difficulty carrying out spatial–sequential tasks. For example, drawing "a square beneath a circle and a triangle beneath a square" (Luria, 1980). Often they may draw the objects in the order described (i.e., square, circle, triangle, square). That is, they have difficulty in conceptualizing how to place the objects in relationship to each other.

Those with left inferior parietal lesions have trouble with more obvious sequential–grammatical relationships (Luria, 1980). For example, they may be unable to understand the question: "John is taller than Jim but shorter that Pete. Who is taller?" In part, this is not only a function of left parietal dysfunction but the right hemisphere's difficulty in dealing with temporal–sequential and grammatical relationships.

Because the right brain does not understand grammatical relationships, a sentence that starts with the name "John" is interpreted by the right parietal area as all about "John"; i.e., the first word of the sentence is understood by the right brain as the "agent," regardless of semantics or grammar (Chernigovaskaya & Deglin, 1986). In this manner, if presented with the sentence, "Give me the book after you give me the pencil," the right brain would respond to the order of presentation rather than to their grammatical relationship; the person would thus present the book, then the pencil. When left parietal input is abolished, proper temporal–sequential and grammatical programming/comprehension suffers.

APRAXIA

Sensory Guidance of Movement

The parietal lobe is highly concerned with the mediation of movement. The primary motor cortex extends well beyond area 4 and includes portions of the somatosensory regions, which in turn contribute almost one third of the fibers that make up the pyramidal tract. (See Chapter 4, The Frontal Lobes.) These areas are in fact richly interconnected (Jones & Powell, 1970). Together, the motor and somesthetic regions comprise a single functional unit, i.e., the sensorimotor cortex. Nevertheless, it is important to emphasize, as pointed out by Luria (1980) that every voluntary movement is in fact composed of a series of movements spatially organized in accordance with successively changing input from other modalities.

That is, in order for a movement to be correctly planned and carried out signals must be directed to the right muscle groups as based on efferent streams of visual, somesthetic, as well as auditory input. This includes information regarding the position of the body and limbs in space. Indeed, movement becomes extremely difficult without sensory feedback and guidance. Because of this, parietal lesions can result in unilateral paresis and even wasting (i.e., parietal wasting), hence the importance of the somesthetic cortex in guiding movement.

Although the entire parietal lobule makes important contributions, the inferior parietal lobule of the left hemisphere appears to be the central region of concern in regard to the performance of skilled temporal–sequential motor acts. This is because the motor engrams for performing these acts appear to be stored in the left angular and supramarginal gyri (Geschwind, 1965; Heilman, 1979). Presumably these engrams assist in programming the motor frontal cortex, where the actions are actually executed. However, the inferior parietal lobule in turn is dependent on input from the primary and association somesthetic areas.

There is some evidence of laterality in regard to all of the above; the right half of the brain may be more concerned with movement of the trunk and the lower extremities. This would include navigational movement through space, running, certain types of dancing, and actions requiring analysis of depth and balance. The left cerebral hemisphere exerts specialized influences on the upper extremities, including the control of certain types of complex, sequenced motor acts, such as those requiring alterations in the orientation and position of the upper limbs (Kimura, 1982).

Apraxic Abnormalities

If the left inferior parietal region is destroyed the patient loses the ability to perform actions in an appropriate temporal sequence or to even appreciate when they have been performed incorrectly. They may also be impaired in their ability to acquire or perform tasks involving sequential changes in the hand or upper musculature (Kimura, 1979, 1982), including well-learned, skilled, and even stereotyped motor tasks, such as lighting a cigarette or using a key. This condition is referred to as apraxia.

Apraxia is a disorder of skilled movement in the absence of impaired motor functioning or paralysis. Apraxic patients usually show the correct intent but perform the movements in a clumsy fashion. Like many other types of disturbances, patients and their families may not notice or complain or apraxic abnormalities. This is particularly true if they're aphasic or paralyzed on the right side. That is, clumsiness with either extremity may not seem significant. Thus, this is something that requires direct evaluation.

Performance deteriorates most significantly when the patient is required to imitate or pantomime certain actions, including the correct usage of some object. For example, the patient may be asked to show the examiner, "how you would use a key to open a door," or "hammer a nail into a piece of wood." In many cases, the patient may use the body, i.e., a finger, as an object (e.g., a key), rather than the finger and thumb holding the key. Although performance usually improves when they use the real objects (Geschwind, 1965; Goodglass & Kaplan, 1972), a rare few may show the disturbance when using the real object as well (Heilman, 1979).

In addition, patients with apraxia may demonstrate difficulty in properly sequencing their actions: they may pretend to stir a cup of coffee, pretend to pour the coffee into the cup, and then take a sip. However, each individual act may be performed accurately.

Broadly speaking, there are several forms of apraxia, which like many of the disturbances already discussed may be attributable to a number of causes or anatomical lesions. These include, ideational apraxia, ideomotor apraxia, buccal facial apraxia, constructional apraxia, and dressing apraxia. With the exception of dressing and constructional apraxia, apraxic abnormalities are usually secondary to left hemisphere damage, in particular, injuries involving the the left frontal and inferior parietal lobes.

For example, Kimura (1982) found that the ability to perform meaningless oral or hand movements was related to the frontal or posterior nature of the lesion, such that those with frontal lesions were impaired on oral movements whereas those with parietal lesions had the most difficulty making hand postures or complex movements of the extremities (Kolb & Milner, 1981). Thus, apraxic abnormalities secondary to left cerebral lesions tend to either involve destruction of the inferior parietal lobule (IFP) or lesions resulting in disconnection of the frontal motor areas (or the right cerebral hemisphere) from this more posterior region of the brain.

If the inferior parietal region is destroyed, the patient loses the ability to appreciate when he has performed an action correctly. If the motor region is destroyed, although the act is still performed inaccurately (due to disconnection from the IFP), the patient is able to recognize the difference (Heilman, 1979).

Ideomotor Apraxia

Ideomotor apraxia is usually associated with lesions within the inferior parietal lobe of the left hemisphere. Rather than problems with temporal sequencing of motor acts per se, these patients tend to be very clumsy when performing an act. They also tend to be very deficient when attempting to perform an action via pantomime or when engaged in meaningful imitation, meaningless imitation, and the meaningful or meaningless use of actual objects (Goodlass & Kaplan, 1972; Kimura & Archibald, 1974; Heilman, 1973). This has been attributed to destruction of the engrams needed for motor performance. Patients will demonstrate apraxic abnormalities in both the right and left hand.

In addition, patients with ideomotor apraxia tend to have difficulty with simple versus complex movements, although various elements within a complex action may be performed somewhat abnormally (Hecaen & Albert, 1978). Such actions as waving goodbye, throwing a kiss, making the "sign of the cross," may be performed deficiently. Moreover, many patients tend to uncontrollably comment on their actions, i.e., "verbal overflow." That is, when asked to "wave goodbye," they may say "goodbye" while waving even when instructed to say nothing. It has been suggested that ideomotor apraxia can occur in the absence of ideational apraxia but that the converse is not true (Hecaen & Albert, 1978). In this regard, ideomotor apraxia may be a less severe form of ideational apraxia.

Ideational Apraxia

Ideational apraxia is usually caused by severe disturbances in the temporal sequencing of motor acts. That is, the separate chain of links that constitutes an entire movement becomes dissociated, such that the overriding idea of the movement in its entirety is lost. Thus, these patients commit a number of temporal and spatial errors when making skilled movements, although the individual elements, in isolation, may be preserved and performed accurately (Hecaen & Albert, 1978; Luria, 1980). For example, a patient may rotate his hand by pantomime before inserting the key, drink from a cup before filling it from a pitcher of water, or puff on a cigarette and then light it. Thus they incorrectly sequence a series of acts. Both hands are affected.

Because of conceptual ideational abnormalities, they may also have difficulty using actual objects correctly. During pantomime, they may use a body part as object such as an index finger for a key. Even so, their actions are out of temporal sequence. Thus, these patients seem to be unable to access the motor engrams (or "memories") which would allow them to perform appropriately (Luria, 1980). In this regard, patients are sometimes hesitant to perform a task, as they have difficulty understanding what has been asked of them. However, they can often describe verbally what they are unable to perform (Heilman, 1979).

Left-Sided or Unilateral Apraxia

Patients with left-sided or unilateral apraxia (also called callosal and frontal apraxia, are unable to imitate or perform certain movements with their left (but not right) hand and are clumsy in their use of objects. Left-sided apraxia is sometimes due to a lesion of the anterior corpus callosum or left frontal motor cortex. This is because lesions of the corpus callosum or premotor and motor region of the left hemisphere can result in a disconnection syndrome; i.e., the motor areas of the right hemisphere cannot gain access to the motor engrams stored within the left inferior parietal lobe. Thus, with a left frontal lesion, an apraxia of the left hand and paralysis of the right result. Often this is secondary to strokes within the distribution of the anterior cerebral artery such that the anterior portion of the corpus callosum is destroyed (Geschwind, 1965).

It is noteworthy that patients may also show deficient finger-tapping performance in the left hand due to apraxic abnormalities secondary to left hemisphere injury (Heilman, 1975). In these instances, reduced finger tapping is bilateral.

Dressing Apraxia

Dressing apraxia is usually secondary to right hemisphere lesions involving the inferior parietal region, and as the name implies, the patient has difficulty putting on their clothes. For example, a patient may attempt to put a shirt on upside down, then inside–out, and then backward. Severe spatial–perceptual abnormalities as well as body image disturbances are usually contributing factors.

Aphasia and Apraxia

Many patients who are aphasic also appear apraxic because they have severe difficulty comprehending language and understanding motor commands. That is, a patient may fail to perform a particular action because he fails to comprehend what is being asked.

To distinguish between receptive aphasic abnormalities and apraxia one must ask "yes" and "no" questions ("Are you in a hospital?"), require them to perform certain actions through pantomime ("Show me how you would throw a ball," or "Show me how a soldier salutes"), as well require pointing response ("Point to the lamp"). If they can answer appropriately "yes" or "no" or point to objects named but are unable to execute commands, they have apraxia. It is important to note that in severe cases apraxic patients may have difficulty even with pointing.

Pantomime Recognition

Patients with damage involving the left inferior parietal lobule make errors not only when performing motor acts but in comprehending, recognizing and discriminating between different types of motor acts such as demonstrated through pantomime (Heilman, Rothi, & Valenstein, 1982). Moreover, patients with lesions in the left inferior occipital lobe have also been shown to have difficulty in verbally understanding, describing, or differentiating between pantomimes (Rothi, Mack, & Heilman, 1986). That is, in the extreme, if one were to pantomime the pouring of water into a glass versus lighting and smoking a cigarette, these patients would demonstrate problems describing what they have viewed or in choosing which was which.

Deficits in pantomime recognition occur frequently among patients with aphasia (Varney, 1978). Moreover, this disturbance is significantly correlated with reading comprehension (Gainotti & Lemmo, 1976; Varney, 1978, 1982). In this regard, patients with alexia frequently suffer from pantomime recognition deficits as well. Because of this relationship it has been suggested that the ability to read may be based on or derived from the ability to understand gestural communication, i.e., the reading of signs (Varney, 1982).

Constructional Apraxia

Constructional apraxia is by no means a unitary disorder (Benton, 1969; Benson & Barton, 1970) and can may be expressed in a number of ways. On a drawing or copying task this may include the addition of unnecessary/nonexistent details or parts, misalignment or inattention to details, disruptions of the horizontal and vertical axis with reversals or slight rotations in reproduction, and scattering of parts. For example, in performing the Block Design subtest from the WAIS-R, the patient may correctly reproduce the model but angle it incorrectly. In drawing or copying figures, the patient may neglect the left half, draw over the model, and misalign details.

Moreover, although constructional deficits are more severe after right hemisphere damage (Arrigoni & DeRenzi, 1964; Black & Strub, 1976; Benson & Barton, 1970; Critchley, 1953; Hier, Mondlock, & Caplan, 1983; Joseph, 1988a; Piercy, Hecaen, & de Ajuriaguerra, 1960), disturbances involving constructional and manipulospatial functioning can occur with lesions to either half of the brain (Arrigoni & DeRenzi, 1964; Mehta *et al.*, 1987; Piercy *et al.*, 1960). Hence, depending on the laterality, as well as the extent and site of the lesion, the deficit may also take different forms. For example, following posterior reight cerebral lesions, rather than apraxic, the patient is spatially agnosic, i.e., suffering from constructional agnosia and a failure to perceive and recognize visual–spatial and object interrelationships. In other cases, such as following left cerebral injury, the disturbance may be secondary to a loss of control over motor programming (Warrington *et al.*, 1966; Warrington, 1969).

Although visual–motor deficits can result from lesions in either hemisphere (Arrigoni & DeRenzi, 1964; Piercy *et al.*, 1960), visual–perceptual disturbances are more likely to result from right hemisphere damage. By contrast, lesions to the left half of the brain may leave the perceptual aspects undisturbed but visual-motor functioning and selective organization compromised (Kim, Morrow, Passafiume, & Boller, 1984; Mehta *et al.*, 1987; Poeck, Kerschensteiner, Hartje, & Orgass, 1973). As such, the patient is likely to recognize that errors have been made.

In general, the size and sometimes the location of the lesion within the right hemisphere have little or no correlation with the extent of the visual–spatial or constructional deficits demonstrated, although right parietal lesions tend to be worst of all. With right parietal involvement, patients tend to have trouble with the general shape and overall organization, the correct alignment and closure of details, and there may be a variable tendency to ignore the left half of the figure or not attend fully to all details. Moreover, the ability to perceive (or care) that errors have been made is usually compromised.

Conversely, constructional disturbances associated with left hemisphere damage are positively correlated with lesion size, and left anterior lesions are worse than left posterior (Benson & Barton, 1970; Black & Bernard, 1984; Black & Strub, 1976; Lansdell, 1970). This is because the capacity to control and program the motor system has been compromised. The larger the lesion, the more extensive the deficit.

Moreover, because the left hemisphere is concerned with the analysis of parts or details and engages in temporal–sequential motor manipulations, lesions result in oversimplification and a lack of detail although the general outline or shape may be retained (Gardner, 1975, Levy, 1974). However, in some cases, when drawing, there may be a tendency to distort the right half of the figure more greatly.

GERSTMANN'S SYNDROME

The Knowing Hand

It has been said that the parietal lobule is an organ of the hand. As noted, the hand appears to be more extensively represented than any other body part, parietal neurons are responsive to hand movements and manipulations, mediate temporal–sequential hand control, and become highly activated in response to objects which are within grasping distance.

It is also by the hand that the parietal lobe gathers information regarding various objects, i.e., stereognosis, and about the Self and the World, so that things and body parts come to be known, named, and identified. Ontogenetically, the hand is in fact primary in this regard. That is, the infant first uses the hand to grasp various objects, so they may be placed in the mouth and orally explored. As the child develops, rather than mouthing, more reliance is placed solely on the hand (as well as the visual system) so that information may be gathered through touch, manipulation, and visual inspection.

As the child and it's brain matures, instead of predominantly touching, grasping, and holding, the fingers of the hand are used for pointing and then naming. It is these same fingers which are later used for counting and the development of temporal–sequential reasoning; i.e., the child learns to count on his or her fingers, then to count (or name) by pointing at objects in space.

In this regard, counting, naming, object identification, finger utilization, and hand control are ontogenetically linked and seem to rely on the same neural substrates for their expression, i.e., the left inferior parietal lobule. Hence, when the more posterior portions of the left hemisphere are damaged, naming (anomia), object and finger identification (agnosia), arithmetical abilities (acalculia), and temporal–sequential control over the hands (apraxia) are frequently compromised.

Hence, a variety of symptoms are associated with left inferior parietal lobe damage. However, a particular constellation of disturbances, i.e., finger agnosia, acalculia, agraphia, and left–right disorientation, when they occur together, have been referred to as Gerstmann's Syndrome (Gerstmann, 1930, 1944; Strub & Geschwind, 1983). Gerstmann's symptom complex is most often associated with lesions in the area of the supramarginal gyrus and superior parietal lobule (Hrbek, 1977; Strub & Geschwind, 1983). However, because this symptom complex does not always occur together, some authors have argued that Gerstmann's syndrome, per se, does not exist. We will not take issue, pro or con on this controversy, but instead will focus on those aspects of Gerstmann's syndrome that have not yet been discussed (finger agnosia, acalculia, left–right disorientation).

Finger Agnosia

Finger agnosia is not a form of finger blindness, as the name suggests. Rather, the difficulty involves naming and differentiating among the fingers of either hand as well as the hands of others (Gerstmann, 1940). This includes pointing to fingers named by the examiner, or moving or indicating a particular finger on one hand when the same finger is stimulated on the opposite hand.

For example, if the examiner touches the patients's finger while his eyes are closed, and asks him to touch the same finger he may have difficulty. If the disturbance is subtle, the examiner may wish to stimulate two fingers and then ask the patient to indicate, in order, the same fingers. Many patients have difficulty on these tests, regardless of their being administered in a verbal (naming) or nonverbal (touching) format (Kinsbourne & Warrington, 1962). In general, it is the middle three fingers which are hardest to recognize and the agnosia is demonstrable in both hands.

Although finger agnosia is only rarely shown with those who have right hemisphere lesions (Hecaen, 1962) many patients also demonstrate some visual-constructive disability (Kinsbourne & Warrington, 1962). Therefore, in testing for this disorder verbal versus nonverbal forms are of assistance in determing the side of lesion.

Often, patients who have difficulty identifying fingers by name or simply by differentiating between them nonverbally also suffer from receptive language abnormalities (Sanquet *et al.*, 1971). Nevertheless, this disorder is not merely a manifestation of aphasia because finger angosia may appear in the absence of language abnormalities (Strub & Geschwind, 1983).

In part, a good way of determining if the disorder is secondary to a right vs. left hemisphere injury is by noting if patients have more problems recognizing fingers on the right versus left hand, or in transferring from the right to left hand (or vice versa), that is, by stimulating a finger (or fingers) on the right hand (while it is out of sight) and then having the patient indicate the same fingers on the left hand. One must rule out deficient attentional functioning in making this diagnoses. Brain damage should not be diagnosed merely on the basis of on poor performance of this one index but should be based on the overall pattern of deficiency.

Acalculia

Problems working with numbers or performing arithmetical operations can be secondary to a number of causes and may result from injuries involving different regions of the brain. For example, a patient may suffer an alexia/agnosia for numbers, or they may have difficulties with spatial–perceptual functioning and thus misalign numbers when adding or subtracting (referred to as spatial acalculia). Therefore, in many instances, a patient may appear to have difficulty performing math problems when, in fact, the basic ability to calculate per se is intact. That is, the apparent difficulty may in fact be attributable to spatial, linguistic, agnosic, or alexic abnormalities.

However, in many instances, patients who are no longer able to perform calculations demonstrate a number of deficiencies. They may erroneously substitute one operation for another, i.e., misreading the sign "+" as "×", such that they multiply rather than add. Or they may reverse numbers, i.e., "16" as "61," substitute counting for calculation, i.e., $21 + 6 = 22$, or inappropriately group $32 + 5 = 325$.

By contrast, with left posterior lesions localized to the vicinity of the inferior parietal lobe, patients may have severe difficulty performing even simple calculations, e.g., carrying, stepwise computation, borrowing (Boller & Grafman, 1983; Hecaen & Albert, 1978). When this occurs in the absence of alexia, aphasia, or visual-spatial abnormalities, and is accompanied by finger agnosia, agraphia, and right–left orientation, it is considered part of Gerstmann's syndrome (Gerstmann, 1930). It has also been referred to as "anarithmetria" (Hecaen & Albert, 1978), or pure acalculia when not accompanied by other abnormalities.

Pure Acalculia/Anarithmetria

Acalculia is an isolated impairment of calculation in the absence of alexia or agraphic or spatial organization problems and involves a disturbance of basic math processes, e.g., carrying, stepwise computation, borrowing (Boller & Grafman, 1983; Levin, 1979). It is manifested as an impairment in the ability to maintain order, to plan correctly in sequence, and to manipulate numbers appropriately.

Indeed, one patient, a former accountant, who had suffered a small circumscribed left parietal subdural hematoma in an auto accident, was unable to add past 10 (e.g., $7 + 4$), although able to read, write, speak appropriately, and recognize objects. However, she did demonstrate severe finger agnosia, and in fact the finger agnosia appeared to be directly related to her inability to perform calculations. In this regard, I was able to work with this patient for a number of months and, by emphasizing finger-recognition tasks, including finger calculations (e.g., taking two fingers on her right hand four on her left, and saying "two times four is?), was able to raise her math ability to the high school level. The normal tendency to recover lost functions partially certainly played a part.

Alexia/Agnosia for Numbers

Alexia for numbers and digits is found in more than 80% of individuals with left temporal-occipital lesions, and in less than 10% of those with right hemisphere lesions. As the name implies, the patient is unable to recognize numbers. Usually these patients also suffer from generalized or literal alexia (Hecaen, 1962), i.e., an inability to recognize letters.

Alexia/Agraphia for Numbers

In some cases acalculia may be associated with an alexia and/or an agraphia for numbers, as well as aphasic abnormalities (referred to as aphasic acalculia (Benson & Weir, 1972). Patients with this disorder are unable to recognize or properly produce numbers in written form. For example, they may be unable to write out or point to the number 4 versus the number 7 or the letter B. The lesion is usually in the left inferior parietal lobule and localized within the angular gyrus. Not all patients are aphasic however (Levin, 1979).

Spatial Acalculia

The right cerebral hemisphere is quite proficient in performing geometrical analysis. (see Chapter 1). However, its basic arithmetical abilities (i.e., the isolated right hemisphere) are limited to the performance of addition, subtraction, and multiplication of simple sums and numbers below 10 (Levy-Agresti, 1968; Sperry, 1968). However, it can also visually recognize correct answers, for small sums, when given a visual choice (Dimond & Beaumont, 1974). Nevertheless, problems with arithmetical reasoning per se, are not usually due to right hemisphere lesions.

However, when the right hemisphere is damaged difficulties in calculation may result due to visual–spatial disturbances (Hecaen & Albert, 1978). For example, figures and digits may not be properly aligned, arranged, or organized on the page when writing out a problem. Or, the patient may ignore the left half of numbers when adding, subtracting, and so forth. If given the opportunity to perform the same calculation verbally, frequently little difficulty is demonstrated indicating that the basic ability to calculate is intact. In general, most patients with spatial acalculia have right hemisphere lesions. However, bilateral disturbances may be present (see Boller & Grafman, 1983; Hecaen & Albert, 1978).

Right–Left Disorientation

Right–left disorientation (e.g., "show me your right hand") is usually associated with left hemisphere and left parieto-occipital damage. It occurs only extremely rarely among individuals with right cerebral injuries (Gerstmann, 1930; McFie & Zangwill, 1960; Sauguet, Benton, & Hecaen, 1971). In general, these patients have difficulty differentiating between the right and left halves of their body or the bodies of others. This may be demonstrated by asking the patient to touch or point to the side named by the examiner, e.g., ''Touch your left cheek,'' or, ''Point to my right ear''; to point on their own body to the body part the examiner has pointed to on his/her body; or in performing crossed commands, ''Touch your left ear with your right hand''. In mild cases only the crossed commands may be performed deficiently (Strub & Geschwind, 1983). Nevertheless, patients with aphasic disorders generally perform most poorly of all brain damaged groups (Sauguet *et al.*, 1971). Interestingly, among presumably neurologically intact adults, approximately 18% of females and 9% of men perform deficiently on right–left orientation tasks (Wolf, 1973).

In part, it seems somewhat odd that right–left spatial disorientation is more associated with left rather than right cerebral injuries, given the tremendous involvement the right half of the brain has in spatial synthesis and geometrical analysis. However, orientation to the left or right transcends geometric space as it relies on language. That is, ''left'' and ''right'' are designated by words and defined linguistically. In this regard, left and right become subordinated to language usage and organization (Luria, 1980). Thus, left–right confusion is strongly related to problems integrating spatial coordinates within a linguistic framework.

ATTENTION AND NEGLECT

Data from a variety of studies have indicated that the parietal lobes are heavily involved in directing and maintaining various aspects of motoric, visual and somesthetic attentional functioning (reviewed above). This includes the maintainance of visual fixation, the guidance of hand and manipulatory activities, or the detection and monitoring of a stimulus moving across the body surface. In part, this is accomplished through interconnections with the various association areas, frontal lobes as well as subcortical structures such as the superior colliculus and the reticular formation—all of which are heavily involved in attention and/or arousal.

In general, however, the parietal lobes of the right and left cerebral hemisphere do not appear to exert similar or equal influences. For example, although many neurons in the secondary somesthetic areas receive contralateral and ipsilateral input whereas many visual neurons in area 7 are responsive to both halves of the visual field, bilateral responsiveness appears to be more characteristic of the right parietal region. The right seems to contain a greater number of bilateral cells.

Thus, visual and somesthetic stimuli exert greater EEG evoked responses over the right half of the brain (Beck, Dustman, & Sakai, 1969; Schenkenberg, Dustman, & Beck, 1971), and the right cerebral hemisphere becomes activated by stimuli applied to the right or left half of the body (Desmedt, 1977; Heilman & Van Den Abell, 1980). Conversely, the left hemisphere becomes aroused only in response to unilateral (right-sided) input.

Reaction times to visual stimuli are also more greatly reduced following right vs. left cerebral injuries (Howes & Boller, 1975). Similarly, among split-brain patients, the right cerebral hemisphere is able to maintain attention for appreciably longer time periods (Dimond, 1976, 1979), whereas the left hemisphere tends to demonstrate attentional lapses as well as unilateral spatial–conceptual neglect (Joseph, 1988b).

Perhaps because of the greater right cerebral monitoring ability across tasks requiring sustained motor–visual attention, performance in the left half of space (with either hand) is superior to performance in the right half of space (Heilman, Bowers, Valenstein, & Watson, 1987).

As is well known, lesions, or even surgical removal of the right parietal lobe (particularly the inferior regions), including the second occipital convolution, can result in unilateral neglect of the left half of visual, somesthetic, and auditory space (Critchley, 1953; Hecaen, Penfield, Bertrand, & Malmo, 1956; Heilman & Valenstein, 1972; Joseph, 1986a, 1988a; Nielson, 1937; Roth, 1944, 1949). In the extreme, these patients may fail to become consciously aware that half the body is in some way dysfunctional, or even that it exists (Bisiach, Luzzati, & Perani, 1979; Critchley, 1953; Denny-Brown, Meyer, & Horenstein, 1952; Joseph, 1986a, 1988a; Roth, 1944, 1949; Sandifer, 1946; Schilder, 1935). They may dress or groom only the right half of their body, eat only off the right half of their plates, etc. Indeed, the left half of the environment is ignored even when the body is aligned in the verticle axis (Calvanio, Petrone, & Levine, 1987); or, when conjuring up mental imagery, i.e., the left half of the image disappears.

Neglect may take the form of hypoarousal or inattentiveness. That is, the patient may not completely ignore the left half of space, but instead, may fail to respond to left sided stimuli only under certain conditions such as when the patient is fatigued or if simultaneously stimulated bilaterally (e.g., to the left and right half of the face, or the right ear and left hand), i.e., extinction.

In addition, rather than the left half of visual–somesthetic space, neglect may encompass the left half of an object, even when the entire object falls to the right (Bisiach, Luzzati, & Perani, 1979). For example, if the word "toothbrush" is presented well to the patient's right, she may report only seeing the word "brush." If presented to her left, she may state that she sees "nothing." This is probably because these patients begin scanning from the right and proceed only a short distance leftward before they stop or are pulled back toward the right.

Similarly, patients may neglect the left half of images they consciously conjure up (Bisiach & Luzzati, 1978) or the left half of words or sentences when reading (Kinsbourne & Warrington, 1962; Barbut & Gazzaniga, 1987). This suggests that neglect is for both internal and external events, and greatly involves the ability to internally generate bilateral perceptions.

Neglect, however, encompasses more than internal and external inattention, but a failure to attend to gravitational influences as well (Gazzaniga & Ladavas, 1987). As noted, the parietal lobule receives and processes information concerning body–positional relationships and integrates this information with visual input regarding objects in space. Through the analysis of proprioceptive and other forms of input, the parietal lobule also takes into account gravitational influences: the position of the body in space.

As pointed out by Gazzaniga and Ladavas, (1987), when the eyes are looking straight forward and the head is in an upright position, the visual frame of reference coincides with the gravitational frame. If the head is turned on its side, however, the left and right side of the gravitational field (which is invariant) no longer coincide with the visual reference; what lies to the right may be groundward, and that to the left may be skyward. If the head is tilted to the right, the left visual field encompasses that which is up, and the right visual field that which is below. When the head is tilted, however, patients with parietal damage and neglect ignore not only the left side of visual space, but the left side of gravitational space as well (Gazzaniga & Ladavas, 1987).

For example, if the head is tilted to the left, the patient would ignore everything which is downward as well as everything falling to the verticle left. Only the right upper quadrant would continue to be perceived and responded to.

Neglect from parietal lesions is probably also secondary to a disconnection of this region from the frontal lobes. That is, the frontal lobes failing to receive input cease to exert activational influences (through its connections with the thalamus, reticular formation), such that information normally processed by the damaged parietal lobe are no longer activated and attended to.

Left Hemisphere Neglect

Although not as common nor as severe, inattention and neglect has also been shown to occur following left-sided lesions (Albert, 1973; Ogden, 1987). However, whereas right hemisphere induced neglect is more profound, attentional disturbances following left cerebral damage tend to be more subtle, e.g., failing to attend to small figures on the right. Or, neglect may only be manifested under procedures employing extinction—when stimulated simultaneously on the right and left halves of the body. Similarly, the right half of drawings, although not neglected per se, may tend to be more distorted and incomplete.

Neglect, following left cerebral injuries, however, is more likely to occur with left anterior rather than left parietal injuries (see Ogden, 1987, for review). Sometimes, however, this is due to motoric abnormalities, such as gaze paralysis, or difficulty moving the head or right arm toward the right; i.e., a hypokinesis. That is, patients may seem not to attend fully to the right half of space because of damage to motor neurons and thus an inability to respond motorically. Moreover, because of a loss of counterbalancing influences, the right hemisphere acting unopposed also causes such patients to favor the left half of space. In addition, if verbal report is required, the left hemisphere being damaged is necessarily at a disadvantage such that what appears to be neglect is really reduced verbalization.

DELUSIONAL DENIAL

Frequently, patients with right parietal lesions, when confronted with their unused or immobile limbs may (at least initially) deny that it belongs to them or swear there is nothing wrong (Joseph, 1986a, 1988a). More often, however, they tend to ignore their left half. In some cases, however, patients may perceive the left half of their body but refer to it using ego-alien language, such as "my little sister," "my better half," "my friend Tommy," "my brother-in-law," and "spirits." For example, Gerstmann (1942) describes a patient with left-sided hemiplegia who "did not realize and on being questioned denied, that she was paralyzed on the left side of the body, did not recognize her left limbs as her own, ignored them as if they had not existed, and entertained confabulatory and delusional ideas in regard to her left extremities. She said another person was in bed with her, a little Negro girl, whose arm had slipped into the patient's sleeve'' (p. 894). Another declared (speaking of her left limbs), "That's an old man. He stays in bed all the time."

One such patient engaged in peculiar erotic behavior with his "absent" left limbs which he believed belonged to a woman. A patient described by Bisiach and Berti (1987, p. 185) "would become perplexed and silent whenever the conversation touched upon the left half of his body; even attempts to evoke memories of it were unsuccessful." Moreover, although "acknowledging that all people have a right and a left side, he could not apply the notion to himself. He would affirm that a woman was lying on his left side; he would utter witty remarks about this and sometimes caress his left arm."

Some patients may develop a dislike for their left limbs, try to throw them away, become agitated when they are referred to, entertain persecutory delusions regarding them, and even complain of strange people sleeping in their beds due to their experience of bumping into their left limbs during the night (Bisiach & Berti, 1987; Critchley, 1953; Gerstmann, 1942). One patient complained that the person tried to push her out of the bed and then insisted that if it happened again she would sue the hospital. Another complained about "a hospital that makes people sleep together." A female patient expressed not only anger but concern lest her husband should find out; she was convinced it was a man in her bed.

Disconnection, Confabulation, and Gap Filling

In some respects, it seems quite puzzling that individuals with right parietal injuries may deny what is visually apparent and what they should easily be able to remember, i.e., the presence of the left half of their body. However, it is possible that when the language dominant left hemisphere denies ownership of the left extremity it is in fact telling the truth. That is, the left arm belongs to the right not the left hemisphere.

Memories are sometimes unilaterally stored (see Chapter 1). In this regard, the left brain may in fact have no memory regarding the left half of the body. All this seems preposterous, and yet patients will deny what is obvious, i.e., the existence or ownership of the left half of their body.

Inevitably, in order for an individual to confabulate, erroneous information must become integrated in some fashion so that the confabulated response can be expressed. When the frontal lobes are compromised there is much flooding of the association and assimilation areas with tangential and irrelevant information much of which is amplified completely out of proportion to more salient details. Consequently, salient and irrelevant, highly arousing and fanciful information are expressed indiscriminantly. The normal filtering process is disrupted. However, when the parietal lobes are compromised, rather than flooding, there results a disconnection and information received in the Language Axis is incomplete and riddled with gaps (Joseph, 1986a).

Assimilation of input from diverse sources is a major feature of left and right parietal (i.e., inferior parietal) activity. When this area is damaged, errors abound in the assimilation of perceptions and ideas as the language axis can no longer access all necessary information.

That is, when the language axis is functionally isolated from a particular source of information about which the patient is questioned (such as in cases of denial), it begins to make up a response based on the information available. To be informed about the left leg or left arm, it must be able to communicate with the cortical area (i.e., the parietal lobe), which is responsible for perceiving and analyzing information regarding the extremities. When no message is received and when the language axis is not informed that no messages are being transmitted, the language zones instead rely on some other source even when that source provides erroneous input (Joseph, 1986a); substitute material is assimilated and expressed and corrections cannot be made (due to loss of input from the relevant knowledge source). The patient begins to confabulate. According to Geschwind (1965), when the speech area is disconnected from a site of perception, then the speech area will be unable to describe what is going on at that site. This is because "the patient who speaks to you is not the 'patient' who is perceiving—they are in fact, separate."

In these instances delusions and confabulatory responses occur as a result of an attempt by the language axis to fill the gaps in the information received with associations and ideas which are in some manner related to the fragments available (Joseph, 1982, 1986a; Joseph *et al.*, 1984; Talland, 1961). In this regard, confabulatory–delusional statements although erroneous, can contain some accurate elements around which erroneous, albeit related, ideations are anchored. Hence, a patient may see his left leg or arm and then state it belongs to the doctor. In general, these disturbances occur most frequently when the right frontal or right parietal lobe is damage. However, neglect, denial, and delusional confabulation may also infrequently result from left parietal injuries (Joseph, 1986a).

Delusional Playmates and Egocentric Speech

Young children not only produce egocentric speech, in which they comment on, explain, and describe their own behavior, but sometimes describe their behavior to others (such as their parents) using ego–alien language. They may claim not to know why they performed certain behaviors, may claim that someone else actually performed the deed for which they are accused, as well as develop imaginary friends with whom they share secrets, play games, or upon whom they may place the blame for some untoward incident. These same "imaginary" friends sometimes urge them to commit certains acts or explain or inform them regarding the actions and motives of others.

Not all children develop elaborate imaginary friends. However, all (or almost all) children develop egocentric speech and at times employ ego–alien descriptions when confronted with their own disagreeable behavior. Largely, much of this is secondary to corpus callosal immaturity. However, among this same age group (up to age 7 and even 10), the parietal lobes are also quite immature, the inferior parietal area in particular.

As seen with adults with destruction of this nuclei, sometimes they uncontrollably comment on their actions when given commands (e.g., "Now I'm waving goodbye"), whereas in other instances they may claim that the person performing the action is someone other than themselves or, they may completely deny that the left half of their body is their own and claim it belongs to another. Although a lesioned parietal lobe is not the same as parietal lobe immaturity (particularly in that immaturity is bilateral and damage is usually unilateral), there remains a curious similarity in the behavior of these adults and children.

Perhaps this is because the ego and self is first identified with the body whereas the image of the body is maintained by the parietal lobe. When one parietal lobe (due to damage or immaturity) is unable to communicate with the other half of the brain, that brain half is unable to recognize a continuity of self. Consequently, behaviors initiated by the opposite (usually right) half of the brain, or the half of the body controlled by right brain are recognize by the speaking half of the cerebrum only from a disconnected (i.e., alien) perspective. When the speaking (i.e., left) hemisphere is questioned about this behavior, or about its left limbs, they are described as initiated or as belonging to someone else, such as "an old man," "my brother-in-law," or an imaginary friend.

SUMMARY

The parietal lobes, although commonly associated with the mediation of somesthetic stimuli, are also concerned with motor and attentional functioning, the perception of spatial relations, including depth, orientation, location, and the identification of motivationally significant auditory, somesthetic, and visual stimuli. It is through the integrative interaction of the parietal lobe that an individual can feel an object and not only determine its physical qualities (e.g., shape, size, weight, texture) but can visualize, verbally lable, and even write out its name. It is also through the interaction of these various cell assemblies that an individual can attend to specific objects in space as well as reach out and manipulate them.

Indeed, the parietal lobe is very important for mediating movement in visual space. That is, in order for a movement to be correctly planned and carried out signals must be directed to the right muscle groups as based on efferent visual, somesthetic, as well as auditory input. Moreover, one requires sensory information as to the position of the body and limbs in space; otherwise, movements will be clumsy. This is accomplished through the dense interconnections linking the primary somesthetic with the motor areas in the frontal lobe and via impulses transmitted down the corticospinal tract. Moreover, parietal neurons appear to guide and monitor movements as they occur in visual space.

Although the entire parietal lobule makes important contributions to movement, the inferior parietal lobule of the left hemisphere appears to be the central region of concern in regard to the performance of skilled temporal–sequential motor acts. These engrams assist in the programming of the motor frontal cortex, where the actions are actually executed.

If the inferior parietal region is destroyed the patient loses the ability to perform actions in an appropriate temporal sequence or even to appreciate when they have performed an action incorrectly. This condition is referred to as apraxia.

By contrast, right parietal injuries are associated with severe disturbances of emotion, constructional deficiencies, as well as a host of visual–spatial perceptual abnormalities including left-sided inattention and neglect. For example, with severe lesions in this area, patients may demonstrate a profound inattention to all forms of stimuli falling to their left. When drawing pictures, they may fail to draw the left half of an object; when writing or reading, they may ignore the left half of words or the left half of the page; and they may fail to perceive and respond to individuals standing to their left, or even the left half of their own body. Largely this condition is secondary to the destruction of neurons that are sensitive to various forms of visual and somesthetic input.

Nevertheless, it is important to emphasize that lesions to the parietal lobe (or any-where within the brain) are seldom localized to one particular quadrant (e.g., inferior, superior) or are even restricted to the parietal lobe. That is, damage may be parietal-occipital, parietal–temporal, frontal–parietal, or even bilateral, such as caused by cere-brovascular disease or compression from a unilateral tumor. Because of this, a patient may display agraphia but normal reading, stereognosis in the absence of apraxia, or conversely a wide mixture of seemingly unrelated symptoms.

REFERENCES

Albert, M. L. (1973). A simple test for visual neglect. *Neurology (New York), 23,* 658–664.

Andersen, R. A., Essics, G. K., & Siegel, R. M. (1985). Encoding of spatial location by posterior parietal neurons. *Science, 230,* 456–458.

Arrigoni, G., & DeRenzi, E. (1964). Constructional apraxia and hemispheric locus of lesion. *Cortex, 1,* 170–197.

Barbut, D., & Gazzaniga, M. S. (1987). Disturbances in conceptual space involving language and speech. *Brain, 110,* 1487–1496.

Beck, E. C., Dustman, R. E., & Sakai, M. (1969). Electrophysiological correlates of selective attention, In C. R. Evans & R. B. Mulholland (Eds.). *Attention in neurophysiology* (pp. 301–320). New York: Appleton.

Benson, D., & Barton, M. (1970). Disturbances in constructional ability. *Cortex, 6,* 19–46.

Benson, D. F., Gardner, H., & Meadows, J. C. (1976). Reduplicative paramnesia. *Neurology (New York), 26,* 147–151.

Benson, D. F., & Geschwind, N. (1969). The alexias. In P. J. Vinken & G. W. Bruyn (Eds.), *Handbook of clinical neurology* (Vol. 4) (pp. 420–455). 4, Amsterdam: North-Holland.

Benson, D. F., Sheremata, W. A., Bouchard, R., Segarram, J. M., Price, D., & Geschwind, N. (1973). Conduction aphasia. *Archives of Neurology, 28,* 339–346.

Benson, D. F., & Weir, W. F. (1972). Acalculia: Acquired anarithmetria. *Cortex, 8,* 465–472.

Benton, A. L. (1969). Disorders of spatial disorientation. In P. J. Vinken & G. W. Bruyn (Eds.), *Handbook of clinical neurology* (Vol. 3,) (pp. 107–120). New York: North-Holland.

Benton, A. L., Hannay, J., & Varney, N. (1975). Arithmetic ability, figner-localization capacity and right–left discrimination in normal and defective children. *American Journal of Orthopsychiatry, 21,* 756–766.

Benton, A. L., & Hecaen, H. (1970). Stereoscopic vision in patients with unilateral cerebral disease. *Neurology (New York), 20,* 1084–1088.

Berkley, K. J., & Parmer, R. (1974). Somatosensory cortical involvement in response to noxious stimulation in the cat. *Experimental Brain Research, 20,* 363–374.

Biemond, A. (1956). The conduction of pain above the level of the thalamus. *Archives of Neurology and Psychiatry, 75,* 231–244.

Bisiach, E., & Berti, A. (1987). Dyschiria. An attempt at its systemic explanation. In M. Jeannerod (Ed.), *Neurophysiological and neuropsychological aspects of spatial neglect* Amsterdam: North-Holland.

Bisiach, E., & Luzzatti, C. (1978). Unilateral neglect of representational space. *Cortex, 14,* 129–133.

Bisiach, E., Luzzati, C., & Perani, D. (1979). Unileteral neglect, representational schema and consciousness. *Brain, 102,* 609–618.

Black, F. W., & Strub, R. L. (1976). Constructional apraxia in patients with discrete missile wounds of the brain. *Cortex, 12,* 212–220.

Blinkov, S. M., & Glezer, I. I. (1968). *The human brain in figures and tables.* New York: Plenum Press.

Blum, J. S., Chow, K. L., & Pribram, K. H. (1950). A behavioural analysis of the organization of the parieto-temporo-preoccipital cortex. *Journal of Comparative Physiology, 93,* 53–199.

Boller, F., & Grafman, J. (1983). Acalculia: Historical development and current significance. *Brain and Cognition, 2,* 205–223.

Bruce, C. J., Desimone, R., & Gross, C. G. (1982). Visual properties of neurons in a polysensory area in superior temporal sulcus of the macaque, *Journal of Neurophysiology, 46,* 369–384.

Bruce, C. J., Desimone, R., & Gross, C. G. (1986). Both striate and superior colliculus contribute to visual properties of neurons in superior temporal polysensory area of *Macaque* monkey. *Journal of Neurophysiology, 58,* 1057–1076.

Burton, H., & Jones, E. G. (1976). The posterior thalamic region and its cortical projection in New world and Old world monkeys. *Journal of Comparative Neurology, 168,* 249–302.

Burton, H., Mitchell, G., & Brent, D. (1982). Second somatic sensory area in the cerebral cortex of cats. *Journal of Comparative Neurology, 210,* 109–135.

Butters, N., & Barton, M. (1970). Effect of parietal lobe damage on the performance of reversible operations in space. *Neuropsychologia, 8,* 205–214.

Calvanio, R., Petrone, P. N., & Levine, D. N. (1987). Left visual spatial neglect is both environment-centered and body-centered. *Neurology (New York), 37,* 1179–1183.

Chernigovskaya, T. V., & Deglin, V. L. (1986). Brain functional asymmetry and neural organization of linguistic competence. *Brain and Language, 29,* 141–153.

Cole, J., & Glees, P. (1954). Effects of small lesions in sensory cortex in trained monkeys. *Journal of Neurophysiology, 17,* 1–13.

Corkin, S., Milner, B., & Rasmussen, T. (1970). Somotosensory thresholds: Contrasting effects of post-central gyrus and posterior parietal-lobe excisions. *Archives of Neurology, 23,* 41–58.

Cowey, A. (1981). Why are there so many visual areas. In F. O. Schmitt, *et al.* (Eds.), *The organization of the cerebral cortex* (pp. 270–299). Cambridge, MA: MIT Press.

Critchley, M. (1953). *The parietal lobes.* New York: Hafner.

Cubelli, R., Caselli, M., & Neri, I. (1984). Pain endurance in unilateral cerebral lesions. *Cortex, 20,* 369–375.

Curtis, E. A., Jacobson, S., & Marcus, E. M. (1972). *An introduction to the neurosciences.* Philadelphia: W. B. Saunders.

Denny-Brown, D., & Chambers, R. A. (1958). The parietal lobe and behavior. *Proceedings of the Association for Rsearch in Nervous and Mental Disease, 36,* 35–117.

Denny-Brown, D., Meyer, J. S., & Horenstein, S. (1952). The significance of perceptual rivalry resulting from parietal lobe lesion. *Brain, 75,* 433–471.

Desmedt, J. E. (1977). Active touch exploration of extrapersonal space elicits specific electrogenesis in the right cerebral hemisphere of intact right handed man. *Proceedings of the National Academy of Sciences, 74,* 4037–4040.

Dimond, S. J. (1976). Depletion of attentional capacity after total commissurotomy in man. *Brain, 99,* 347–356.

Dimond, S. J. (1979). Tactual and auditory vigilance in split-brain man. *Journal of Neurology, Neurosurgery and Psychiatry, 42,* 70–74.

Dimond, S. J., & Beaumont, J. G. (1974). Experimental studies of hemisphere function in the human brain. In S. J. Dimond & J. G. Beaumont (Eds.), *Hemisphere function in the human brain.* New York: John Wiley & Sons.

Evarts, E. V. (1969). Activity of pyramidal tract neruons during postural fixation. *Journal of Neurophysiology, 32,* 375–385.

Gainotti, G., & Lemmo, M. (1976). Comprehension of symbolic gestures in aphasia. *Brain and Language, 3,* 451–460.

Garcha, H. S., Ettlinger, G., & MacCabel, J. J. (1982). Unilateral removal of the second somatosensory projection cortex in the monkey. *Brain, 105,* 787–810.

Gardner, H. (1975). *The shattered mind.* New York: Vintage Books.

Gardner, H., Brownell, H. H., Wapner, W., & Michelow, D. (1983). Missing the point: The role of the right hemisphere in the processing of complex linguistic materials. In E. Perceman (Ed.), *Cognitive processing in the right hemisphere* (pp. 270–301). Orlando, FL: Academic Press.

Gazzaniga, M. S., & Ladavas, E. (1987). Disturbances in spatial attention following lesion or disconnection of the right parietal lobe. In M. Jeannerod (Ed.), *Neurophysiological and neuropsychological aspects of spatial neglect.* Amsterdam: North-Holland.

Gerstmann, J. (1930). Syndrome of finger agnosia, disorientation for right and left, agraphia and acalculia. *Archives of Neurology and Psychiatry, 44,* 398–408.

Gerstmann, J. (1942). Problem of imperception of disease and of impaired body territories with organic lesions. *Archives of Neurology and Psychiatry, 48,* 890–913.

Geschwind, N. (1965). Disconnexion syndromes in animals and man. *Brain, 88,* 585–644.

Goodlass, H., & Kaplan, E. (1972). *The assessment of aphasia and related disorders.* Philadelphia: Lea & Febiger.

Gross, C. G., Rocha-Miranda, C. E., & Bender, D. B. (1972). Visual properties of neruons in inferotemporal cortex of the macaque. *Journal of Neurophysiology, 35,* 96–111.

Gross, C. G., Bender, D. B., & Rocha-Miranda, C. E. (1974). Inferotemporal cortex. A single unit analysis. In F. O. Schmitt & F. G. Worden (Eds.), *The neurosciences: Third study program.* Cambridge: MA: MIT Press.

Hannay, H. J., Varney, N. R., & Benton, A. L. (1976). Visual localization in paitenrts with unilateral brain disease. *Journal of Neurology, Neurosurgery and Psychiatry, 39,* 307–313.

Haslam, D. R. (1970). Lateral dominance in the perception of size and pain. *Quarterly Journal of Experimental Psychology, 22,* 503–507.

Hecaen, H. (1962). Clinical symptomology in right and left hemispheric lesions. In V. B. Mountcastle (Ed.), *Interhemispheric relations and cerebral dominance.* Baltimore: Johns Hopkins Press.

Hecaen, H., & Albert, M. L. (1978). *Human neuropsychology.* New York: John Wiley & Sons.

Hecaen, H., & De Ajuriaguerra, J. (1954). Balint's syndrome (psychic paralysis of visual fixation) and its minor forms. *Brain, 77,* 373–400.

Hecaen, H., & Kremin, H. (1976). Neurolinguistic research on reading disorders from left hemisphere lesions. In H. A. Whitkaer & H. Whitaker (Eds.), *Studies in neurolinguistics* (pp. 22–40). New York: Academic Press.

Hecaen, H., Penfield, W., Bertand, C., & Malmo, R. (1956). The syndromes of apractoognosia due to lesions of the minor cerebral hemisphere. *Archives of Neurology and Psychiatry, 75,* 400–434.

Heilman, K. M. (1973). Ideational apraxia. *Brain, 96,* 861–864.

Heilman, K. M. (1975). Reading and writing disorders caused by central nervous system defects. *Geriatrics, 30,* 115–118.

Heilman, K. M. (1979). Neglect and related disorders. In K. M. Heilman & E. Valenstein (Eds.), *Clinical neuropsychology* (pp. 268–307). New York: Oxford University Press.

Heilman, K. M., Bowers, D., Valenstein, E., & Watson, R. T., (1987). Hemispace and hemispatial neglect. In M. Jeannerod (Ed.), *Neurophysiological and neuropsychological aspects of spatial neglect* (pp. 320–332). Amsterdam: North-Holland.

Heilman, K. M., Rothi, L. J., & Valenstein, E. (1982). Two forms of ideomotor apraxia. *Neurology (New York), 32,* 342–346.

Heilman, K. M., & Valenstein, E. (1972). Frontal lobe neglect in man. *Neurology (New York), 22,* 660–664.

Heilman, K. M., & Van Den Abell, T. (1980). Right hemisphere dominance for attention. The mechanism underying hemispheric asymmetries of inattention (neglect). *Neurology (New York), 30,* 327–330.

Heilman, K. M., & Watson, R. T. (1977). The neglect syndrome. In S. Harnad, *et al.* (Eds.), *Lateralization in the nervous system.* New York: Academic Press.

Hier, D. B., Mondlock, J., & Caplan, L. R. (1983). Behavioral abnormalities after right hemisphere stroke. *Neurology (New York), 33,* 337–344.

Hom, J., & Reitan, R. (1982). Effects of lateralized cerebral damage on contralateral and ipsilateral sensorimotor performance. *Journal of Clinical Neuropsychology, 3,* 47–53.

Howes, D., & Boller, F. (1975). Simple reaction times: Evidence for focal impairment from lesions of the right hemisphere. *Brain, 98,* 317–322.

Hrbek, V. (1977). Pathophysiologic interpretation of Gerstmann's syndrome. *Neuropsychologia, 11,* 377–388.

Humphrey, M. E., & Zangwill, O. L. (1951). Cessation of dreaming after brain injury. *Journal of Neurology, Neurosurgery, and Psychiatry, 14,* 322–325.

Hyvarinen, J. (1982). *The parietal cortex of monkey and man.* Berlin: Springer-Verlag.

Hyvarinen, J., & Poranen, A. (1974). Function of the parietal associative area 7 as revealed from cellular discharges in alert monkeys. *Brain, 97,* 673–692.

Hyvarinen, J., & Shelepin, Y. (1979). Distribution of visual and somatic fucntions in the parietal association area of the monkey. *Brain Research, 169,* 561–564.

Iwamura, Y., & Tanaka, M. (1978). Postcentral neruons in hand region of area 2. *Brain Research, 150,* 662–666.

Jampel, R. S. (1960). Convergence, divergence, pupillary reactions and accomodatin of the eyes from faradic stimulation of the macaque brain. *Journal of Comparative Neurology, 115,* 371–397.

Jennings, V. A., Lamour, Y., Solis, H., & Fromm, C. (1983). Somatosensory cortex activity related to position and force. *Journal of Neurophysiology, 49,* 1216–1229.

Jones, E. G., & Powell, T. P. S. (1970). An anatomical study of converging sensory pathways within the cerebral cortex of the monkey. *Brain, 93,* 793–820.

Joseph, R. (1982). The neuropsychology of development: Hemispheric laterality, limbic language, and the origin of thought. *Journal of Clinical Psychology, 44,* 3–33.

Joseph, R. (1986). Confabulation and delusional denial: Frontal lobe and lateralized influences. *Journal of Clinical Psychology, 42,* 845–860.

Joseph, R. (1988a). The right cerebral hemisphere *Journal of Clinical Psychology, 44,* 630–673.

Joseph, R. (1988b). Dual mental functioning in a split-brain patient. *Journal of Clinical Psychology, 44,* 770–779.

Joseph, R., & Gallagher, R. E. (1985). Interhemispheric transfer and the completion of reversible operations in non-conserving children. *Journal of Clinical Psychology, 41,* 796–800.

Joseph, R., Gallagher, R. E., Holloway, W., & Kahn, J. (1984). Two brains—one child. Interhemispheric transfer deficits and confabulation in children aged 3,7,10. *Cortex, 20,* 317–331.

Kaas, J. H., Nelson, R. J., Sur, M., & Merzenich (1981). Mutliple representations of the body in the post central somatosenory cortex of primates. In C. N. Woolsey (Ed.), *Cortical sensory organization.* (Vol. 1) (pp. 214–240). New Jersey: Humana Press.

Kawamura, S., Spraguwe, J. M., & Niimi, K. (1974). Corticofugal projections from the visual corotices to the thalamus and superior colliculus. *Journal of Comparative Neurology, 158,* 339–362.

Kawano, K., & Sasaki, M. (1984). Resposne properties of neurons in posterior parietal cortex of monkey during visual–vestibular stimulation. *Journal of Neurophysiology, 51,* 352–360.

Kawano, K., Sasaki, M., & Yamashita, M. (1984). Response properties of neurons in posterior parietal cortex of monkey during visual–vestibular stimulation. *Journal of Neurophysiology, 51,* 340–351.

Kim, Y., Morrow, L., Passafiume, D., & Boller, F. (1984). Visuoperceptual and visuomotor abilities and locus of lesion. *Neuropsychologia, 2,* 177–185.

Kimura, D. (1979). Neuromotor mechanmisms in the evolution of human communication. In H. D. Steklis, & M. J. Raleigh (Eds.), *Neurobiology of social communication in primates* (pp. 401–420). Orlando, FL: Academic Press.

Kimura, D. (1982). Left-hemisphere control of oral and brachial movement and their relation to communication. *Philosophical Transactions of the Royal Society of London, 298,* 135–149.

Kimura, D., & Archibald, Y. (1974). Motor functions of the left hemisphere. *Brain, 97,* 337–350.

Kinsbourne, M., & Warrington, E. K. (1962). A variety of reading disabilities associated with right hemisphere lesions. *Journal of Neurology, Neurosurgery and Psychiatry, 25,* 339–344.

Kinsbourne, M., & Warrington, E. K. (1964). Disorders of spelling. *Journal of Neurology, Neurosurgery, and Psychiatry, 27,* 224–228.

Knuezle, H., & Akert, K. (1977). Efferent connections of cortical area 8. *Journal of Comparative Neurology, 173,* 147–164.

Kolb, B., & Milner, B. (1981). Performance on complex arm and fascial movement after focal brain lesions. *Nreuropsychologia, 19,* 491–503.

Lamotte, R. H., & Acuna, C. (1978). Defects in accuracy of reaching after removal of posterior parietal cortex in monkeys. *Brain Research, 139,* 309–326.

Lamotte, R. H., & Mountcastle, V. B. (1979). Disorders in somesthesis following lesions of the parietal lobe. *Journal of Neurophysiology, 42,* 400–419.

Lansdell, H. (1970). Relation of extent of temporal removal to closure and visuomotor factors. *Perceptual and Motor Skills, 31,* 491–498.

Leinonen, L., Hyvarinen, J., Nyman, & Linnakoski, D. (1979). Functional properties of neurons in the lateral part of associative area 7 of awake monkeys. *Experimental Brain Research, 34,* 299–320.

Levin, H. S. (1979). The acalculias. In K. M. Heilman & E. Valenstein (Eds.), *Clinical neuropsychology* (pp. 128–140). New York: Oxford University Press.

Levitt, M., & Levitt, J. (1968). Sensory hind-limb representation in cortex of cat after spinal tractotomies. *Experimental Neurology, 22,* 276–302.

Levy, J. (1974). Psychological implications of bilateral asymmetry. In S. Diomond & J. G. Beaumont (Eds.), *Hemisphere function in the human brain.* London: Paul Elek, Ltd.

Levy-Agresti, J., & Sperry, R. W. (1968). Differential perceptual capacities in major and minor hemispheres. *Proceedings of the U.S. National Academy of Sciences, 61,* 1151.

Luria, A. R. (1980). *Higher cortical functions in man*. New York: Basic Books.

Lynch, J. C. (1980). The functional organization of posterior parietal association cortex. *Behavioral Brain Sciences, 3,* 485–499.

Lynch, J. C., Mountcastle, V. B., Talbot, W. H., & Yin, T. C. T. (1977). Parietal lobe mechanisms for directed visual attention. *Journal of Neurophysiology, 40,* 362–389.

McFie, J., & Zangwill, O. L. (1960). Visual–constructive disabilities associated with lesions of the left cerebral hemisphere. *Brain, 83,* 243–260.

Mehta, Z., Newcombe, F., & Damasio, H. (1987). A left hemisphere contribution to visuospatial processing. *Cortex, 23,* 447–461.

Mesulam, M.-M., & Mufson, E. J. (1982). Insula of the Old World Monkey. III. *Journal of Comparative Neurology, 212,* 38–52.

Mesulam, M-M., Van Hoesen, G. W., Pandya, D. N., & Geschwind, N. (1977). Limbic and sensory connections of the inferior parietal lobule in the rhesus monkey. *Brain Research, 136,* 393–414.

Milner, B. (1968). Visual recognition and recall after right temporal lobe excision in man. *Neuropsychologia, 6,* 191–209.

Motter, B. C., & Mountcastle, V. B. (1981). The functional properties of the light sensitivity neruons of the posterior parietal cortex studies in waking monkey. *Journal of Neuroscience, 1,* 3–26.

Mountcastle, V. B. (1957). Modalities and topographic properties of single neurons of cat's sensory cortex. *Journal of Neurophysiology, 20,* 408–434.

Mountcastle, V. B. (1976). The world around us: Neural command functions for selective attention. *Neurosciences Research Progress Bulletin, 14,* 1–47.

Mountcastle, V. B., Lynch, J. C., Georgopoulos, A., (1975). Posterior parietal assocation cortex of the monkey. *Journal of Neurophysiology, 38,* 871–908.

Mountcastle, V. B., Motter, B. C., & Andersen, R. A. (1980). Some further observations on the functional properties of neurons in the parietal lobe of the waking monkey. *Brain Behavioral Sciences, 3,* 520–529.

Mountcastle, V. B., & Powell, T. P. S. (1959). Central nervous mechanisms subserving position sense and kinesthesis. *Bulletin of the Johns Hopkins Hospital, 105,* 173–200.

Newcombe, F., & Russell, W. R. (1969). Dissociated visual perceptual and spatial deficits in focal lesions of the right hemisphere. *Journal of Neurology, Neurosurgery and Psychiatry, 32,* 73–81.

Nielsen, J. M. (1937). Unilateral cerebral dominance as related to mind blindness. *Archives of Neurology and Psychiatry, 38,* 108–135.

Ogden, J. A. (1987). The 'neglected' left hemisphere and its contributions to visuo-spatial neglect. In M. Jeannerod (Ed.), *Neurophysiological and neuropsychological aspects of spatial neglect*. Amsterdam: North-Holland.

Pandya, D. N., & Kuypers, H. G. J. M. (1969). Corticocortical connections in the rhesus monkey. *Brain Research, 13,* 13–36.

Penfield, W., & Jasper, H. (1954). *Epilepsy and the functional anatomy of the human brain*. Boston: Little-Brown.

Penfield, W., & Rasmussen, T. (1950). *The cerebral cortex of man: A clinical study of localization of function*. New York: Macmillan.

Piercy, M., Hecaen, H., & de Ajuriaguerra, J. (1960). Constructional apraxia associated with unilateral cerebral lesions, left and right cases compared. *Brain, 83,* 225–242.

Poeck, K., Kerschensteiner, M., Hartje, W., & Orgass, B. (1973). Impairment in visual recognition of geometric figures in patients with circumscribed retrorolandic brain lesions. *Neuropsychologia, 11,* 311–319.

Randolf, M., & Semmes, J. (1974). Behavioral consequences of selective subtotal ablations in the posterior gyrus of *Macaca mulatta*. *Brain Research, 70,* 55–70.

Ratcliff, D. A., & Davies-Jones, G. A. B. (1972). Defective visual localization in focal brain wounds. *Brain, 95,* 49–60.

Ridley, R. M., & Ettlinger, G. (1976). Impaired tactile learning and retention after removals of the second somatic sensory projection cortex (SII). in the monkey. *Brain Research, 109,* 656–660.

Robinson, D. L. (1973). Electrophysiological analysis of interhmispheric relations in the second somatosensory cortex of the cat. *Experimental Brain Research, 18,* 131–144.

Robinson, D. L., Goldberg, M. E., & Stanton, G. B. (1978). Pairetal association cortex in the priamte: Sensory mechanisms and behavioral modulation. *Journal of Neurophysiology, 41,* 910–932.

Roland, P. E. (1976). Astereognosis. *Archives of Neurology, 33,* 543–550.

Rolls, E. T., Perret, D., Thorpe, S. J., *et al.* (1979). Responses of neurons in area 7 of the parietal cortex to objects of different significance. *Brain Research, 169,* 194–198.

Roth, M. (1949). Disorders of the body image caused by lesions of the right parietal lobe. *Brain, 72,* 89–111.

Roth, N. (1944). Unusual types of anosognosia and their relation to the body-image. *Journal of Nervous and Mental Disease, 100,* 35–43.

Rothi, L. J. G., Mack, L., & Heilman, K. M. (1986). Pantomime agnosia. *Journal of Neurology, Neurosurgery and Psychiatry, 49,* 451–454.

Russell, W. R. (1945). Transient disturbances following gunshot wounds of the head. *Brain, 68,* 79–97.

Russo, M., & Vignolo, L. (1967). Visual figure-ground discrimination in patients with unilateral cerbral disease. *Cortex, 3,* 111–127.

Sakata, H., & Iwamura, Y. (1978). Cortical procssing of tactile information in the first somatosensory and pareital association areas in the monkey. In G. Gordon (Ed.), *Active touch* (pp. 110–137). Oxford: Pergamon Press.

Sakata, H., Shibutani, H., & Kawano, K. (1980). Spatial properties of visual fixation neurons in posterior parietal association cortex of the monkey. *Journal of Neurophysiology, 43,* 1654–1672.

Sandifer,. P. H. (1946). Anosognosia and disorders of body scheme. *Brain, 69,* 122–137.

Sauguet, J., Benton, A. L., & Hecaen, H. (1971). Disturbances of the body schema in relation to language impairment and hemispheric locus of lesion. *Journal of Neurology, Neurosurgery and Psychiatry, 34,* 496–501.

Schenkenberg, P. H., Dustman, R. E., & Beck, E. C. (1971). Changes in evoked responses related to age, hemisphere and sex. *Electroencephalography and Clinical Neurophysiology, 30,* 163.

Schilder, P. (1935). *The image and appearance of the human body.* London: Routledge, Kegan Paul.

Schwarz, D. W. F., Deecke, L., & Fredrickson, J. M. (1973). Cortical projection of group 1 muscle afferents to areas 2, 3a, and the vestibular fields in teh rhesus monkey. *Experimental Brain Research, 17,* 516–526.

Seltzer, B., & Pandya, D. N. (1978). Afferent cortical connections and architectonics of the superior temporal sulcus and surround cortex in the rhesus monkey. *Brain Research, 149,* 1–24.

Semmes, J. (1965). A non-tactual factor in astereognosis. *Neuropsychologia, 3,* 295–315.

Semmes, J. (1973). Somesthetic effects of damage to the central nervous system. In A. Iggo (Ed.), *Handbook of sensory physiology.* Berlin: Springer-Verlag.

Semmes, J., & Turner, B. (1977). Effects of cortical lesions on somatosensory tasks. *Journal of Investigative Dermatology, 69,* 181–189.

Sperry, R. W. (1968). Hemisphere disconnection and unity in conscious awareness. *American Psychologist, 23,* 723–733.

Sur, M., Nelson, R. J., & Kaas, J. H. (1982). Representations of the body surface in cortical areas 3b and 1 of squirrel monkeys. *Journal of comparative neurology, 211,* 177–192.

Talland, G. A. (1961). Confabulation in the Wernicke–Korsakoff syndrome. *Journal of Nervous and Mental Disease, 132,* 772–791.

Tucker, D., Watson, R. T., & Heilman, K. M. (1977). Affective discrimination and evocation of affectively toned speech in patients with right parietal disease. *Neurology (New York), 27,* 947–950.

Varney, N. R. (1978). Linguistic correlates of pantomime recognition in aphasic patients. *Journal of Neurology, Neurosurgery and Psychiatry, 41,* 564–568.

Vignolo, L. A. (1983). Modality specific disorders of written language. In A. Kertesz (Ed.), *Localization in neuropsychology* (pp. 140–167). Orlando, FL: Academic Press.

Wall, J. T., Symonds, L. L., & Kaas, J. H. (1982). Cortical and subcortical projections of the middle temporal area (MT) and adjacent cortex in galagos. *Journal of Comparative Neurology, 211,* 193–214.

Warren, S., Hamalainen, H. A., & Gardner, E. (1986*a*). Coding of the spatial period of gratings rolled across receptive fields of somatosensory neurons in awake monkeys. *Journal of Neurophysiology, 56,* 623–639.

Warren, S., Hamalainen, H. A., & Gardner, E. (1986*b*). Objective classification of motion and direction sensitive neurons in primary somatosensory cortex of awake monkeys. *Journal of Neurophysiology, 56,* 598–622.

Warrington, E. K. (1969). Constructional apraxia. In P. Vinken & G. Bruyn (Eds.), *Handbook of clinical neurology* (pp. 301–330). Amsterdam: North-Holland.

Warrington, E. K., James, M., & Kinsbourne, M. (1966). Drawing disability in relation to laterality of lesion. *Brain, 89,* 53–92.

Warrington, E. K., James, M., & Maciejewski, C. (1986). The WAIS as a lateralizing and localizing instrument: A case study of 656 patients with unilateral cerebral lesions. *Neuropsychologia, 24,* 223–239.

Warrington, E. K., & Rabin, P. (1971). Visual span of apprehension in patients with unilateral cerebral lesions. *Quarterly Journal of Experimental Psychology, 23,* 423–431.

Weber, E. H. (1834/1978). Weber on sensory asymmetry (by J. D. Mollon). In M. Kinsbourne (Ed.), *Asymmetrical function of the brain* (pp. 318–327). Cambridge: Cambridge University Press.

Weinstein, S. (1978). Functional cerebral hemispheric asymmetry. In M. Kinsbourne (Ed.), *Asymmetrical function of the brain* (pp. 17–48). Cambridge: Cambridge University Press.

Whitsel, B. L., & Petrucelli, L. M., & Werner, G. (1969). Symmetry and connectivity in the map of the body surface in somatosensory area II of primates. *Journal of Neurophysiology, 32,* 170–183.

Whitsel, B. L., Roppolo, J. R., & Werner, G. (1972). Cortical information processing of stimulus motion on primate skin. *Journal of Neurophysiology, 35,* 691–717.

Wolf, S. M. (1973). Diufficulties in right–left discrimination in a normal population. *Archives of Neurology, 29,* 128–129.

Yin, T. C. T., & Mountcastle, V. B. (1977). Visual input to the visuomotor mechanisms of the monkey's parietal lobe. *Science, 197,* 1381–1383.

Zeki, S. M. (1974). Functional organization of a visual area in the posterior bank of the superior temporal sulcus of the rhesus monkey. *Journal of Physiology, 236,* 549–573.

6

The Occipital Lobe

Like the frontal, temporal, and parietal lobes, which respond to and process information from a number of modalities, the occipital lobe contains neurons that, although predominantly concerned with the analysis of visual stimuli (i.e., areas 17, 18, and 19), respond to vestibular, acoustic, or somesthetic input as well (Jung, 1961).

The visual cortex consists of a primary receptive area (i.e., striate cortex, area 17), located predominantly within the medial wall; of association cortices (areas 18 and 19), which are located medially and along the lateral convexity; and of higher-order association areas within the parietal (area 7) and inferior and middle temporal lobes. In this regard, the visual cortex extends well beyond the occipital lobe and includes the posterior third of both cerebral hemispheres.

PRECORTICAL VISUAL ANALYSIS

There is much processing of visual input prior to its reception in the occipital lobe. Initially, visual information analysis takes place in the receptor cells (rods and cones) within the retina and then undergoes successive hierarchical stages of analysis as it is passed through the sequential cell layers of which the retina is composed, i.e., horizontal cells, bipolar cells, amacrine cells, ganglion cells. Information is then relayed via the optic nerve to the lateral geniculate nucleus of the thalamus (Casagrande & Joseph, 1978, 1980), where yet further forms of analysis are performed. From the lateral geniculate, visual stimuli are then transmitted via the optic radiations to the primary visual receiving area, the striate cortex. In addition, visual information is transmitted to the superior colliculus and then the pulvinar of the thalamus and is then relayed to the visual cortex (Doty, 1983; Snyder & Diamond, 1968; Tigges, Walker, & Tigges, 1983).

In general, a strict topographical relationship is maintained throughout the visual projection system and the visual cortex. Within the visual cortex, immediately adjacent groups of neurons respond to visual information from neighboring regions within the retina. Also, at the neocortical level information is generally first received in the primary visual receiving area, 17. From the visual cortex this information is then transferred back to the lateral geniculate nucleus of the thalamus (from which it was first relayed), to the superior colliculus (Kawamura, Sprague, & Niimi, 1974) and to the association areas 18

233

and 19 as well as the middle temporal lobe (Doty, 1983; Lin, Weller, & Kaas, 1982) where higher-order processing occurs.

This same arrangement seems to characterize information reception and transfer in the auditory and somesthetic cortices as well. That is, information transferred from the thalamus to the neocortex is then transferred back to the thalamus as well as to the adjacent association areas. In this manner, a feedback loop is constructed such that information transmission from the thalamus to the cortex can be enhanced, diminished, or altered, depending on neocortical requirements.

Once visual stimuli are relayed to association areas 18 and 19 (where further analyses take place), this information is transmitted back to area 17 and to the temporal and parietal lobe, where polymodal associations are performed (Martinez-Millan & Hollander, 1975; Tigges *et al.*, 1983; Zeki, 1978*a,b*).

NEOCORTICAL COLUMNAR ORGANIZATION

Throughout the striate cortex, neurons with similar receptive properties are stacked in columns. Indeed, one column of cells may respond to a certain visual orientation, and the cells in the next column to an orientation of a slightly different angle. Moreover, columns exist for color (Zeki, 1974), location, movement, and so forth. In addition, since certain cells respond predominantly to input from one eye, there are ocular (eye) dominance columns as well (Hubel & Wiesel, 1968, 1974). A similar columnar arrangement in regard to somesthetic input is maintained in the parietal lobe.

Nevertheless, although these neurons seem to communicate predominantly with those in the same or immediately adjacent columns, it is likely that considerable parallel communication occurs (Dow, 1974). That is, information is analyzed both vertically and horizontally, so as to create a series of superimposed mosaics of the visual word.

SIMPLE, COMPLEX, AND HYPERCOMPLEX CELLS

The visual cortex is made up of a variety of cell types each of which is concerned with the analysis of different visual features (Hubel & Wiesel, 1959, 1962, 1968). These include simple, complex, and (higher- and lower-order) hypercomplex cells distributed disproportionately throughout areas 17,18, and 19.

To summarize briefly, simple cells appear to be involved in the initial analysis of incoming visual cortical input and are most sensitive to moving stimuli. They are found predominantly within area 17. Some are sensitive to stimuli moving in one direction, whereas others may respond to stimuli moving in any direction. In addition, simple cells are responsive to the particular position and orientation a stimulus may take. However, for a simple cell to fire, a stimulus must assume a specific orientation and position.

Simple cells relay this processed information to the far more numerous complex cells. Each complex cell receives input from several simple cells. Complex cells are also concerned with the orientation of the stimulus. However, these cells are more flexible and will respond to and analyze a stimulus, regardless of its particular orientation. Through the combined input from simple cells, these cells are probably involved in the earliest stages of actual form perception, i.e., the determination of the outline of an object. A considerable number of complex cells receive converging input from both eyes, the remainder being monocular. Complex cells are found predominantly within area 18.

Hypercomplex cells are concerned with the analysis of discontinuity, angles, and corners, as well as movement, position, and orientation. That is, these cells respond selectively to certain visual configurations and thus act so as to determine precise geometrical form. It is also through the action of these cells (in conjunction with visual neurons in the temporal lobe) that the first stages of visual closure are initiated. This in part requires that the functional activity of these cells be suppressed such that when presented with an incomplete figure these cells are overridden and the brain is able to "fill in the gaps" in stimuli perceived. It is also for this reason that one does not notice a "blind spot"—it is filled in. Hypercomplex cells are found predominantly within area 19.

STRIATE CORTEX: AREA 17

The primary visual cortex, area 17, is located predominantly within the medial walls of the cerebral hemispheres, extending only minimally along the lateral convexity. This area is often referred to as striate because the incoming fibers from the optic radiations form a stripe along the cortical surface that can be seen by the naked eye. Areas 18 and 19 do not have this striped appearance.

Like the primary motor and somesthetic cortices, a greater degree of cellular representation is maintained for those areas which are the most densely innervated and of the most sensory importance, i.e., the fovea (Daniel & Whitteridge, 1961; Hubel & Wiesel, 1979) (Figs. 44 and 45). Indeed, the central part of the retina has a cortical representation 35 times more detailed than that of the periphery. This is particularly important in that the fovea contains cells that are most sensitive to the detection and representation of form.

Although all neuron types are found within the striate cortex, simple and complex cells predominate. Thus, the primary receiving area is predominantly involved in the analysis of color, movement, position, and orientation, the most elementary aspects of form perception.

The primary visual cortex, however, receives fibers from nonvisual brain areas as well. These include brainstem nuclei, the pontine and mesencephalic reticular formation, the lateral amygdala, and the lateral hypothalamus (Doty, 1983; Tigges et al., 1983). Processing in the primary region can thus be enhanced or diminished through reticular influences and emotional–motivational concerns. In this manner, if a stimulus is emotionally significant, greater visual attention will be directed toward the object.

Hallucinations

Electrical stimulation, tumors, seizures, or trauma involving the striate cortex may produce simple visual hallucinations, such as sparks, tongues of flames, colors, and flashes of lights (Penfield and Jasper, 1954; Tarachow, 1941). Objects may seem to become exceedingly large (macropsia) or small (micropsia), blurred in terms of outline, or stretched out in a single dimension; colors may become modified or even erased (see Hecaen & Albert, 1978, for review). Sometimes simple geometrical forms may be re-

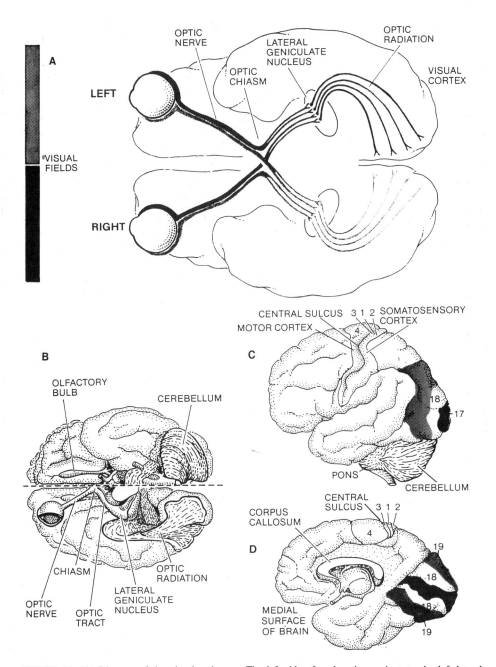

FIGURE 44. (A) Diagram of the visual pathways. The left side of each retina projects to the left lateral geniculate nucleus of the thalamus and then to left visual cortex. (B) Visual pathways in partially dissected brain, depicting the optic nerve, chiasm, optic tract, lateral geniculate nucleus, optic radiations. (C) Lateral view of visual cortex. (D) Medial view of visual cortex. From *From neuron to brain* by S. W. Kuffler & J. G. Nicholls, 1976. Courtesy of Sinauer Associates.

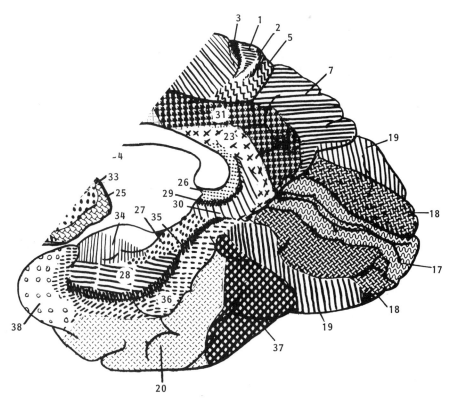

FIGURE 45. Medial view of the posterior portion of right cerebral hemisphere. Numbers refer to Brodmann's areas. Note extensive medial representation of the visual areas.

ported. The hallucination is usually restricted to one half the visual field. That is, if the seizure is in the right occipital lobe, the hallucination will appear in the left visual field.

Although elementary hallucinations are usually associated with abnormalities involving the occipital lobe, they may occur with temporal lobe lesions or electrical stimulation (Penfield & Rasmussen, 1950; Tarachow, 1941).

ASSOCIATION AREAS 18 AND 19

Areas 18 and 19 are involved in the translation and interpretation of visual impressions transmitted from area 17. Although simple and complex cells are found in the association cortex, this region is populated predominantly by hypercomplex (both higher- and lower-order) neurons, most of which are concerned with the determination of precise geometrical form as well as the assimilation of signals transmitted from the primary cortex.

In contrast to the neurons within area 17, many of the cells within area 18 receive binocular input and can be activated by either eye (Hubel & Wiesel, 1970). This same pattern of bincularity is evident in the parietal association area. It is through the action of these cells that one is able to gather information regarding distance and discrepancies in stimulus location and thereby determine depth and achieve stereoscopic vision (Blakemore, 1970; Hubel & Wiesel, 1970). Indeed, some association neurons will only fire when a target is a definite distance from the eye.

Many of the neurons in this region, particularly area 19, receive higher-order converging input from the parietal and temporal lobe. For example, in addition to visual input, neurons in the superior portions of area 19 respond to tactile and proprioceptive stimuli, whereas those in the inferior portions respond to auditory signals. It is probably in this manner (in conjunction with subcortical connections with, for example, the superior colliculus) that one is able to orient toward and gaze on an auditory stimulus as well as maintain stabilization of the head (via proproceptive–vestibular input) while engaged in visual search.

Thus, overall, the visual association area appears to be involved in the initial analysis of form, distance, and depth perception, as well as in the performance of visual closure. It is thus heavily involved in the association of various visual attributes, so that a variety of qualities may be ascertained. This would include an object's shape, length, thickness, and color.

It is important to emphasize that the visual association areas also maintain intimate relationships with the parietal visual regions (area 7) as well as with the visual areas in the middle and inferior temporal lobes. The temporal-visual areas are in turn reciprocally interconnected with area 7. Thus, a complex interactional visual loop is maintained, the inferior–medial temporal lobe, being concerned with form perception and the analysis of emotional–motivational significance; area 7 being involved in visual attention, visual fixation, and the analysis of distance, depth, and objects within grasping distance; and areas 18 and 19 both providing (and receiving) required visual input.

In this regard, when an object is recognized (through the interaction of the the visual areas in the temporal–occipital lobe), the parietal visual areas are alerted so that the object may be selectively fixated on, its distance determined, and then, once within grasping distance, grasped and tactually explored. If it is a potential food item (signaled by limbic structures within the temporal lobe), it can then be orally explored and eaten.

Hallucinations

Electrical stimulation of or lesions involving areas 18 and 19 can produce complex visual hallucinations (Foerster, 1929, cited by Brodal, 1981; Hecaen & Albert, 1978; Tarachow, 1941), such as images of men, animals, various objects and geometrical figures, liliputian-type individuals, including micropsias and macropsias (see Luria, 1980, and Hecaen & Albert, 1978, for review). Sometimes objects may seem to become telescoped and far away, whereas in other situations, when approached, objects may seem to loom and become exceedingly large.

Complex hallucinations are usually quite vivid and fully formed, and the patient may think what he sees is a real (Hecaen & Albert, 1978). Foerester (1928, cited by Hecaen & Albert, 1978) reported a patient who hallucinated a butterfly and then attempted to catch it when area 19 was electrically stimulated. Another hallucinated a dog and then called to it, denying the possibility that it was not real.

Complex hallucinations, although usually associated with tumors or abnormal activation of the visual association area, have also been reported with parietal–occipital involvement (Russell & Whitty, 1955), occipital–temporal, or inferior–temporal damage (Mullan & Penfield,, 1959; Tarachow, 1941; Teuber, Battersby & Bender, 1960), or with lesions of the occipital pole and convexity (Hecaen & Albert, 1978).

Laterality

According to Hecaen and Albert (1978), based on their review of the international literature, although simple hallucinations are likely following damage to either hemisphere, complex hallucinations are usually associated with right rather than left cerebral lesions (Teuber *et al.*, 1960; Mullan & Penfield, 1959; Hecaen & Albert, 1978).

CORTICAL BLINDNESS

Lesions of the occipital lobe, especially if the entire visual cortex is ablated, result in cortical blindness, such that pattern and form vision is lost. Rather, what is left is the ability to discriminate only between different fluxes in luminous energy, i.e., lightness and darkness (Brindley, Smith, & Lewin, 1969; Brodal, 1981; Hecaen & Albert, 1978; Weiskrantz, 1963). If damage is restricted to the occipital lobe of only one of the hemispheres, the patient will lose patterned vision for the opposite half of the visual field (i.e., a *hemianopsia*). This is not the same as unilateral neglect or inattention. However, if the lesion is sufficiently large and involves the right parietal area as well, the patient may suffer from both hemianopsia and neglect.

Nevertheless, if only a portion of the visual cortex is destroyed, vision is lost only for the corresponding quadrant of the visual field, referred to as a *scotoma*. However, in cases of partial cortical blindness, patients are able to make compensatory eye movements and are not terribly troubled by their disability (Luria, 1980). Indeed, patients frequently have no awareness that they have lost a quadrant or even half of their visual field, so this must be tested for.

"Blind Sight"

Although considered somewhat controversial, it has been reported that although blind (due to destruction of a portion of the visual cortex), some patients are able to indicate the presence or absence of a stimulus within the "blind" portion of their visual field and even differentiate between various objects, although not knowing what they are. This has been referred to as "blind sight" (Weiskrantz, Warrington, Sanders, & Marshall, 1974). Possibly, although cortically blind, patients are able to accomplish this through intact subcortical nuclei involved in visual orientation, i.e., the superior colliculus (Schneider, 1969).

Denial of Blindness

More frequently, however, patients with cortical blindness (such as following massive lesions of the visual cortex) initially seem quite confused and indifferent regarding their condition and report a variety of hallucinatory experiences that may be complex or elementary in form. Moreover, frequently these patients will deny initially that they are blind (Redlich & Dorsey, 1945)—a condition referred to as Anton's syndrome. For example, a number of patients described by Redlich and Dorsey (1945), although bumping into furniture and unable to recognize objects held before them, invented elaborate excuses for their errors and failure to see, e.g., claiming that it was a little dark and that they needed their glasses or, conversely, that they saw better at home, i.e., these patients confabulated.

These confabulatory abnormalities are attributable to a disconnection such that the language axis, failing to receive information from the visual cortex (i.e., that it cannot see), responds instead to associations from intact areas which concern "seeing" (Chapters 1 and 5; and Joseph, 1986). That is, the language axis does not know that it is blind because information concerning blindness is not being received from the proper neural channels. It is also possible that these patients deny being blind, because subcortically they are still able to see. Although at a neocortical level there is no sight, subcortically there remains an unconscious awareness of the visual world.

VISUAL AGNOSIA

Visual agnosia is a condition in which the patient loses the capacity to recognize objects visually, although visual sensory functioning is largely normal. This condition often arises with lesions involving the inferior medial occipital lobe. In general, objects are detected, but they lose the ability to evoke meaning and cannot be identified (Critchley, 1964; Teuber, 1968). The percept becomes stripped of its meaning. For example, if shown a comb, the patient might have no idea as to what it is or what it might be used for. If asked to guess, she might call it a harmonica or a tiny box. If shown a pair of spectacles, she might call it a bicycle, or two spoons. A picture of a dial telephone might be described as a clock (Luria, 1980).

Many patients are unable to sort pictures or objects into categories or match pictures with the actual object, such that there appears to be a deficit in the ability to not only recognize but to classify visual percepts (Hecaen & Albert, 1978). Moreover, they are unable to point to objects that are named.

Nevertheless, this is not a naming disorder, because regardless of modality, anomics continue to have word finding and naming difficulties. By contrast, those with agnosia show enhanced recognition if an object is presented through a second intact modality (e.g., if they palpate it by hand). Thus, agnosia can often be limited to a single input channel, i.e., visual versus tactual. Moreover, if an object is used in context, recognition can be greatly enhanced (Rubens, 1979). Some patients may complain that objects change while they are looking at them and/or that they disappear, a condition that suggests optic ataxia. Usually, however, the deficit is conceptual rather than perceptual.

Although recognition is abolished, they may be able to describe, draw, or copy various aspects of the object they are shown accurately (Albert, Reches, & Silverberg, 1975; Mack & Boller, 1977; Rubens & Benson, 1971). However, they fail to draw the entire object correctly. Moreover, if asked to trace rather than copy, these patients may trace over and over the outlines of objects or drawing but cannot recognize where they started. Thus they seem unable to synthesize visual details into an integral whole (Luria, 1980). That is, patients may recognize an isolated detail (e.g., the dial of a phone) but are unable to relate it to the headset, and so forth. If asked what they have been shown, they may erroneously extrapolate from the detail perceived and thus confabulate a concept.

With increasing complexity, if surrounded by other objects, if it is presented in pictorial (versus actual) form, or if unnecessary lines are drawn across the picture, the abilty to recognize the object deteriorates even further (Luria, 1980; Rubens & Benson, 1971).

Agnosic patients also often have difficulty with reading (Albert *et al.*, 1975; Mack & Boller, 1977; Rubens & Benson, 1971) and may suffer from prosopagnosia and/or impaired color naming (Mack & Boller, 1977). Interestingly, in some cases visual memory may be intact (Rubens, 1979).

Like alexia, agnosia can occur following lesions to the medial and deep mesial portion of the left occipital lobe. The left inferior temporal lobe and posterior hippocampus may also be damaged in some cases. In some respects, it is likely that agnosia is due not so much to tissue destruction as to tissue disconnection. That is, if the visual form-recognition neurons in the temporal lobe are no longer able to receive input from the visual association areas, this particular region becomes cortically blind, preventing form recognition. However, like some other disconnection syndromes, if a different input channel is employed, i.e., if the object is verbally described or tactually explored, recognition is enhanced.

PROSOPAGNOSIA

Prosopagnosia is a severe disturbance in the ability to recognize the faces of friends, loved ones, or pets (DeRenzi, 1986; DeRenzi, Faglioni, & Spinnler, 1968; DeRenzi & Spinnler, 1966; Hecaen & Angelergues, 1962; Landis, Cummings, Christen, Bogen, & Imhof, 1986; Levine, 1978; Whitely & Warrington, 1977). Some patients may in fact be unable to recognize their own face in the mirror. Nevertheless, they usually realize that a face is a face; they just don't know to whom the face belongs. In this regard, prosopagnosia is not a visual agnosia as described above, in which the patient cannot recognize that a chair is a chair or a clock is a clock.

A number of investigators have argued that prosopagnosia is caused by bilateral injuries involving the inferior and medial occipital lobe, hence the visual association areas (see Damasio & Damasio, 1983, for review). Nevertheless, although frequently such patients do indeed suffer from bilateral injuries, in many cases the lesions are restricted to the right hemisphere and involve the occipital and inferior temporal regions (DeRenzi, 1986; DeRenzi *et al.*, 1968; DeRenzi & Spinnler, 1966; Hecaen & Angelergues, 1962; Landis *et al.*, 1986; Levine, 1978; Whitely & Warrington, 1977). Prosopagnosia does not usually result from lesions restricted to the left half of the brain.

Although prosopagnosia could be explained from a disconnection perspective, it is likely that the actual face-identification neurons have been destroyed, whereas neurons involved in the recognition of facial parts have been preserved (see Chapter 7).

SIMULTANAGNOSIA

Simultanagnosia occurs with left hemisphere damage and is an inability to see more than one thing at a time (Kinsbourne & Warrington, 1962, 1964). This condition is sometimes accompanied by abnormal eye movements (Luria, 1980). In fact, by surrounding the object with other objects, perceptual recognition deteriorates even further. These patients often have difficulty shifting gaze and/or performing visual search tasks such that their ability to scan and visually explore the environment is drastically reduced. As described by Luria (1980), this is caused by a breakdown in the ability to perform serial feature-by-feature visual analysis. Visual attention is largely limited to the central visual field, whereas the periphery is ignored (Hecaen & De Ajuriaguerra, 1954; Luria, 1973, 1980). However, patients complain that even objects in the central visual field tend to disappear as they stare at them.

Simultagnosia has been described following lesions to the frontal eye fields and following bilateral superior occipital lobe lesions (Rizzo & Hurtig, 1987). In many cases, the lesion may be localized to the superior occipital–parietal region (area 7). Thus, the patient is no longer able to maintain visual fixation and cannot adequately focus on an object or explore its parts. This disorder has also been referred to as Balint's syndrome as well as optic ataxia, paralysis of gaze, and concentric narrowing of the visual field.

IMPAIRED COLOR RECOGNITION

In impaired color recognition, although sometimes able to name objects correctly, patients are unable to name, match, and identify colors or point to colors named by the examiner correctly. No, this is not color blindness. Frequently patients with color imperception also display prosopagnosia (Green & Lessel, 1977; Meadows, 1974b).

DeRenzi and Spinnler (1967) found that 23% of those with right cerebral damaged and 12% of those with left-sided destruction had difficulty with color matching. Other investigators note that impairment of color perception is frequently secondary to bilateral inferior occiptial lobe damage (Green & Lessell, 1977; Meadows, 1974a). In addition, almost 50% of those with aphasia demonstrate deficient color naming and color identification (DeRenzi & Spinnler, 1967; DeRenzi et al., 1972). However, color perception per se is largely intact among aphasic patients.

SUMMARY

The primary visual cortex is located predominantly within the medial walls of the cerebral hemispheres and is concerned with the elementary aspects of form peception. Damage limited to this area will usually affect foveal vision and/or give rise to simple hallucinations. From the primary area, information is then relayed to the association areas, 18 and 19, where complex analysis including form recognition, position, and analysis of depth takes place. Damage involving these areas and the primary region can cause cortical blindness or hemianopsia if only one hemisphere is lesioned. Destruction or abnormal activity in areas 18 and 19 is associated with the formation of complex hallucinations.

Visual information is next relayed to area 7 in the parietal lobe and to the inferior temporal lobule, where higher-order analysis and multimodal processing occurs. Damage to the parietal–occipital borders may result in abnormalities involving depth and form perception. Destruction of the temporal–occipital regions can give rise to visual agnosias and an inability to rcognize faces, i.e., prosopagnosia.

The occipital lobes also appear to be lateralized in regard to certain capabilities such as facial recognition. For example, destruction of the right occipital region is associated with prosopagnosia, and abnormal activity in this area is more likely to give rise to complex visual hallucinations.

REFERENCES

Albert, M. L., Reches, A., & Silverberg, R. (1975). Associative visual agnosia without alexia. *Neurology (New York), 25,* 322–326.

Blakemore, C. (1970). The representation of three-dimensional space in the cat's striate cortex. *Journal of Physiology, 209,* 155–178.

Brindley, G. S., Smith, G. P. C., & Lewin, W. (1969). Cortical blindness and the functions of the nongeniculate fibers of the optic tracts. *Journal of Neurology, Neurosurgery and Psychiatry, 32,* 259–264.

Brodal, A. (1981). *Neurological anatomy.* New York: Oxford University Press.

Casagrande, V. A., & Joseph, R. (1978). Effects of monocular deprivation on geniculostriate connections in prosimian primates. *Anatomical Record, 190,* 359.

Casagrande, V. A., & Joseph, R. (1980). Morphological effects of monocular deprivation and recovery on the dorsal lateral geniculate nucleus in galago. *Journal of Comparative Neurology, 194,* 413–426.

Critchley, M. (1964). The problem of visual agnosia. *Journal of Neurological Sciences, 1,* 274–290.

Damasio, A. R., & Damasio, H. (1983). Localization of lesions in achromatopsia and prosopagnosia. In A. Kertesz (Ed.), *Localization in neuropsychology* (pp. 110–123). Orlando, FL: Academic Press.

Daniel, P. M., & Whitteridge, L. (1961). The representation of the visual field on the cerebral cortex in monkeys. *Journal of Physiology, 159,* 203–221.

DeRenzi, E. (1986). Prosopagnosia in two patients with CT-scan evidence of damage confined to the right hemisphere. *Neuropsychologia, 24,* 385–389.

DeRenzi, E., Faglioni, P., & Spinnler, H. (1968). The performance of patients with unilateral brain damage on face recognition tasks. *Cortex, 4,* 17–34.

DeRenzi, E., & Spinnler, H. (1966). Facial recognition in brain-damaged patients. An experimental approach. *Neurology (New York), 16,* 145–152.

DeRenzi, E., & Spinnler, H. (1967). Impaired performance on color tasks in patients with hemispheric damage. *Cortex, 3,* 194–216.

Doty, R. W. (1983). Nongeniculate afferents to striate cortex in macaques. *Journal of Comparative Neurology, 218,* 159–173.

Dow, B. M. (1974). Functional classes of cells and their laminar distribution in monkey visual cortex. *Journal of Neurophysiology, 37,* 927–946.

Green, G. L., & Lessel, S. (1977). Acquired cerebral dyschromatopsia. *Archives of Ophthamology, 95,* 121–128.

Hecaen, H., & Albert, M. L. (1978). *Human neuropsychology.* New York: John Wiley & Sons.

Hecaen, H., & Angelergues, R. (1962). Agnosia for faces (prosagnosia). *Archives of Neurology, 7,* 92–100.

Hecaen, H., & De Ajuriaguerra, J. (1954). Balint's syndrome (psychic paralysis of visual fixation) and its minor forms. *Brain, 77,* 373–400.

Hubel, D. H., & Wiesel, T. N. (1959). Receptive fields of single neurons in the cat's striate cortex. *Journal of Physiology, 148,* 574–591.

Hubel, D. H., & Wiesel, T. N. (1962). Receptive fields, binocular perception and functional architecture in the cat's visual cortex. *Journal of Physiology, 160,* 106–154.

Hubel, D. H., & Wiesel, T. N. (1968). Receptive fields and functional architecture of monkey striate cortex. *Journal of Physiology, 195,* 215–243.

Hubel, D. H., & Wiesel, T. N. (1970). The period of susceptibility to the physiological effects of unilateral eye closure in kittens. *Journal of Physiology, 206,* 419–436.

Hubel, D. H., & Wiesel, T. N. (1974). Sequence regularity and geometry of orientation columns in monkey striate cortex. *Journal of Comparative Neurology, 158,* 267–293.

Hubel, D. H., & Wiesel, T. N. (1979). Brain mechanisms of vision. *Scientific American, 241,* 150–163.

Joseph, R. (1986). Confabulation and delusional denial. Frontal lobe and lateralized influences. *Journal of Clinical Psychology, 42,* 507–519.

Jung, R. (1961). Neuronal integration in the visual cortex and its significance for visual information. In W. A. Rosenblith (Ed.), *Sensory communication* (pp. 112–137). Canmbridge, MA: MIT Press.

Kawamura, S., Sprague, J. M., & Niimi, K. (1974). Corticofugal projections from the visual cortices to the thalamus and superior colliculus. *Journal of Comparative Neurology, 158,* 339–362.

Kinsbourne, M., & Warrington, E. K. (1962). A variety of reading disabilities associated with right hemisphere lesions. *Journal of Neurology, Neurosurgery and Psychiatry, 25,* 339–344.

Kinsbourne, M., & Warrington, E. K. (1964). Disorders of spelling. *Journal of Neurology, Neurosurgery and Psychiatry, 27,* 224–228.

Landis, T., Cummings, J. L., Christen, L., Bogen, J. E., & Imhof, H.-G. (1986). Are unilateral right posterior cerebral lesions sufficient to cause prosopagnosia? Clinical and radiological findings in six additional patients. *Cortex, 22, 243,* 252–587.

Levine, D. N. (1978). Prosopagnosia and visual object agnosia: A behavioral study. *Brain and Language, 5,* 341–365.

Lin, C.-S., Weller, R. E., & Kaas, J. H. (1982). Cortical connections of striate cortex in the owl monkey. *Journal of Comparative Neurology, 211,* 165–176.

Luria, A. (1973). *The working brain.* New York: Basic Books.

Luria, A. (1980). *Higher cortical functions in man.* New York: Basic Books.

Mack, J. L., & Boller, F. (1977). Associative visual agnosia and its related deficits. *Neuropsychologia, 15,* 345–349.

Martinez-Millan, L., & Hollander, H. (1975). Cortico-cortical projections from striate cortex of the squirrel monkey. *Brain Research, 83,* 405–417.

Meadows, J. C. (1974a). Disturbed perception of colours associated with localized cerebral lesions. *Brain, 97,* 615–632.

Meadows, J. C. (1974b). The anatomical basis of prosopagnosia. *Journal of Neurology, Neurosurgery and Psychiatry, 37,* 489–501.

Mullan, S., & Penfield, W. (1959). Epilepsy and visual halluciantions. *Archives of Neurology and Psychiatry, 81,* 269–281.

Penfield, W., & Jasper, H. (1954). *Epilepsy and the functional anatomy of the human brain.* Boston: Little, Brown.

Penfield, W., & Rasmussen, T. (1950).*The cerebral cortex of man: A clinical study of localization of function.* New York: Macmillan.

Redlich, F. C., & Dorsey, J. E. (1945). Denial of blindness by patients with cerebral disease. *Archives of Neurology and Psychiatry, 53,* 407–417.

Rizzo, M., & Hurtig, R. (1987). Looking but not seeing. *Neurology (New York), 37,* 1642–1648.

Rubens, A. B. (1979). Agnosia. In K. M. Heilman & E. Valenstein (Eds.), *Clinical neuropsychology* (pp. 141–200). New York: Oxford University Press.

Rubens, A. B., & Benson, D. F. (1971). Associative visual agnosia. *Archives of Neurology, 24,* 305–316.

Russell, W. R., & Whitty, W. M. (1955). Studies in traumatic epilepsy. *Journal of Neurology, Neurosurgery and Psychiatry, 18,* 79–96.

Schneider, G. E. (1969). Two visual systems. *Science, 163,* 895–902.

Snyder, M., & Diamond, I. T. (1968). The organization and function of the visual cortex in the gtree shrew. *Brain Behavior and Evolution, 1,* 244–288.

Tarachow, S. (1941). The clinical value of hallucinations in localizing brain tumors. *American Journal of Psychiatry, 97,* 1434–1443.

Teuber, H. L. (1968). Disorders of memory following penetrating missile wounds of the brain. *Neurology (New York), 18,* 287–288.

Teuber, H. L., Battersby, W. S., & Bender, M. B. (1960). *Visual field defects after penetrating missile wounds of the brain.* Cambridge, MA: Harvard University Press.

Tigges, J., Walker, L. C., & Tigges, M. (1983). Subcortical projections to the occipital and parietal lobes of the chimpanzee brain. *Journal of Comparative Neurology, 220,* 106–115.

Weiskrantz, L. (1963). Contour discrimination in a young monkey with striate cortex ablation. *Neuropsychologia, 1,* 145–164.

Weiskrantz, L., Warrington, E. K., Sanders, M. D., & Marshall, J. (1974). Visual capacity in the hemianopic field following a restricted occipital ablation. *Brain, 97,* 709–728.

Whiteley, A. M., & Warrington, E. K. (1977). Prosopagnosia: A clinical, psychological and anatomical study of three patients, *Journal of Neurology, Neurosurgery and Psychiatry, 40,* 395–403.

Zeki, S. M. (1974). Functional organization of a visual area in the posterior bank of the superior temporal sulcus of the rhesus monkey. *Journal of Physiology, 236,* 549–573.

Zeki, S. M. (1978a). Functional specialisation in the visual cortex of the rhesus monkey. *Nature (London), 274,* 423–428.

Zeki, S. M. (1978b). The cortical projections of foveal striate cortex in the rhesus monkey. *Journal of Physiology, 277,* 227–244.

The Temporal Lobes

The temporal lobes are usually associated with the processing of auditory stimuli; indeed, the primary and association auditory areas are localized within the superior temporal gyrus. Nevertheless, the temporal lobe also receives extensive projections from the somesthetic and visual association areas 18 and 19 (Jones & Powell, 1970; Seltzer & Pandya, 1978); receives and processes gustatory, visceral, and olfactory sensations; harbors the amygdala and hippocampus within its inferior depths; and contains a considerable number of neurons that are heavily involved in the performance of complex visual integrative activities, including visual closure and the recognition of specific meaningful forms. Indeed, it has been argued that the temporal lobe evolved from visual cortex (Diamond, 1943), and it is apparent based on a variety of neurophysiological, neuroanatomical, and behavioral studies that the middle, inferior, and posterior–superior temporal lobe are indeed cortical visual areas.

TEMPORAL TOPOGRAPHY

The temporal lobes are composed of a number of cytoarchitectural–functional regions, which, unfortunately, are not well demarcated through the use of Brodmann's maps. Nevertheless, it is possible to very loosely define the anterior–middle and superior–temporal lobes as auditory cortex, whereas the inferior, posterior–middle temporal zones are visual cortices. The posterior–superior temporal lobule (coextensive with the inferior parietal region) is a multimodal association area, as it contains both auditory and visually responsive nuclei and receives fibers from somesthetic cortex. In addition, buried within the depths of the inferior temporal lobe are the amygdala and hippocampus, two limbic nuclei intimately involved in emotion, learning, and memory. These latter regions act to assign emotional and motivational significance to visual somesthetic and auditory perceptions. (See Chapter 3 for details.) Lastly, located around and behind the superior temporal lobe is the insular region. The insular cortex maintains extensive interconnections with the limbic system, as well as the somesthetic, visual, and auditory association areas, and contains neurons specialized for the reception and analysis of gustatory, olfactory, visceral sensations.

AUDITORY FUNCTIONING

Primary Auditory Receiving Area

Once auditory stimuli are received in the cochlea of the ear, a series of transformations follows as the information is relayed to various nuclei, e.g., the cochlear nucleus, superior olivary complex, and lateral lemniscus of the brainstem, inferior colliculus, and medial geniculate nucleus of the thalamus before reception in the primary auditory cortex. Auditory information is relayed from the medial geniculate nucleus of the thalamus to a neocortical region referred to as Heschl's gyrus, i.e., the primary auditory receiving area (Brodmann's areas 41 and 42), all located within the superior temporal gyrus and buried within the depths of the Sylvian fissure. In general, the primary auditory cortex appears to be larger on the left (Geschwind & Levitsky, 1968; Wada, Clark, & Hamm, 1975).

Unlike the primary visual and somesthetic areas, the primary auditory region receives some bilateral input. This is because there is so much cross-talk between different subcortical nuclei as information is relayed to and from various regions prior to transfer to the neocortex. Predominantly, however, the right ear transmits to the left cerebral cortex and vice versa (Figs. 46–48).

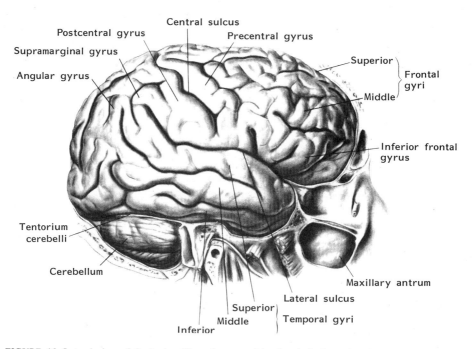

FIGURE 46. Lateral view of the brain still partly encased by the skull. Reproduced, by permission, from *Neuroanatomy*, 2nd Ed., by F. A. Mettler, 1948, C. V. Mosby Company, St. Louis, MO.

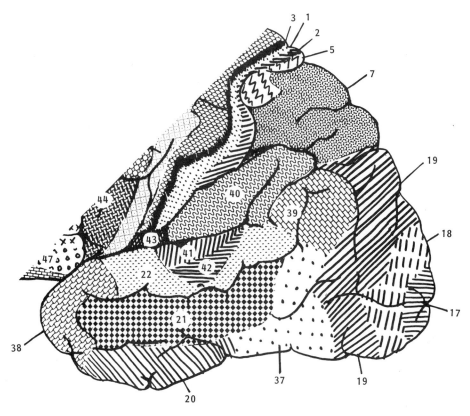

FIGURE 47. Lateral view of the posterior portion of the left hemisphere. Numbers refer to Brodmann's areas.

Anatomical–Functional Organization

There is some indication that the primary auditory area is tonotopically organized (Woolsey & Fairman, 1946), such that different auditory frequencies are progressively anatomically represented. High frequencies are received and analyzed in the anterior–medial portions and low frequencies in the posterior–lateral regions of the superior temporal lobe (Merzenich & Brugge, 1973).

Sustained Activity

One of the main functions of the primary receptive area appears to be the retention of sounds for brief time periods (up to 1 second), so that temporal and sequential features may be extracted and discrepancies in spatial location identified. This allows comparisons to be made with previously received and incoming auditory input. Moreover, through their sustained activity, these neurons are able to prolong (perhaps via a perseverative feedback loop with the thalamus) the duration of certain sounds such that they are more amenable to analysis (Luria, 1980). In this manner, even complex sounds can be broken

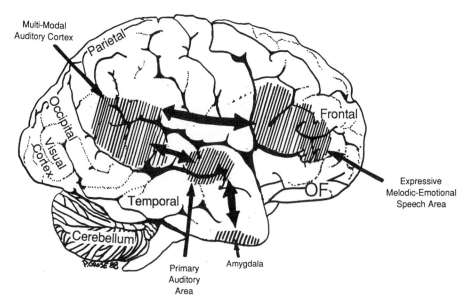

FIGURE 48. Auditory pathways within the right hemisphere.

down into components that are then separately anlayzed; i.e., sounds can be perceived as sustained temporal sequences.

Temporal–Sequential and Linguistic Sensitivity

Nevertheless, although it is apparent that the auditory regions of both cerebral hemispheres are capable of discerning and extracting temporal–sequential rhythmic acoustics (Milner, 1962), the left temporal lobe apparently contains a greater concentration of neurons specialized for this purpose as the left brain is clearly superior in this capacity.

For example, the left hemisphere has been repeatedly shown to be specialized for sorting, separating, and extracting in a segmented fashion, the phonetic and temporal–sequential or linguistic–articulatory features of incoming auditory information so as to identify speech units. It is also more sensitive to rapidly changing acoustic cues, be they verbal or nonverbal, as compared with the right hemisphere (Shankweiler & Studdert-Kennedy, 1967; Studdert-Kennedy & Shankweiler, 1970). Moreover, through dichotic listening tasks, the right ear (left temporal lobe) has been shown to be dominant for the perception of real words, word lists, numbers, backwards speech, Morse code, consonants, consonant–vowel syllables, nonsense syllables, the transitional elements of speech, single phonemes, and rhymes (Blumstein & Cooper, 1974; Bryden, 1967; Cutting, 1974; Kimura, 1961; Kimura & Folb, 1968; Levy, 1974; Mills & Rollman, 1979; Papcun, Krashen & Ter Beek, 1974; Shankweiler & Studert-Kennedy, 1966, 1967; Studdert-Kennedy & Shankweiler, 1970).

Spatial Localization, Attention, and Environmental Sounds

In conjunction with the inferior colliculus, and because the neurons in this region receive input from both ears, the primary auditory area plays a significant role in orienting to and localizing the source of various sounds (Sanchez-Longo & Forster, 1958), e.g., by comparing time and intensity differences in the neural input from each ear. A sound arising from one's right will reach and sound louder to the right ear as compared with the left.

Indeed, among mammals, a considerable number of auditory neurons respond or become highly excited only in response to sounds from a particular location (Evans & Whitfield, 1968). Moreover, some of these neurons become excited only when the subject looks at the source of the sound. Thus, these neurons act so that location may be identified and fixated upon. These complex interactions probably involve the parietal area (7), as well as the midbrain colliculi. As based on lesions studies in humans, the right temporal lobe is more involved than the left in discerning location (Penfield & Evans, 1934; Shankweiler, 1961).

There is also some indication that certain cells in the auditory area are highly specialized and will respond only to certain meaningful vocalizations (Wollberg & Newman, 1972). In this regard they seemed to be tuned to respond only to specific auditory parameters so as to identify and extract certain meaningful features, i.e., feature detector cells. For example, some cells will respond to cries of alarm and sounds suggestive of fear or indicating anger, whereas others will react only to specific sounds and vocalizations.

Nevertheless, although the left temporal lobe appears to be more involved in extracting certain linguistic features, the right temporal region is more adept at identifying and recognizing nonverbal environmental acoustics (e.g., wind, rain, animal noises), prosodic–melodic nuances, sounds that convey emotional meaning, as well as most aspects of music (Joseph, 1988) (see also Chapter 1).

Indeed, the right temporal lobes spatial localization sensitivity coupled with its ability to perceive and recognize environmental sounds no doubt provided great survival value to early primitive man. That is, in response to a specific sound (e.g., a creeping predator), one is able to identify, localize, locate, and fixate immediately on the source and thus take appropriate action. Even modern humans relie upon the same mechanisms to escape being run over by cars when walking across streets or riding bicycles, or to ascertain and identify approaching individuals.

Hallucinations

Electrical stimulation of Heschyl's gyrus produces elementary hallucinations (Penfield & Jasper, 1954; Penfield & Perot, 1963). These include buzzing, clicking, ticking, humming, whispering, and ringing, most of which are localized as coming from the opposite side of the room. Tumors involving this area also give rise to similar albeit transient hallucinations, including tinnitus (Brodal, 1981). Patients may complain that sounds seem louder and/or softer than normal, closer and/or more distant, strange, or even unpleasant (Hecaen & Albert, 1978). There is often a repetitive quality, which makes the experience even more disagreeable. In some instances, the hallucination may become meaningful, such as the sound of footsteps, clapping hands, or music, most of which seem (to the patient) to have an actual external source.

Laterality

Penfield and Perot (1963) reported that electrical stimulation of the superior temporal gyrus, the right temporal lobe in particular results in musical hallucinations. Patients with tumors and seizure disorders, particularly those involving the right temporal region, may also experience musical hallucinations. Frequently the same melody is heard over and over. In some instances, patients have reported the sound of singing voices, and individual instruments may be heard (Hecaen & Albert, 1978).

Conversely, it has been frequently reported that lesions or complete surgical destruction of the right temporal lobe significantly impairs the ability to name or recognize melodies and musical passages. It also disrupts time sense, the perception of timbre, loudness, and tonal memory (Chase, 1967; Joseph, 1988; Milner, 1962; Shankweiler, 1966).

Auditory verbal hallucinations seem to occur with right or left temporal destruction or stimulation (Hecaen & Albert, 1978; Penfield & Perot, 1963; Tarachow, 1941), although left temporal involvement is predominant. The hallucination may involve single words, sentences, commands, advice, or distant conversations that cannot quite be made out. According to Hecaen and Albert (1978), verbal hallucinations may precede the onset of an aphasic disorder, such as due to a developing tumor or other destructive process. Patients may complain of hearing "distorted sentences," "incomprehensible words," and so forth.

Cortical Deafness

In some instances, such as in middle cerebral artery stroke, the primary auditory receiving areas of the right or left cerebral hemisphere may be destroyed. This results in a disconnection syndrome such that sounds relayed from the thalamus cannot be received or analyzed by the temporal lobe. In some cases, however, the strokes may be bilateral. When both primary auditory receiving areas have been destroyed, the patient is said to be suffering from cortical deafness. However, sounds continue to be processed subcortically—much like cortical blindness. Thus, the ability to hear sounds per se, is retained. Nevertheless, since the sounds that are heard are not received neocortically, they cannot be transmitted to the adjacent association areas, and sounds become stripped of meaning. That is, meaning cannot be extracted or assigned. Rather, only differences in intensity are discernible—much like cortical blindness.

Patients cannot respond to questions, do not show startle responses to loud sounds, lose the ability to discern the melody for music, cannot recognize speech or environmental sounds, and tend to experience the sounds they do hear as distorted and disagreeable, e.g., the banging of tin cans, buzzing, and roaring (Albert, Sparks, von Strockert, & Sax, 1972; Auerbach, Allard, Naeser, *et al.*, 1982; Earnest, Monroe, & Yarnell, 1977; Mendez & Geehan, 1988; Reinhold, 1950).

Such patients also commonly experience difficulty discriminating sequences of sound, detecting difference in temporal patterning, and determining sound duration, whereas intensity discriminations are better preserved. Such patients may display auditory inattention (Hecaen & Albert, 1978) and a failure to respond to loud sounds.

Nevertheless, patients who are cortically deaf are not aphasic or agnosic. They can read, write, speak, and comprehend pantomime and are fully aware of their deficit. Nevertheless, although not aphasic, per se, speech is sometimes noted to be hypophonic and contaminated by occasional literal paraphasias.

In some instances, rather than bilateral, a destructive lesion may be limited to the primary receiving area of just the right or left cerebral hemisphere. These patients are not considered cortically deaf. However, when the auditory receiving area of the left temporal lobe is destroyed, the patient suffers from a condition referred to as *pure word deafness*. If the lesion is in the right temporal receiving area, the disorder is described as an *auditory agnosia*.

Pure Word Deafness

With a destructive lesion involving the left auditory receiving area, Wernicke's area becomes disconnected from almost all sources of acoustic input, and patients are unable to recognize or perceive the sounds of language, be they sentences, single words, or even single letters (Hecaen & Albert, 1978). All other aspects of comprehension are preserved, including reading, writing, and expressive speech. Moreover, because of sparing of the right temporal region, the ability to recognize musical and environmental sounds is preserved. However, the ability to name or verbally describe them is impaired as a result of disconnection and the inability of the right hemisphere to talk.

Pure word deafness also occurs with bilateral lesions, in which case environmental sound recognition is also affected. In these instances, the patient is considered cortically deaf.

Pure word deafness, when caused by a unilateral lesion of the left temporal lobe, is partly a consequence of an inability to extract temporal–sequential features from incoming sounds. Thus, linguistic messages cannot be recognized. However, pure word deafness can be partly overcome if the patient is spoken to in an extremely slowed manner (Albert & Bear, 1974). The same is true of those with Wernicke's aphasia.

Auditory Agnosia

A patient with cortical deafness caused by bilateral lesions suffers from a generalized auditory agnosia involving words and nonlinguistic sounds. However, in many instances, an auditory agnosia, with preserved perception of language may occur with lesions restricted to the right temporal lobe. In these instances, a patient loses the capability to discern environmental sounds correctly (e.g., birds singing, doors closing, keys jangling), emotional–prosodic speech, as well as music (see Chapter 1).

These problems are less likely to come to the attention of a physician unless accompanied by secondary emotional difficulties. That is, most patients with this disorder, being agnosic, would not know that they have a problem and therefore would not complain. If they are their families notice (e.g., if a patient does not respond to a knock on the door) the likelihood is that the problem will be attributed to faulty hearing or even forgetfulness.

However, because such patients may also have difficulty discerning emotional–

melodic nuances, it is likely that they will misperceive and fail to comprehend a variety of paralinguistic social–emotional messages. This includes difficulty discerning what others may be implying or in appreciating emotional and contextual cues, including such variables as sincerity or mirthful intonation. Thus, a host of behavioral difficulties may arise.

For example, a patient may complain that his wife no longer loves him and that he knows this from the sound of her voice. In fact, a patient may notice that the voices of friends and family sound in some manner different, which, when coupled with difficulty discerning such nuances as humor and friendliness may lead to the development of paranoia and what appears to be delusional thinking. Indeed, unless appropriately diagnosed, it is likely that the patients problem will feed on and reinforce itself and grow more severe.

It is important to note that rather than completely agnosic or word deaf, patients may suffer from only partial deficits. In these instances, they may seem to be hard of hearing, frequently misinterpret what is said to them, and/or slowly develop related emotional difficulties.

AUDITORY ASSOCIATION AREA

The auditory area although originating in the depths of the superior temporal lobe extends in a continuous beltlike fashion posteriorly from primary and association (e.g., Wernicke's) area toward the inferior parietal lobule and through the arcuate fasciculus onward toward Broca's area. Indeed, in the left hemisphere, this massive rope of interconnections forms an axis such that Wernicke's area, the inferior parietal lobule, and Broca's area are able together to mediate the perception and expression of most forms of language and speech.

The ropelike arcuate fasciculus is a bidirectional fiber pathway, however, that runs not only from Wernicke's through to Broca's area but extends inferiorly deep into the temporal lobe, where contact is established with the amygdala. In this manner, auditory input comes to be assigned emotional–motivational significance, whereas verbal output becomes emotionally–melodically colored. Within the right hemisphere, these interconnections, which include the amygdala, appear to be more extensively developed.

Wernicke's Area

Following the analysis performed in the primary auditory receiving area, auditory information is transmitted to the immediately adjacent association cortex (Brodmann's area 22), where more complex forms of processing take place. In both hemispheres, this region partly surrounds the primary area and then extends posteriorly, merging with the inferior parietal lobule with which it maintains extensive interconnections. Within the left hemisphere, the more posterior portion of area 22, and part of area 42 corresponds to Wernicke's area.

Wernicke's area and the corresponding region in the right hemisphere are not merely auditory association areas, as they also receive a convergence of fibers from the somesthetic and visual association cortices (Jones & Powell, 1970; Zeki, 1978b). Thus, it is involved in multimodal as well as auditory associational analyses. The auditory association area (area 22) also receives fibers from the contralateral auditory association area via the corpus callosum and anterior commissure and projects to the frontal convexity and orbital region, the frontal eye fields, and cingulate gyrus (Jones & Powell, 1970), so that a considerable number of multimodal linkages are maintained by the auditory association area. In fact, this region appears to be responsible for the integration and assimilation of a diverse number of informational variables (Luria, 1980) and probably acts in close conjunction with the frontal and inferior parietal lobe in this regard. Indeed, the richness of language and the ability to use a mutlitude of words and images to describe a single object or its use is very much dependent on these interconnections.

Receptive Aphasia

When the posterior portion of the left auditory association area is damaged, severe receptive aphasia results, i.e., Wernicke's aphasia. Individuals with Wernicke's aphasia, in addition to severe comprehension deficits (see Chapter 2 for details) usually suffer abnormalities involving expressive speech, reading, writing, repeating, word finding, and so forth. Spontaneous speech is often fluent, however, and sometimes is hyperfluent such that they speak at an increased rate and seem unable to bring sentences to an end—as if the temporal–sequential separations between words have been extremely shortened or in some instances abolished. In addition, many of the words spoken are contaminated by neologistic and paraphasic distortions. As such, what these patients say is often incomprehensible (Hecaen & Albert, 1978). This disorder has also been referred to as *fluent aphasia*.

Patients with Wernicke's aphasia, however, are still able to perceive the temporal–sequential pattern of incoming auditory stimuli to some degree (due to preseveration of the primary region). Nevertheless, they are unable to perceive spoken words in their correct order, cannot identify the pattern of presentation (e.g. two short and three long taps) and become easily overwhelmed (Hecaen & Albert, 1978; Luria, 1980). Patients with Wernicke's aphasia, in addition to other impairments, are often ''word deaf.'' As these individuals recover from their aphasia, word deafness is often the last symptom to disappear (Hecaen & Albert, 1978).

The Melodic–Intonational Axis

It has been consistently demonstrated among normals (such as in dichotic listening studies), that the right temporal lobe (left ear) predominates in the perception of timbre, chords, tone, pitch, loudness, melody, and intensity—the major components (in conjunction with harmony) of a musical stimulus (Joseph, 1988). Both the right and left hemisphere seem to process the rhythmic features of music with equal facility.

When the right temporal lobe is damaged (e.g., right temporal lobectomy, right amygdalectomy), time sense, rhythm, and the ability to sing, carry a tune, perceive, recognize or recall tones, loudness, timbre, and melody are disrupted. Similarly, the ability to recognize even familiar melodies and the capacity to obtain pleasure while listening to music is abolished or significantly reduced, a condition referred to as *amusia*.

In addition, lesions involving the right temporal–parietal area have been reported to impair significantly the ability to perceive and identify environmental sounds, comprehend or produce appropriate verbal prosody, emotional speech, or to repeat emotional statements (Joseph, 1988*a*). Indeed, when presented with neutral sentences spoken in an emotional manner, right temporal–parietal damage has been reported to disrupt the perception and comprehension of emotional prosody, regardless of its being positive or negative in content. (See Chapter 1 and references cited therein.)

Hence, the right temporal–parietal area is involved in the perception, identification, and comprehension of environmental and musical sounds and various forms of melodic and emotional auditory stimuli; it probably acts to prepare this information for expression via transfer to the right frontal convexity, which is dominant regarding the expression of emotional–melodic and even environmental sounds. Indeed, it appears that an emotional–melodic–intonational axis, somewhat similar to the language axis in anatomical design, is maintained within the right hemisphere (Ross, 1981; Gorelick & Ross, 1987).

When the posterior portion of the melodic–emotional axis is damaged, the ability to comprehend or repeat melodic–emotional vocalizations in disrupted. Such patients are thus agnosic for nonlinguistic sounds. With right frontal convexity damage speech becomes bland, atonal, and monotone.

The Amygdala

The right cerebral hemisphere appears to maintain more extensive as well as bilateral interconnections with the limbic system (Joseph, 1982, 1989). (See also Chapters 1, 3, and 4.) Indeed, the limbic system also appears to be lateralized in regard to certain aspects of emotional functioning such that the right amygdala, hippocampus, and hypothalamus seem to exert dominant influences.

As noted, the arcuate fasciculus extends from the amygdala (which is buried within the anterior–inferior temporal lobe) through the auditory association area and inferior parietal region and into the frontal convexity. It is possibly through these interconnections that emotional colorization is added to neocortical acoustic perceptions as well as sounds being prepared for expression. Thus, when the right amygdala has been destroyed or surgically removed, the ability to sing as well as to intonate properly is altered (see Chapter 3). In this regard, the amygdala should be considered part of the melodic–intonational axis of the right hemisphere, as it not only subcortically responds to and analyzes environmental sounds and emotional vocalizations but imparts emotional significance to auditory input and output processed and expressed at the level of the neocortex.

Nevertheless, it is possible that emotional–prosodic intonation is imparted directly to speech variables as they are being organized for expression within the left hemisphere. That is, although the right hemisphere is dominant in regard to melodic–emotional vocalizations, the two amygdalas are in direct communication through the anterior commissure. Thus, although originating predominantly within the right amygdala/hemisphere, these influences can be directly transmitted to the left half of the brain via the anterior commissure and then via the arcuate fasciculus into the linguistic stream of the language axis.

MIDDLE TEMPORAL LOBE

The middle temporal region is a complex multifunctional zone that is functionally lateralized and has both extensive visual and auditory capabilities. In general, the anterior middle region is more involved in auditory functioning, whereas the posterior middle temporal lobe is more intimately concerned with the processing of higher level visual information.

Anterior Middle Temporal Lobe: Audition

The anterior middle temporal region (AMT) maintains extensive interconnections with the superior and inferior temporal lobe, the auditory association area, frontal convexity, and orbital region (Jones & Powell, 1970; Pandya & Kuypers, 1969). In its journey from Wernicke's area to to the amygdala, the arcuate fasciculus passes through this cortical territory. The AMT appears to play a role in auditory memory as well as in the discrimination and organization of speech and other auditory sounds (Dewson, Pribram, & Lynch, 1969; Weiskrantz & Mishkin, 1958).

Left ATM Language Capabilities

As based on the electrical stimulation studies of Penfield and Rasmussen (1950), it appears that the auditory capabilities of the ATM are more extensively represented within the left hemisphere and that this area plays a significant role in speech output. Thus when the middle temporal lobe is stimulated there can result aphasic abnormalities (Penfield & Rasmussen, 1950).

Lesions involving this area are also associated with subtle disturbances involving language, including word-finding difficulty, confrontive naming deficits, abnormalities in the maintenance of temporal order and sequence, as well as verbal memory impairments (Luria, 1980). Patients may have difficulty recalling word lists or order of word presentation; the longer the list, the greater the difficulty. Hence, if a list of four words were read, the patient cannot repeat the correct order even after repeated presentations, although individual words may be recalled correctly (Luria, 1980). If the same material is presented visually, however, i.e., in a written format, the patient is able to perform without difficulty.

Thus, the disorder is caused by a failure to store auditory–linguistic rather than visual–linguistic material and is presumably secondary to disconnection. That is, a lesion involving the middle temporal region results in a severance of the fibers linking the memory centers in the inferior temporal region (e.g., the amygdala and hippocampus) with the auditory receiving areas. By presenting material visually, the intact pathway is used and the region of disconnection circumvented. Moreover, because the inferior temporal lobule is also specialized for the visual recognition of forms, disconnection may result in an inability to associate verbal labels with visual images, hence the confrontive naming difficulties associated with lesions to the left middle temporal lobe.

Hallucinations

Tumors involving the middle temporal lobe have been associated with the development of auditory and visual hallucinations, dream states, and alterations in emotional functioning—particularly as the lesion encroaches on the inferior regions (Luria, 1980). Electrical stimulation also initiates the development of complex hallucinations and alterations in consciousness (Penfield & Roberts, 1959).

Posterior Middle Temporal Lobe: Vision

The middle temporal gyrus (MTG), like other structures throughout the brain, appears to be functionally lateralized such that the right temporal region is more involved in visual functioning, whereas the left MTG is more concerned with auditory–linguistic capabilities. Whereas the auditory–linguistic zones appear to be more extensive within the left temporal lobe (and include portions of the posterior temporal region), the right MTG seems to be more associated with visual responsiveness. In general, however, the posterior middle temporal gyrus of both hemispheres appear to contain visually responsive neurons. Nevertheless, since there have been relatively few published studies of the effects of lesions or the functional capabilities of the middle temporal lobes in humans, notions regarding the extensiveness of auditory vs. visual lateralized representation are admittedly speculative.

Visual Functioning

Visual cells in the MTG receive direct projections from the striate cortex, area 17, and the association area 18 (Wall, Symonds, & Kass, 1982). This area in turn projects to the MTG of the opposite hemisphere via the corpus callosum, ipsilaterally to areas 17, 18, and 19, the inferior temporal and the parietal–occipital cortex (Tigges, Tigges, & Anschell, 1981; Wall, Symonds, & Kaas, 1982), and maintains interconnections with the pulvinar, superior colliculus, and pontine nuclei of the brainstem (Wall *et al.*, 1982) (Fig. 49). Thus this region has connections with areas concerned with visual and visual-attentional capabilities.

MTG neurons are sensitive to speed and direction of stimulus movement, motion, orientation, width, and disparity (Felleman & Kaas, 1984; Maunsell & Van Essen, 1983).

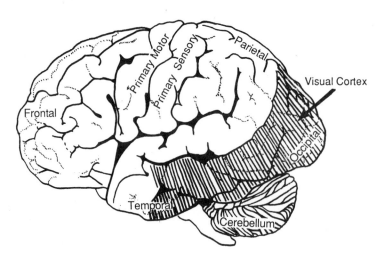

FIGURE 49. Schematic representation of visual cortex within the parietal, occipital, and temporal regions of the left cerebral hemisphere.

However, most MTG neurons are not particular sensitive to the form of a stimulus—most preferring narrow stimuli (Albright, Deimone, & Gross, 1984; Maunsell & Van Essen, 1983). A large number of cells have binocular capabilities and respond to stimuli from either or both eyes. Thus, these cells are significantly involved in stereoscopic vision as well as in determining distance.

Although not specialized for perception of form per se, by means of the combined analysis of width, orientation, speed, and direction of movement, these cells can process visual stimuli in a three-dimensional fashion, particularly in regard to trajectory, depth, and position, i.e., if an object is near or far, approaching or withdrawing (Maunsell & Van Essen, 1983).

Through its interconnections with the parietal–occipital lobe (an area involved in depth perception, visual fixation, and the visual–somesthetic guidance of movement), the MTG appears to provide visual guidance in regard to interactional object and body movement. That is, through the analysis of the flow of movement, local direction, and speed, as well as the relative distances of objects, these neurons (in conjunction with area 7 cells) are important in guiding the movements of the body as well as the individual's limbs toward the object (Maunsell and Van Essen, 1983).

The MTG maintains extensive interconnections with the inferior region and thus with limbic nuclei. It is probably via these connections that objects or conspecies of motivational significance can be discerned and attended to. That is, not only are the speed, movement, distance, and so forth, of a stimulus determined, but so are its emotional attributes (e.g., should it be feared, chased, eaten?).

INFERIOR TEMPORAL LOBE

Inferior temporal neurons receive highly processed input from the visual association areas in the occipital lobes of both cerebral hemispheres (via the corpus callosum), and from the superior colliculus by way of the pulvinar of the thalamus (Chow, 1950; Kuypers, Szwarcbart, Mishkin, & Rosvold, 1965; Rocha-Miranda, Bender, Gross, & Mishkin, 1975). Also, within the depths of the inferior temporal lobe (ITL) are the amygdala and hippocampus, with which extensive interconnections are maintained (see Chapter 3).

Visual Capabilities and Form Recognition

The neocortex of the ITL is specialized for receiving, analyzing, discriminating, recognizing, and recalling complex visual information and is involved in attention and visually guided behavior (Gross, Rocha-Miranda, & Bender, 1972), including the recollection and learning of visual discriminations (Gross, 1972). Cells in the ITL have very large, bilateral visual receptive fields, which include the fovea.

Many ITL neurons are involved in the supramodal analysis of information already processed in the association areas and are sensitive to the direction of stimulus movement, color, contrast, size, shape, orientation, and the perception of three-dimensional objects (Gross, Rocha-Miranda, & Bender, 1972). Indeed, a single neuron can respond to a combination of these features and many will fire selectively in response to particular shapes (Gross *et al.,* 1972; Richmond, Wurtz, & Sato, 1983).

Visual Attention

Attention and visual fixation involves the activation of neurons in the superior parietal lobe (area 7)—a region with which the ITL maintains interconnections. Attention, however, generally requires that visual fixation be focused. Since many ITL neurons maintain large bilateral visual fields, when engaged in visual fixation these cells appear to become partly suppressed. That is, the area of the visual field they respond to becomes restricted to the fovea (Richmond, Wurtz, & Sato, 1983). In this manner, ITL neurons become less responsive to other objects such as those in the periphery as the receptive field contracts around the object attended to.

Thus, ITL neurons seems to scan the entire visual field so as to alert the organism to objects of interest or motivational importance (through interconnections with limbic nuclei). When detected, area 7 neurons are activated triggering visual fixation. Simultaneously, ITL visual form recognition neurons are activated whereas those with wide nonspecific visual fields are inhibited. In this manner, objects of interest are detected and fixated on. Of adjunctive importance is the middle temporal lobe, which in turn can analyze the velocity and direction of the objects movement so that the individual may approach and, through interaction with cells in area 7, grasp and manipulate the object.

Form and Facial Recognition

Overall, the ITL appears to be involved in the highest level of visual integration, containing highly developed neurons that seem to be the end station of a hierarchical system that mediates the perception and recognition of specific and particular shapes and forms (cf. Desimone & Schein, 1987). Indeed, there is a pathway, beginning in the primary visual cortex, that passes through areas 18 and 19 and terminates in the ITL (Kuypers *et al.*, 1965). As information is passed from the primary visual cortex to these association areas, various features important in the identification of specific objects become progressively and hiarchically analyzed and increasingly complex associations are formed.

In fact, based on single cell recordings, some of these ITL neurons have been found to become particularly excited when presented with two-dimensional patterns or three-dimensional objects, such as hands, brushes, and, in particular, faces (Desimone & Gross, 1979; Gross *et al.*, 1972; Richmond *et al.*, 1983; Richmond, Optican, Podell, & Spitzer, 1987). A variety of different feature detectors were found. Some cells are responsive to particular facial orientations, such as a profile. In addition, some respond to only parts of the face, such as eyes or a mouth, whereas others respond only to the entire face, i.e., a correctly organized facial gestalt. Interestingly, the ITL also contains neurons that will fire even to a scrambled face, as long as all the features are present.

None of these cells which are selective to faces, hands, etc., will respond to other objects, including those with high emotional value. Face neurons only respond to faces. Thus, a minority of ITL neurons are in effect, facial neurons, hand neurons, etc., activated only when these items are viewed. Most cells in this area, however, were found to be selective for aspects of shapes, colors, or texture. These particular neurons probably act collectively so as to code and assemble a particular shape, including the formation of gestalts and thus the performance of visual closure.

Prosopagnosia and Visual Discrimination Deficits

Damage or removal of the inferior temporal lobe results in severe disturbances involving visual discrimination learning and retention (Gross & Mishkin, 1977; Mishkin, 1972) and severe difficulty performing visual closure and recognizing incomplete figural stimuli (Lansdell, 1968,1970). For example, primates with lesions in this vicinity have severe difficulty learning to discriminate between different shapes and patterns and objects which differ in regard to size or color, although visual acuity is normal.

With damage to the right occipital–temporal region, a severe disturbance in the ability to recognize the faces of friends, loved ones, or pets can result (DeRenzi, 1986; DeRenzi, Faglioni, & Spinnler, 1968; DeRenzi & Spinnler, 1966; Hecaen & Angelergues, 1962; Landis, Cummings, Christen, Bogen, & Imhof, 1986; Levine, 1978; Whitely & Warrington, 1977); a condition referred to as prosopagnosia. Some patients may in fact be unable to recognize their own face in the mirror. For example, one patient was unable even to discriminate between people on the basis of sex but instead had to rely on the presence of details, such as lipstick, rouge, hair length, a moustache, so as to make discriminations (Levine, 1978).

Presumably, the inability to recognize faces is a function of the destruction of facial (gestalt) recognition neurons. Because these cells are in a minority, whereas those specialized for analyzing facial parts are more numerous, the ability to recognize facial details is therefore more likely to be preserved.

Lateralization and Facial Recognition

Although patients with prosopagnosia often suffer from bilateral injuries, in many cases the lesions are restricted to the right hemisphere (DeRenzi, 1986; DeRenzi et al., 1968; DeRenzi & Spinnler, 1966; Hecaen & Angelergues, 1962; Landis et al., 1986; Levine, 1978; Whitely & Warrington, 1977). Disturbances involving facial recognition do not usually occur with isolated left cerebral lesions. Indeed, the right hemisphere appears to be dominant in regard to the recognition of both familiar and unfamiliar faces as has been well demonstrated in numerous studies of brain injured as well as normal, intact individuals (Bradshaw, Taylor, Patterson, & Nettleton, 1980; DeRenzi, 1982; DeRenzi, Faglione, & Spinnler, 1968; DeRenzi & Spinnler, 1966; Geffen, Bradshaw, & Wallace, 1971; Levy, Trevarthen, & Sperry, 1972; Ley & Bryden, 1977; Hecaen & Angelergues, 1962). There is some suggestion, however, that the left hemisphere is involved in the recognition of famous faces (Marzi & Berlucchi, 1977).

Among neurosurgical patients, it has also been reported that electrical stimulation of the posterior right temporal gyrus disrupts visual–spatial memory for faces in general (Fried, Mateer, Ojemann, Wohns, & Fedio, 1982). Electrical stimulation of the posterior portion of the right middle temporal gyrus also results in an inability to label emotional faces correctly.

It has also been reported that right temporal lobectomy or damage involving the inferior regions results in difficulty matching smells (Abraham & Mathai, 1983), although the ability to detect odor is intact.

Agnosias

When the ITL is damaged, in addition to prosopagnosia there may occur difficulty identifying various familiar stimuli and objects, e.g., utensils, cars, as well as differentiating among similar visual stimuli (Damasio & Damasio, 1983). Many patients also have difficulty with color recognition (Green & Lessell, 1977; Meadows, 1974). Frequently these types of agnosic disturbances are related to left cerebral or bilateral dysfunction.

MEMORY

Although a variety of neurochemical and neuroanatomical regions are involved in the formulation of memory (see Squire, 1987, for a recent detailed review), it has long been known that damage or the neurosurgical removal of the temporal lobes can produce profound disturbances in the learning and recollection of verbal and visual stimuli (Milner, 1958; Kimura, 1963). For example, left temporal lobectomy, seizures, or lesions involving the inferior temporal areas can moderately disrupt immediate memory and severely impair delayed memory for verbal passages, and significantly interfere with the recall of verbal paired associates, consonant trigrams, word lists, and number sequences (Delaney, Rosen, Mattson & Novelly, 1980; Meyer, 1959; Meyer & Yates, 1955; Milner, 1958, 1968, Milner & Teuber, 1968; Weingartner, 1968). Similarly, severe anterograde and retrograde memory loss for verbal material has been noted when the anterior and posterior temporal regions (respectively) are electrically stimulated (Ojemann, Fedio, & van Buren, 1968; Ojemann, Blick, & Ward, 1971).

In contrast, right temporal lesions or lobectomy significantly impair recognition memory for tactile and recurring visual stimuli such as faces and meaningless designs, as well as memory for object position and orientation, and visual–pictorial stimuli (Corkin, 1965; Delaney, Rosen, Mattson, & Novelly, 1980; Kimura, 1963; Milner, 1968; Taylor, 1969). Electrical stimulation of the right anterior and posterior temporal region also causes, respectively, severe anterograde and retrograde memory loss for designs and geometric stimuli, and impairs memory for faces (Fried *et al.*, 1982; Ojeman *et al.*, 1968).

With bilateral removal of the inferior temporal region, a condition variably referred to as psychic blindness and the Kluver–Bucy syndrome results. However, as explained in Chapter 3, this is caused by destruction of the amygdala. If the mesial regions are removed, severe memory disturbances involving visual and auditory stimuli result such that the patient suffers a permanent anterograde amnesia.

Based on lesion, temporal lobectomy, and electrical stimulation studies it appears that the anterior temporal region is more involved in initial consolidation storage phase of memory, whereas the posterior region is primarily involved in memory retrieval and recall. Overall, however, it appears important that the amygdala and hippocampus be in some manner compromised and/or at least disconnected from the source of input for these deficiencies involving memory to arise (Milner, 1974; Mishkin, 1978).

HALLUCINATIONS

The functional integrity of the temporal lobes, the inferior regions in particular, are highly important in regard to the memorization and recollection of various auditory, visual, olfactory, and emotional experiences. When destroyed, disconnected from sources of input, or compromised in some fashion, the ability to store information and to draw visual–verbal mnemonic imagery from memory is severely attenuated.

Conversely, when the temporal lobes and/or the limbic nuclei buried within its depths (i.e., the amygdala and hippocampus) are artificially or abnormally activated, it sometimes occurs that visual–auditory imagery as well as a variety of emotional reactions are evoked involuntarily. These may take the form of complex hallucinations, dreamlike states, confusional episodes, or may involve the abnormal attribution of emotional significance to otherwise neutral thoughts and external experiences.

Hallucinations and the Interpretation of Neural "Noise"

Hallucinations may occur secondary to tumors or seizures involving the occipital, parietal, frontal, and temporal lobe or may arise secondary to toxic exposure, high fevers, general infections, exhaustion, starvation, extreme thirst, partial or complete hearing loss including otosclerosis, and with partial or complete blindness such as due to glaucoma (Bartlet, 951; Flournoy, 1923; Pesme, 1939; Rhein, 1913; Ross, Jossman, Bell, *et al.*, 1975; Rozanski & Rosen, 1952; Semrad, 1938; Tarachow, 1941). Interestingly, when secondary to peripheral hearing loss, patients frequently report hearing certain songs and melodies from their childhood—melodies that they had usually long forgotten. In addition, patients suffering from cortical blindness, i.e., Anton's syndrome (Redlich & Dorsey, 1945), and deafness (Brown, 1972), as well as those recovering from Wernicke's aphasia, frequently experience hallucinations.

In general, hallucinations secondary to loss of visual or auditory input appears to be secondary to the interpretation of neural noise. That is, with loss of input, various brain regions begin to extract or assign meaningful significance to random neural events or to whatever input may be received. Thus, we find that subjects will hallucinate when placed in sensory reduced environments or even when movement is restricted (Lilly, 1956, 1972; Lindsley, 1961; Shurley, 1962; Zuckerman & Cohen, 1964).

Conversely, hallucinations can occur due to increased levels of neural noise as well. For example, if an area of the neocortex is abnormally activated that area in turn may act to interpret its own neural activity. However, the degree of interpretive activity depends on the type of processing performed in the region involved. In this regard, we find that hallucinations become increasingly complex as the disturbance expands from primary to association areas and as involvement moves from the occipital to anterior temporal regions (Critchley, 1939; Penfield & Perot, 1963; Tarachow, 1941), which is one of the major interpretive regions of the neocortex (Gibbs, 1951; Penfield & Perot, 1963). That is, in the primary regions, neural noise is given a simple interpretation (simple hallucinations), whereas in the association and multiassociational areas, neural noise is given a complex interpretation.

For example, tumors or electrical stimulation of the occipital lobe produce simple hallucinations such as colors, stars, spots, balls of fire, flashes of light, whereas with superior temporal involvement the patient may experience crude noises, such as buzzing, roaring sounds, bells, and an occasional voice or sounds of music. However, with anterior and inferior temporal abnormalities, the hallucinations become increasing complex consisting of both auditory and visual features, including faces, people, objects, and animals (Critchley, 1939; Penfield & Perot, 1963; Tarachow, 1941). However, the anterior– inferior temporal region may give rise to the most complex forms of imagery because cells in this area are specialized for the perception and recognition of specific and complex forms.

Indeed, it has frequently been reported that as compared with other cortical areas, the most complex and most forms of hallucination occur secondary to temporal lobe involvement (Critchley, 1939; Malh, Rothenberg, Delgado, & Hamlin, 1964; Horowitz, Adams & Rutkin, 1968; Penfield & Perot, 1963; Tarachow, 1941) and that the hippocampus and amygdala (in conjunction with the temporal lobe) appear to be the responsible agents (Gloor, Olivier, Quesney, et al., 1982; Horowitz et al., 1968; Halgren, Babb, & Crandall, 1978). For example, Halgren et al. (1978) and Horowitz and colleagues (1968) note that hippocampal stimulation was predominantly associated with either fully formed and/or memorylike hallucinations including feelings of familiarity, and secondarily dreamlike hallucinations, whereas stimulation limited to the neocortex had little effect (Gloor et al., 1982). In this regard, it appears that limbic activation is necessary in order to bring to a conscious level percepts that are being processed in the temporal lobes.

LSD

This does not mean, however, that neocortical involvement is not necessary for frequently it is the interpretive interaction of the temporal lobe that gives rise to certain types of hallucinations, i.e., bringing them to a conscious level. For example, it is well known that the ingestion of LSD will trigger the formation of vivid and complex auditory and visual hallucinations. Following LSD administration, electrophysiological abnormalities are noted in the amygdala and hippocampus (Chapman, Walter, Ross, et al., 1963). However, if the temporal lobes are surgically removed there is a significant decrease, with unilateral removal (Serafetinides, 1965), or complete abolition, with bilateral lateral removal, of LSD-induced hallucinatory activity (Baldwin, Lewis, & Bach, 1959), even when the amygdala and hippocampus are spared. Again, this is presumably a function of form recognition neurons being located as well as activated within the inferior temporal region. Interestingly, the hallucinatory effect of LSD appears to be greatest in the right temporal lobe (Serafetinides, 1965).

Dreaming

Vivid, visual–auditory, and sometimes intensely emotional hypnogic dream imagery is clearly associated with rapid eye movement (REM) sleep (Foulkes, 1962; Goodenough, Shapiro, Holden, & Steinschriber, 1959; Monroe, Rechtschaffen, Foulkes, & Jensen, 1965). As discussed in detail in Chapter 1, Electrophysiological studies or measures of cerebral blood flow have indicated that the right hemisphere becomes highly active during REM, whereas conversely the left brain becomes more active during non-REM (N-REM) sleep (Goldstein, Stolzfus, & Gardocki, 1972; Hodoba, 1986; Meyer, Ishikawa, Hata, & Karacan, 1987).

It has also been reported that abnormal and seizurelike activity in the right temporal and temporal–occipital area acts to increase dreaming and REM sleep for an atypically long time period. Similarly, REM sleep increases activity in this same region much more than in the left hemisphere (Hodoba, 1986) indicating that there is a specific complementary relationship among REM sleep, dreaming, and right temporal–occipital electrophysiological activity.

In this regard, although not conclusive, there seems to be a convergence of evidence which suggests that the right temporal lobe may be more involved than the left in the production of visual–auditory hallucinations and dreamlike mental states be they produced secondary to LSD, electrical stimulation, abnormal seizure activity, or occurring naturally during sleep.

As pertaining to right versus left cerebral involvement in the production and recollection of hallucinations and dreams, it is interesting to note that Horowitz et al. (1968), reported that electrically induced hallucinated events were usually forgotten by patients within 10–15 minutes after the experience, and when questioned the next day, memory was not improved. Similar forgetting patterns are characteristic of memory for normal sleep induced dreams as well (Joseph, 1988). That is, it becomes progressively more difficult to recall one's dreams as one spends time in or awakens during N-REM (Wolpert & Trosman, 1958)—which is associated with high left hemisphere and low right brain activation (Goldstein et al., 1972).

TEMPORAL LOBE (PARTIAL COMPLEX) SEIZURES

Personality and Psychiatric Disturbances

Personality and psychiatric disorders have frequently been reported as a common associated complication among a small percentage of individuals with seizure-disorders localized to the temporal lobe. Such patients may appear depressed, paranoid, hysterical, or suffering from schizophreniclike symptomology. Some investigators have argued that, like hallucinations, the nearer the seizure foci to the anterior temporal lobe, the greater the probability of significant psychiatric abnormality (Gibbs, 1951). Presumably this is a function of hyperactivation of underlying limbic structures and thus abnormal attribution of emotional significance to different afferent streams of perceptual experience (Bear, 1979).

Nevertheless, the disturbance in emotional functioning waxes and frequently wanes, such that in some cases there are islands of normality, whereas in others there are islands of psychosis. These changes are possibly a function in variations in subclinical seizure activity.

In some instances, the psychiatric disturbance may develop over days as a prelude to the actual onset of a seizure, presumably due to increasing levels of abnormal activity until the seizure is triggered. In other cases, particularly in regard to depression, the alterations in personality and emotionality may occur following the seizure and may persist for weeks or even months.

In yet other instances, patients may act increasingly bizzare for weeks, experience a seizure, and then behave in a normal fashion for some time only to again begin acting increasingly bizzarre. This has been referred to as an interictal (between seizure) psychosis and is possibly secondary to a buildup of abnormal activity in the temporal lobes and limbic system (cf. Bear, 1979). Thus, once the seizure occurs, the level of abnormal activity is decreased and the psychosis goes away only to gradually return as abnormal activity again builds up.

Behavioral Manifestations of Seizures

Usually, during the course of a temporal lobe seizure, there are no abrupt and drastic alterations in motor activity such as tonic–clonic spasms. However, some patients may simply cease to respond and stare blankly straight ahead, make licking or smacking movements of the lips, and/or fiddle with their clothing, as if picking up pieces of lint. Although conscious-awareness is lost, these patients are not unconscious. Rather, their mental state is one of absence. In fact, they may appear awake and conscious, although unable to speak or respond to questions, and behaviorally their actions seem semipurposeful. Nevertheless, it is sometimes extremely obvious that they are experiencing a seizure, whereas in other cases an inexperienced observer may only have the impression that the person is acting somewhat odd.

Some patients also note an *aura* immediately before seizure onset. This may involve feelings of fear or anxiety, alterations in gastric motility, or unpleasant tastes or in particular, odors (e.g., burning rubber or feces), i.e., an olfactory aura. Presumably, the experience of olfactory hallucinations is due to abnormal activation of the rhinencephalon (the "nose brain") and thus limbic nuclei such as the amygdala. Possibly the licking and smacking movements are also due to activation of the amygdala and other limbic structures associated with food consumption. Changes in gastric motility may be secondary to insular activation and/or limbic participation. Nevertheless, unless the patient has several different seizure foci, the same characteristic behavioral manifestations are elicited every time a patient has a seizure. The patient does not simply stare on one occasion and on the next begin rolling his eyes and crying out.

Running, Laughing, and Crying Seizures

In some instances, patients with temporal lobe seizures (triggered perhaps by tumor) may display extremely odd and bizzare behaviors during the course of the seizure (Chen & Forster, 1973). For example, a number of authors have presented case reports of patients who developed laughing (*gelastic epilepsy*), crying (*dacrystic epilepsy*), and/or running seizures (*cursive epilepsy*).

One patient's seizure consisted of suddenly bursting into laughter, rubbing his upper abdomen, and running wildly about the room with an expression of fear on his face (Sethi & Rao, 1976). Another patient displayed paroxysmal attacks of weeping, sobbing, and mournful moaning (Offen, Davidoff, Troost, & Richey, 1976). These behaviors were involuntary, however, and part of the seizure. Once consciousness returned, the patients would have no recollection of their actions.

Emotion

The most common emotional reactions and sensations that occur secondary to or during the course of a temporal lobe seizure include feelings of fear, anxiety, depression, depersonalization, pleasure, unpleasure, and familiarity (Bear, 1979; Herman & Chhabria, 1980; Gloor *et al.*, 1982; Perez & Trimble, 1980; Strauss, Risser, & Jones, 1982; Weil, 1956; Williams, 1956), fear being the most frequently experienced. Many of these same feelings are also triggered by electrical stimulation of the temporal lobes, amygdala and hippocampus (Gloor, 1972; Gloor *et al.*, 1982; Heath, 1964; Mullan & Penfield, 1959).

Depression (lasting from hours to weeks) may occur as an immediate sequela to the seizure, many patients also experiencing confusion. A depressive aura may also precede and thus hearld the coming of a seizure by hours or even days (Williams, 1956).

Rather than increased emotionality, some patients complain of emotional blocking, and feelings of emptiness: "feelings don't reach me anymore" (Weil, 1956). Presumably this is a consequence of limbic disconnection. That is, the seizure foci (or lesion) acts to deconnect the limbic areas from the temporal (or orbital frontal) lobes. In consequence, percepts and thoughts no longer come to be assigned emotional or motivational significance.

Between Seizure Psychoses

Estimates of psychosis and affective disorders among individuals suffering from temporal lobe epilepsy, be it a single episode or chronic psychiatric condition have varied at 2–81% (Falconer, 1973; Gibbs, 1951; Jensen & Larsen, 1979; Sherwin, 1977, 1981; Taylor, 1972). Probably a more realistic figure is about 11–17%. The range of disturbances among temporal lobe epileptics includes a strikingly high rate of sexual abberation as well as hyposexuality, aggressiveness, paranoia, depression, deepening of emotion, intensification of religious concerns, disorders of thought, depersonalization, hypergraphia, complex visual and auditory hallucinations, and schizophrenia (Bear, 1982; Bear *et al.*, 1982; Flor-Henry, 1969, 1983; Sherwin, 1977, 1981; Schiff *et al.*, 1982; Stevens *et al.*, 1979; Taylor, 1975).

SCHIZOPHRENIA

A variety of anatomical as well as biochemical disturbances have been found in various populations of individuals diagnosed as suffering from schizophrenia. These include impaired interhemispheric transfer of visual, auditory, and somesthestic information (Beaumont & Dimond, 1973; Carr, 1980; Green & Kotenko, 1980), increased corpus callosum thickness (Rosenthal & Bigelow, 1972), pathological abnormalities in the amygdala, hippocampus, and hypothalamus (Berman *et al.*, 1987; Brown, Levin, & Blumer, *et al.*, 1986; Bogerts, Meertz, Schonfeldt-Bausch, 1985), reduced prefrontal cortical metabolic activity (Ingvar & Franzen, 1974; Ariel, Golden, Berg, *et al.*, 1983; Weinberger, Berman, & Zec, 1986; Berman Zec, & Weinberger, 1986), increased lateral ventricular size (Berman, Weinberger, Shelton, & Zec, 1987), and disturbances involving the dopamine neurotransmitter system (see Swerdlow & Koob, 1987, for review).

Nevertheless, in almost every study published that has addressed the issue of laterality and "schizophrenia," left frontal and in particular left temporal lobe abnormalities have been reported (Abrams & Taylor, 1980; Flor-Henry, 1983; Morihisa, Duffy, & Wyatt, 1983; Morstyn, Duffy, & McCarley, 1983*b*). Although bilateral abnormalities have been observed, unilateral dysfunction of the right half of the brain has not been demonstrated. Thus, disturbances of the left hemisphere and the left temporal lobe are indicated in a sizeable minority of patients diagnosed with schizophrenia.

Seizures and Psychosis

Similarly, it has been consistently reported that those suffering from temporal lobe seizures and schizophreniclike abnormalities have bilateral damage or seizure foci lateralized to the left half of the brain (Falconer & Taylor, 1970; Flor-Henry, 1983; Sherwin, 1977, 1981; Sherwin et al., 1982; Taylor, 1975). Conversely, those with affective disturbances, e.g., mania, depression, etc. have been found to suffer from seizures involving the right temporal lobe (Bear et al., 1982; Falconer & Taylor, 1970; Flor-Henry, 1969).

There are several distinct neurological explanations for the association between temporal lobe damage and psychotic and affective disorders. As discussed in detail in previous chapters, the right hemisphere is dominant for most aspects of emotional functioning. Hence, when damaged or abnormally activated, such as from a seizure or chronic subclinical seizure activity, emotional functioning becomes altered and disturbed. Moreover, since the amygdala and hippocampus are often secondarily aroused (or hyperaroused), the possibility of abnormal emotionality is enhanced even further.

In this regard, Gloor et al., (1982), in a depth electrode stimulation study of patients suffering from epilepsy, presented evidence indicating that all experiential and emotional alterations were encountered following right amygdala and hippocampal activation. The limbic system seems to be lateralized and the right amygdala and hippocampus appear to be more involved in emotional functioning (Joseph, 1989) (see Chapter 3). Thus, abnormal activation of these nuclei (such as during the course of a temporal lobe seizure) are more likely to give rise to abnormal emotional reactions. Nevertheless, some patients with temporal lobe seizures may complain of emotional blunting. Hence, rather than a limbic hyperconnection, these individuals suffer from a disconnection.

Aphasia and Psychosis

Conversely, as the left temporal lobe is intimately involved in all aspects of language comprehension as well as the organization of linguistic expression, altered neocortical activity involving this region is likely to result in significant disruptions in language functioning and the formulation of linguistic thought. Patients with left temporal lobe damage and Wernicke's aphasia are at some risk of being misdiagnosed as suffering from a formal thought disorder because of to their fluent aphasic language disturbances and in particular their failure to comprehend (see Chapter 2). Indeed, some authorities have noted significant similarities between schizophrenic discourse and aphasia (Faber, Abrams, Taylor, Kasprisin, Morris, & Weisz, 1983; Hillbom, 1951), such that the semantic, temporal–sequential, and lexical aspects of speech organization and comprehension are disturbed and deviantly constructed (Chaika, 1982; Flor-Henry, 1983; Hoffman, 1986; Hoffman, Stopek, & Andreasen, 1986; Rutter, 1979). Similar findings have been reported for individuals developing post-traumatic schizophreniclike symptoms following head injury and missile wounds (Hillbom, 1951).

Patients with left temporal seizures commonly become globally aphasic during the course of their seizure. When spoken to or if their name is repeatedly called they may make only fleeting eye contact, grunt or utter partial words such a "huh?" Some patients remain aphasic for seconds to minutes after seizure termination as well.

Between seizures, language impairments, verbal memory disorders, and associated linguistic deficiencies are usually apparent if adequately assessed. Moreover, patients with left-sided foci tend to have lower (WAIS-R) verbal IQs as compared with their performance IQs and as compared with those with right-sided foci. This is not surprising, as language is represented in the left hemisphere.

Thus, it is possible that abnormal activity in the left temporal lobe, as well as the presence of an active lesion, can result in significant alterations in not only language, but the organization of linguistic thought such that the patient appears psychotic. In this regard, abnormal thought formation may become a characteristic pattern. In fact, even the neurological representation of language can be drastically altered due to left cerebral damage (Joseph, 1986; Novelly & Joseph, 1983). Moreover, if the left temporal region is periodically disconnected from centers mediating emotion, patients may demonstrate what appears to be emotional blunting as well as a formal thought disorder.

Caveats

Some investigators have argued that there is no significant relationship between these psychotic disorders and temporal lobe epilepsy (Stevens & Hermann, 1981), whereas others have drawn attention to possible social–developmental contributions (Matthews, Barbas, & Ferrari, 1982). That is, growing up with a seizure disorder, feeling victimized, not knowing when a seizure may strike, loss of control over one's life, and so on, can independently create significant emotional aberrations.

Probably only a subpopulation of persons with temporal lobe epilepsy come to the attention of most researchers, e.g., those persons with the most serious or intractable problems. What this means is that one should not immediately view a patient with temporal lobe (or any type of epilepsy) as immediately suspect for emotional–psychotic abnormalities.

REFERENCES

Abraham, A., & Mathai, K. V. (1983). The effect of right temporal lesions on matching of smells. *Neuropsychologia, 21,* 277–282.

Abrams, R., & Taylor, M. A. (1980). Psychopathology and the electroencephalogram. *Biological Psychiatry, 15,* 871–878.

Albert, M. L., & Bear, D. (1974). Time to understand. A case study of word deafness with reference to the role of time in auditory comprehension. *Brain, 97,* 383–394.

Albert, M. L., Sparks, R., von Strockert, T., & Sax, D. (1972). A case of auditory agnosia. Linguistic and nonlinlguistic processing. *Cortex, 8,* 427–443.

Albright, T. D., Desimone, R., & Gross, C. G. (1984). Columnar organization of directionally selective cells in visual area MT of the macaque. *Journal of Neurophysiology, 51,* 16–31.

Ariel, R. N., Golden, C. J., Berg, R. A., et al. (1983). Regional blood flow in schizophrenia. *Archives of General Psychiatry, 40,* 258–263.

Auerbach, S. H., Allard, T., Naeser, M., et al. (1982). Pure word deafness. *Brain, 105,* 271–300.

Baldwin, M., Lewis, S. A., & Bach, S. A. (1959). The effects of lysergic after cerebral ablation. *Neurology (New York), 9,* 469–474.

Bartlet, J. E. A. (1951). A case of organized visual halluciantion in an old man with cataract, and their relation to the phenomena of the phantom limb. *Brain, 84,* 363–373.

Bear, D. (1977). The significance of behavior change in temporal lobe epilepsy. *McLean Hospital Journal, 9,* 11–23.

Bear, D. M. (1979). Temporal lobe epilepsy: A syndrome of sensory–limbic hyperconnexion. *Cortex, 15,* 357–384.

Bear, D. M., Levin, K., Blumer, D., *et al.* (1982). Interictal behaviour in hospitalized temporal lobe epileptics. *Journal of Neurology, Neurosurgery and Psychiatry, 45,* 481–488.

Beaumont, J. G., & Dimond, S. J. (1973). Brain disconnection and schizophrenia. *British Journal of Psychiatry, 23,* 661–662.

Berman, K. F., Weinberger, D. R., Shelton, R. C., & Zec, R. F. (1987). A relationship between anatomical and physiological brain pathology in schizophrenia. *American Journal of Psychiatry, 144,* 1277–1282.

Berman, K. F., Zek, R. F., & Weinberger, D. R. (1986). Physiological dysfucntion of dorsolateral prefrontal cortex in schizophrenia. *Archives of General Psychiatry, 43,* 126–143.

Blumstein, S., & Cooper, W. E. (1974). Hemispheric processing of intonational contours, *Cortex, 10,* 146–158.

Bogerts, B., Meertz, E., & Schonfeldt-Bausch, R. (1985). Basal ganglia and limbic system pathology in schizophrenia. *Archives of General Psychiatry, 42,* 784–791.

Bradshaw, J. L., Taylor, M. J., Patterson, K., & Nettleton, N. (1980). Upright and inverted faces, and housefronts, in the two visual fields: A right and a left hemisphere contribution. *Journal of Clinical Neuropsychology, 2,* 245–257.

Brodal, A. (1981). *Neurological anatomy.* New York: Oxford University Press.

Brown, J. W. (1972). *Aphasia, apraxia and agnosia.* Springfield, IL: Charles Thomas.

Brown, R., Colter, N., Corsellis, J. A. N., *et al.* (1986). Postmortem evidence of structural brain changes in schizophrenia. *Archives of General Psychiatry, 43,* 36–42.

Bryden, M. P. (1967). A model for the sequential organization of behaviour. *Canadian Journal of Psychology, 21,* 36–56.

Carr, S. A. (1980). Interhmispheric transfer of stereognostic information in chronic schizophrenics. *British Journal of Psychiatry, 136,* 53–58.

Chapman, L. F., & Walter, R. D. (1965). Actions of lysergic acid dienthalamid on averaged human cortical evoked rsposnes to light flash. *Recent Advances in Biological Psychiatry, 7,* 23–36.

Chapman, L. F., Walter, R. D., Ross, W. (1963). Altered electrical activity of human hippocampus and amygdala induced by LSD-25. *Physiologist, 5,* 118.

Chase, R. A. (1967). Discussion. In F. L. Darley (Ed.), *Brain mechanisms underlying speech and language* (pp. 136–139). New York: Grune & Stratton.

Chaika, E. (1982). A unified explanation for the diverse structural deviations reported for adult schizophrenics with disrupted speech. *Journal of Communication Disorders, 15,* 167–189.

Chen, R., & Forster, F. M. (1973). Cursive and gelastic epilepsy. *Neurology (New York), 23,* 1019–1029.

Chow, K. L. (1950). A retrograde cell degeneration study of the cortical projection field of the pulvinar of the monkey. *Journal of Comparative Neurology, 93,* 313–340.

Corkin, S. (1965). Tactually guided maze learning in man. *Neuropsychologia, 3,* 339–352.

Critchley, M. (1939). Neurological aspect of visual and auditory hallucinations. *British Medical Journal, 33,* 634–639.

Cutting, J. E. (1974). Two left hemisphere mechanisms in speech perception. *Perception and Psychophysics, 16,* 601–612.

Damasio, A. R., & Damsio, H. (1983). Localization of lesions in achromatopsia and prosopagnosia. In A. Kertesz (Ed.), *Localization in neuropsychology* (pp. 182–197). Orlando, FL: Academic Press.

Delaney, R. C., Rosen, A. J., Mattson, R. H., & Novelly, R. A. (1980). Memory function in focal epilepsy: A comparison of non-surgical unilateral temporal lobe and frontal lobe samples. *Cortex, 16,* 103–117.

DeRenzi, E. (1982). *Disorder of space exploration and cognition.* Chichester: John Wiley & Sons.

DeRenzi, E. (1986). Prosopagnosia in two patients with CT-scan evidence of damage confined to the right hemisphere. *Neuropsychologia, 24,* 385–389.

DeRenzi, E., Faglioni, P., & Spinnler, H. (1968). The performance of patients with unilateral brain damage on face recognition tasks. *Cortex, 4,* 17–34.

DeRenzi, E., & Spinnler, H. (1966). Facial recognition in brain-damaged patients. An experimental approach. *Neurology (New York), 16,* 145–152.

Desimone, R., & Gross, C. G. (1979). Visual areas in the temporal cortex of the macaque. *Brain Research, 178,* 363–380.

Desimone, R., & Schein, S. J. (1987). Visual properties iof neruons in area V4 of the Macaque: Sensitivity to stimulus form. *Journal of Neurophysiology, 57,* 835–867.

Dewson, J. H., Pribram, K., & Lynch, J. C. (1969). Effects of ablations of temporal cortex upon speech sound discrimination in the monkey. *Experimental Neurology, 24,* 579–591.

Diamond, I. T. (1973). The evolution of the tectal–pulvinar system in mammals: Structural and behavioural studies of the visual system. *Symposium of the Zoological Society of London, 33,* 205–233.

Earnest, M. P., Monroe, P. A., & Yarnell, P. R. (1977). Cortical deafness. *Neurology (New York), 27,* 1172–1175.

Faber, R., Abrams, R., Taylor, M., Kasprisin, A., Morris, C., & Weisz, R. (1983). Comparison of schizophrenic patients with formal thought disorder and neurologically impaired patients with aphasia. *American Journal of Psychiatry, 140,* 1348–1351.

Felleman, D. J., & Kaas, J. H. (1974). Receptive field properties of neruons in middle temporal visual area (MT) of owl monkeys. *Journal of Neurophysiology, 52,* 488–513.

Flor-Henry, P. (1969). Psychosis and temporal lobe epilepsy. *Epilepsia, 10,* 363–395.

Flor-Henry, P. (1983). *Cerebral basis of psychopathology.* Boston: John Wright.

Flournoy, H. (1923). Hallucinations. *Encephale, 2,* 566–572.

Foulkes, W. D. (1962). Dream reports from different stages of sleep. *Journal of Abnormal and Social Psychology, 65,* 14–25.

Freedman, S. J. (1961). Perceptual changes in sensory deprivation. *Journal of Nervous and Mental Disease, 132,* 17–21.

Fried, I., Mateer, C., Ojemann, G., Wohns, R., & Fedio, P. (1982). Organization of visuospatial functions in human cortex. *Brain, 105,* 349–371.

Geffen, G., & Bradshaw, J. L., & Wallace, G. (1971). Interhemispheric effects on reaction time to verbal and nonverbal visual stimuli. *Journal of Experimental Psychology, 87,* 415–422.

Geschwind, N., & Levitsky, W. (1968). Human brain: Left–right asymmetries in temporal speech regions. *Science, 161,* 186–187.

Gibbs, A. F. (1951). Ictal and non-ictal psychiatric disorders in temporal lobe epilepsy. *Journal of Nervous and Mental Disease, 113,* 522–528.

Gloor, P. (1972). Temporal lobe epilepsy. In B. E. Elftheriou (Ed.), *The neurobiology of the amygdala* (pp. 212–275). New York: Plenum.

Gloor, P., Olivier, A., Quesney, L. F., *et al.* (1982). The role of the limbic system in experimental phenomena of temporal lobe epilepsy. *Annals of Neurology, 12,* 129–144.

Goldstein, L., Stoltzfus, N. W., & Gardocki, J. F. (1972). Changes in interhemispheric amplitude relationships in the EEG during sleep. *Physiology and Behavior, 8,* 811–815.

Goodenough, D. R., Shapiro, A., Holden, M., & Steinschriber, R. (1959). Comparison of "dreamers" and "non-dreamers". *Journal of Nervous and Mental Disease, 59,* 295–302.

Gorelick, P. B., & Ross, E. D. (1987). *Journal of Neurology, Neurosurgery and Psychiatry, 37,* 727–737.

Green, G. L., & Lessel, S. (1977). Acquired cerebral dyschromatopsia. *Archives of Ophthamology, 95,* 121–128.

Gross, C. G., & Mishkin, M. (1977). The neural basis of stimulus equivalence across retinal translation. In S. Harnad, *et al.* (Eds.), *Lateralization in the nervous system.* New York: Academic Press.

Gross, C. G., Rocha-Miranda, C. E., & Bender, D. B. (1972). Visual properties of neurons in inferotemporal cortex of the macaque. *Journal of Neurophysiology, 35,* 96–111.

Halgren, E., Babb, T. L., & Crandall, P. H. (1978). Activity of human hippocampal formation and amygdala neurons during memory tests. *Electroencephalography and Clinical Neurophysiology, 45,* 585–601.

Heath, R. (1954). *Studies in schizophrenia.* Cambridge, MA: Harvard University Press.

Heath, R. (1964). Pleasure response of human subjects to direct stimulation of the brain. In R. G. Heath (Ed.), *The role of pleasure in behavior* (pp. 121–170). New York: Harper & Row.

Hecaen, H., & Albert, M. L. (1978). *Human neuropsychology.* New York, John Wiley & Sons.

Hecaen, H., & Angelergues, R. (1962). Agnosia for faces (prospagnosia). *Archives of Neurology, 7,* 92–100.

Hermann, B. P., & Chambria, S. (1980). Interictal psychopathology in patients with ictal fear. *Archives of Neurology, 37,* 667–668.

Hillbom, E. (1951). Schizophrenia-like psychoses after brain trauma. *Acta Psychiatrica, 60,* 36–47.

Hillbom, E. (1960). After-effects of brain injuries. *Acta Psychiatrica Scandinavica (Suppl.) 142,* 1–183.

Hodoba, D. (1986). Paradoxic sleep facilitation by interictal epileptic activity of right temporal origin. *Biological Psychiatry, 21,* 1267–1278.

Hoffman, R. E. (1986). Verbal hallucinations and language production processes in schizophrenia. *Behavioral and Brain Sciences, 9,* 503–548.

Hoffman, R., Stopek, S., & Andreasen, N. (1986). A discourse analysis comparing manic versus schizophrenic speech disorganization. *Archives of General Psychiatry, 43,* 831–838.

Horowitz, M. J., Adams, J. E., & Rutkin, B. B. (1968). Visual imagery on brain stimulation. *Archives of General Psychiatry, 19,* 469–486.

Hubel, D. H., Calvin, O. H., Rupert, A., & Galambos, R. (1959). Attention units in the auditory cortex. *Science, 129,* 1279–1280.

Ingvar, D. H., & Franzen, G. (1974). Abnormalities of cerebral blood flow distribution in patients with chronic schizophrenia. *Acta Psychiatrica Scandinavica, 50,* 425–462.

Jensen, I., & Larsen, J. K. (1979). Psychoses in drug-resistant temporal lobe epilepsy. *Journal of Neurology, Neurosurgery and Psychiatry, 42,* 948–954.

Jones, E. G., & Powell, T. P. S. (1970). An antomical study of converging sensory pathways within the cerebral cortex of the monkey. *Brain, 93,* 793–820.

Joseph, R. (1982). The neuropsychology of development: Limbic language, hemispheric laterality, and the origin of thought. *Journal of Clinical Psychology, 38,* 4–33.

Joseph, R. (1986). Reversal of cerebral dominance for language and emotion in a corpus callostomy patient. *Journal of Neurology, Neurosurgery and Psychiatry, 49,* 628–634.

Joseph, R. (1988). The right cerebral hemisphere. *Journal of Clinical Psychology, 44,* 630–673.

Joseph, R. (1989). The limbic system. Emotion, laterality, unconscious mind. *Psychoanalytic Review,*

Kimura, D. (1961). Cerebral dominance and the perception of verbal stimuli. *Canadian Journal of Psychology, 15,* 156–171.

Kimura, D. (1963). Right temporal lobe damage: Perception of unfamiliar stimuli after damage. *Archives of Neurology, 18,* 264–271.

Kimura, D., & Folb, S. (1968). Neural processing of backward speech sounds. *Science, 161,* 395–396.

Kuypers, H. G. J. M., Szwarcbart, M. K., Mishkin, M., & Rosvold, H. E. (1965). Occipitotemporal cortico-cortical connections in the Rhesus monkey. *Experimental Neurology, 11,* 245–262.

Landis, T., Cummings, J. L., Christen, L., Bogen, J. E., & Imhof, H-G (1986). Are unilateral right posterior cerebral lesions sufficient to cause prosopagnosia? Clinical and radiological findings in six additional patients. *Cortex, 22,* 243–252.

Lansdell, H. (1968). Extent of temporal lobe albations on two lateralized deficits. *Physiology and Behavior, 3,* 271–273.

Lansdell, H. (1970). Relation of extent of temporal removal to closure and visuomotor factors. *Perceptual and Motor Skills, 31,* 491–498.

Levine, D. N. (1978). Prosopagnosia and visual object agnosia: A behavioral study. *Brain and Language, 5,* 341–365.

Levy, J. (1974). Psychological implications of bilateral asymmetry. In S. Diamond & J. G. Beaumont (Eds.), *Hemisphere function in the human brain* (pp. 127–183). London: Paul Elek.

Levy, J., Trevarthen, C., & Sperry, R. W. (1972). Perception of bilateral chimeric figures following hemi-spheric deconnection. *Brain, 95,* 61–78.

Ley, R. G., & Bryden, M. P. (1979). Hemispheric differences in processing emotions and faces. *Brain and Language, 7,* 127–138.

Lilly, J. C. (1956). Mental effects of reduction of ordinary levels of physical stimuli on intact, healthy persons. *Psychiatric Research Reports, 5,* 1–9.

Lilly, J. C. (1972). *The center of the cyclone.* New York: Julian Press.

Lindsley, D. (1961). Common factors in sensory deprivation. In P. Solomon (Ed.), *Sensory deprivation* (pp. 27–52). Cambridge, MA: Harvard University Press.

Luria, A. (1973). *The working brain.* New York: Basic Books.

Luria, A. (1980). *Higher cortical functions in man.* New York: Basic Books.

Malh, G. F., Rothenberg, A., Delgado, J. M. R., & Hamlin, H. (1964). Psychological resposne in the human to intracerebral electrical stimulation. *Psychosomatic Medicine, 26,* 337–368.

Marzi, I. A., & Berlucchi, G. (1977). Right visual field superiority for accuracy of recognition of famous faces in normals. *Neuropsychologia, 15,* 751–756.

Matthews, W. S., Barbas, G., & Ferrari, M. (1982). Emotional concomitants of childhood epilepsy. *Epilepsia, 23,* 671–681.

Maunsell, J. H. R., & Van Essen, D. C. (1983). Functional properties of neurons in middle temporal visual area of the macaque. *Journal of Neurophysiology, 49,* 1127–1165.

Meadows, J. C. (1974). The anatomical basis of prosopagnosia. *Journal of Neurology, Neurosurgery and Psychiatry, 37,* 489–501.

Mendez, M. F., & Geehand, G. R. (1988). *Journal of Neurology, Neurosurgery and Psychiatry, 51,* 1–9.

Merzenich, M. M., & Brugge, J. F. (1973). Representation of the cochlear partition of the superior temporal plan of teh macaque monkey. *Brain Research, 50,* 275–296.

Meyer, J. S., Ishikawa, Y., Hata, T., & Karacan, I. (1987). Cerebral blood flow in normal and abnormal sleep and dreaming. *Brain and Cognition, 6,* 266–294.

Meyer, V., & Yates, A. (1955). Intellectual changes following temporal lobecotomy for pschomotor epilepsy. *Journal of Neurology, Neurosurgery and Psychiatry, 18,* 44–52.

Mills, L., & Rollman, G. B. (1980). Hemispheric asymmetry for auditory perception of temporal order. *Neuropsychologia, 18,* 41–47.

Milner, B. (1958). Psychological defects produced by temporal lobe excisions. *Research Publication of the Association for Research in Nervous and Mental Disease, 36,* 244–257.

Milner, B. (1962). Laterality effect in audition. In V. Mountcastle (Ed.), *Interhemispheric relations and cerebral dominance* (pp. 44–82). Baltimore: John Hopkins University Press.

Milner, B. (1968). Visual recognition and recall after right temporal lobe excision in man. *Neuropsychologia, 6,* 191–209.

Milner, B. (1974). Hemispheric specialization: Scope and limits. In F. E. Schmitt & F. G. Worden (Eds.), *The neurosciences. Third study program* (pp. 215–231). Cambridge, MA: MIT Press.

Milner, B., & Teuber, H. L. (1968). Alteration of perception and memory in man. In L. Weiskrantz (Ed.), *Analysis of behavioral changes* (pp. 107–130). New York: Harper & Row.

Mishkin, M. (1972). Cortical visual areas and their interaction. In A. G. Karczman & J. C. Eccles (Eds.), *Brain and human behavior* (pp. 57–93). Berlin: Springer-Verlag.

Mishkin, M. (1978). Memory in monkeys severely impaired by combined but not by separate removal of amygdala and hippocampus. *Nature (London) 273,* 297–299.

Morihisa, A., Duffy, F. H., & Wyatt, R. J. (1983). Brain electrical activity mapping (BEAM) in schizophrenic patients. *Archives of General Psychiatry, 40,* 719–728.

Monroe, B., Rechtschaffen, A., Foulkes, D., & Jensen, J. (1965). Discriminability of REM and NREM reports. *Personality and Social Psychology, 2,* 456–460.

Morstyn, R., Duffy, F. H., & McCarley, R. (1983). Altered topography of EEG spectral content in schizophrenia. *Electroenecephalograpy and Clinical Neurophysiology, 56,* 263–271.

Mullan, S., & Penfield, W. (1959). Epilepsy and visual hallucinations. *Archives of Neurology and Psychiatry, 81,* 269–281.

Myers, R. E. (1959). Interhemispheric communication through the corpus callosum: Limitations under conditions of conflict. *Journal of Comparative and Physiological Psychology, 52,* 6–9.

Novelly, R. J., & Joseph, R. (1983). Complex partial epilepsy of early development: Gender specific effects on IQ with right hemisphere speech, In *15th Annual Epilepsy International Symposium, September* (p. 53).

Offen, M. L., Davidoff, R. A. Troost, B. T., & Richey, E. T. (1976). Dacrystic epilepsy. *Journal of Neurology, Neurosurgery and Psychiatry, 39,* 829–834.

Ojemann, G. A., Blick, K. I., & Ward, A. A. (1971). Improvement and disturbance of short-term verbal memory with human ventrolateral stimulation. *Brain, 94,* 225–240.

Ojemann, G. A. Fedio, P., & van Buren, J. (1968). Anomia from pulvinar and subcortical parietal stimulation. *Brain, 91,* 99–116.

Ojemann, G. A., & Fedio, P. (1968). Effect of stimulation of the human thalamus, parietal, and temporal white matter on short-term memory. *Journal of Neurosurgery, 29,* 51–59.

Pandya, D. N., & Kuypers, H. G. J. M. (1969). Corticocortical connections in the rhesus monkey. *Brain Research, 13,* 13–36.

Papcun, G., Krashen, S., Terbeek, D. (1974). Is the left hemisphere specialized for speech, language and/or something else. *Journal of the Acoustical Society of America, 55,* 319–327.

Penfield, W., & Evans, J. (1934). Functional defects produced by cerebral lobectomies. *Publication of the Association for Research in Nervous and Mental Disease, 13,* 352–377.

Penfield, W., & Jasper, H. (1954). *Epilepsy and the functional anatomy of the human brain.* Boston: Little, Brown.

Penfield, W., & Perot, P. (1963). The brain's record of auditory and visual experience. *Brain, 86,* 595–696.

Penfield, W., & Rasmussen, T. (1950). *The cerebral cortex of man: A clinical study of localization of function.* New York: Macmillan.

Perez, M. M., & Trimble, M. R. (1980). Epileptic psychosis—Diagnostic comparison with process schizophrenia. *British Journal of Psychiatry, 137,* 245–249.

Pesme, P. (1939). Auditory hallucinations in a deaf person. *Review of Neuropathology and Ophthamalogy, 17,* 280–291.

Redlich, F. C., & Dorsey, J. E. (1945). Denial of blindness by patients with cerebral disease. *Archives of Neurology and Psychiatry, 53,* 407–417.

Reinhold, M. (1950). A case of pure auditory agnosia. *Brain, 73,* 203–223.

Rhein, J. H. W. (1913). Hallucinations of hearing and diseases of the ear. *New York Medical Journal, 97,* 1236–1238.

Richmond, B. J., Optican, L. M., Podel, M., & Spitzer, H. (1987). Temporal encoding of two-dimensional patterns by single units in primate inferior temporal cortex. *Journal of Neurophysiology, 57,* 132–162.

Richmond, B. J., Wurtz, R. H., & Sato, T. (1983). Visual responses of inferior temporal neurons in awake rhesus monkey. *Journal of Neurophysiology, 50,* 1415–1432.

Rocha-Miranda, C. E. Bender, D. B., Gross, C. G., & Mishkin, M. (1975). Visual activation of nerúons in the inferior–temporal cortex depends on striate cortex and forebrain commissures. *Journal of Neurophysiology, 38,* 475–491.

Ross, E. (1981). The aprosodias: Functional–anatomic organization of the affective components of language in the right hemisphere. *Archives of Neurology, 38,* 561–589.

Ross, E. D., Jossman, P. B., Bell, B. *et al.* (1975). Musical halucinations in deafness. *Journal of the American Medical Association, 231,* 620–622.

Rozanski, J., & Rosen, H. (1952). Musical hallucinosis in otosclerosis. *Cinfina Neurologica, 12,* 49–54.

Rutter, D. (1979). The reconstruction of schizophrenic speech. *British Journal of Psychiatry, 134,* 356–359.

Sanchez-Longo, L. P., & Forster, F. M. (1958). Clinical significance of impairment of sound localization. *Neurology (New York), 8,* 119–125.

Schiff, H. B., Sabin, T. D., Geller, A., *et al.* (1982). Lithium in aggressive behaivor. *American Journal of Psychiatry, 139,* 1346–1348.

Seltzer, B., & Pandya, D. N. (1978). Afferent cortical connections and architectonics of the superior temproal sulcus and surrounding cortex in the rhesus monkey. *Brain Research, 149,* 1–24.

Semrad, E. V. (1938). Study of the auditory apparatus in patients experiencing auditory hallucinations. *American Journal of Psychiatry, 95,* 53–63.

Serafetinides, E. A. (1965). The significance of the temporal lobes and of hemisphere dominance in the production of the LSD-25 symptomology in man. *Neuropsychologia, 3,* 69–79.

Sethi, P. K., & Rao, S. T. (1976). Gelastic, quiritarian, and cursive epilepsy. *Journal of Neurology, Neurosurgery and Psychiatry, 39,* 823–828.

Shankweiler, D. (1961). Performance of brain-damaged patients on two tests of sound localization. *Journal of Comparative and Physiological Psychology, 54,* 375–381.

Shankweiler, D. (1966). Effects of temporal lobe damage on the perception of dichotically prsented melodies. *Journal of Comparative and Physiological Psychology, 62,* 115–122.

Shankweiler, D., & Studdert-Kennedy, M. (1966). Lateral differences in perception of dichotically presented synthetic consonant–vowel syllables and steady-state vowels. *Journal of the Acoustic Society of America, 39,* 1256A.

Shankweiler, D., & Studdert-Kennedy, M. (1967). Identification of consonants and vowels presented to left and right ears. *Quarterly Journal of Experimental Psychology, 19,* 59–63.

Sherwin, I. (1977). Clinical and EEG aspects of temporal lobe epilepsy with behavior disorder. *McLean Hospital Journal, 12,* 40–50.

Sherwin, I. (1981). Psychosis associated with epilepsy. *Journal of Neurology, Neurosurgery and Psychiatry,* *44,* 83–85.

Sherwin, I., Peron-Magnana, P., Bancard, J. (1982). Prevalence of psychosis in epilepsy as a function of the laterality of the epileptogenic lesion. *Archives of Neurology, 39,* 621–625.

Shurley, J. (1960). Profound experimental sensory isolation. *American Journal of Psychiatry, 117,* 539–545.

Squire, L. (1987). *Memory and brain.* New York: Oxford University Press.

Stevens, J. R., Bigelow, L., Denney, D. (1979). TeleMetered EEG in schizophrenia. *Journal of Neurology, Neurosurgery and Psychiatry, 36,* 251–262.

Strauss, E., Risser, A., & Jones, M. W. (1982). Fear responses in patients with epilepsy. *Archives of Neurology, 39,* 626–630.

Studdert-Kennedy, M., & Shankweiler, D. (1970). Hemispheric specialization for speech perception. *Journal of the Acoustical Society of America, 48,* 579–594.

Swerdlow, N. R., & Koob, G. F. (1987). Dopamine, schizophrenia, mania, and depression. *Behavioral and Brain Sciences, 10,* 197–245.

Tarachow, S. (1941). The clinical value of hallucinations in localizing brain tumors. *American Journal of Psychiatry, 99,* 1434–1442.

Taylor, D. C. (1969). Aggression and epilepsy. *Journal of Psychosomatic Research, 13,* 229–236.

Taylor, D. C. (1972). Mental state and temporal lobe epilepsy. *Epilepsia, 13,* 727–765.

Taylor, D. C. (1975). Factors influencing the occurrence of schizophrenia-like psychosis in patients with temporal lobe epilepsy. *Psychological Medicine, 5,* 429–254.

Tigges, J., Tigges, M., Anschell, S. (1981). Areal and laminar distribution of neurons interconnecting the central visual cortical areas, 17, 18, 19 and MT. *Journal of Comparative Neurology, 202,* 539–560.

Wada, J., Clarke, R., & Hamm, A. (1975). Cerebral hemispheric asymmetry in humans. Cortical speech zones in 100 adults and 100 infant brains. *Archives of Neurology, 32,* 239–246.

Wall, J. T., Symonds, L. L., & Kaas, J. H. (1982). Cortical and subcortical projections of the middle temporal area (MT) and adjacent cortex in galagos. *Journal of Comparative Neurology, 211,* 193–214.

Weil, A. A. (1956). Ictal depression and anxiety in temporal lobe disorders. *American Journal of Psychiatry, 113,* 149–157.

Weinberger, D. R., Berman, K. F., & Zek, R. F. (1986). Physiological dysfunction of dorsolateral prefrontal cortex in schizophrenia. *Archives of General Psychiatry, 114,* 114–125.

Weingartner, H. (1968). Verbal learning in patients with temporal lobe lesions. *Journal of Verbal Learning and Verbal Behavior, 7,* 520–526.

Weiskrantz, L., & Mishkin, M. (1958). Effect of temporal and frontal cortical lesions on auditory functions in monkey. *Brain, 81,* 233–275.

Whiteley A. M., & Warrington, E K. (1977). Prosopagnosia: A clinical, psychological and anatomical study of three patients. *Journal of Neurology, Neurosurgery and Psychiatry, 40,* 395–403.

Williams, D. (1956). The structure of emotions reflected in epileptic experience. *Brain, 79,* 29–67.

Wollberg, Z., & Newman, V. D. (1972). Auditory cortex of squirrel monkey. *Science, 175,* 212–214.

Woolsey, C. N., & Fairman, D. (1946). Contralteral, ipsilateral, and bilateral representation of cutaneous receptors in somatic areas I and II of the cerebral cortex. *Surgery, 19,* 684–702.

Wolpert E. A., & Trosman, H. (1958). Studies in psychophysiology of dreams. I. Experimental evocation of sequential dream episodes. *Archives of Neurology, 79,* 603–606.

Zeki, S. M. (1978b). The cortical projections of foveal striate cortex in the rhesus monkey. *Journal of Physiology, 277,* 227–244.

Zuckerman, M., & Cohen, N. (1964). Sources of reports of visual and auditory sensations in perceptual-isolation experiments. *Psychological Bulletin, 62,* 1034–1956.

8

Cerebral and Cranial Trauma
Anatomy and Pathophysiology of Mild, Moderate, and Severe Head Injury

THE MENINGES

The living brain is a soft, delicate tissue with a rather compact gelatinous consistency. Because the brain is so fragile, it is protected by several outercoatings (i.e., membranes) that act as a cushion between it and the hard inner shell of the cranium. The innermost membrane is a sheer sheet of translucent material that actually adheres to the brain surface. This is called the pia mater. Lying above the pia mater is yet another very thin weblike fibrous membrane referred to as the arachnoid. The space between the arachnoid and pia mater is called the subarachnoid space, through which circulates cerebrospinal fluid (CSF). Collectively, the arachnoid and pia mater are called the leptomeninges.

Sitting above the leptomeninges and partially adhering to the inside of the skull is a thick, tough, leathery membrane, the dura mater (i.e., "tough mother"). The dura mater is richly innervated by blood vessels, including the middle meningeal artery, which is sometimes subject to laceration following skull fractures, creating an epidural hemorrhage.

The dura not only acts as a hard shield protecting the brain from the skull, but forms a number of compartments that partly encompass and support various portions of the cerebrum. One major compartment formed by the dura is the falx cerebri, which juts down between the cerebral hemispheres. The falx in turn gives rise (in fanlike fashion) to the tentorium cerebelli, on which sits the occipital lobes and below which is the cerebellum. With certain types of head trauma, movement of the brain against the falx and tentorium can causes contusions and shearing of cortical tissue (Figs. 50–52).

THE SKULL

Completely encasing and supporting the brain is a thick bony covering that protects it from damage, i.e., the skull. The cranium is composed of several bony sheets, e.g., the frontal, parietal, temporal, and occipital bones. The frontal bone constitutes the skeletal framework for the forehead (including the orbits for the eyes) and is joined to the parietal bones (the bulging topsides of the skull) by the coronal sutures. Comprising the lower and lateral portion of the cranium, including parts of its floor, are the temporal bones which also house the structures of the inner ear. The occipital bone makes up the lower posterior portion of the cranium (Figs. 53–56).

Although seemingly smooth on the outside, the skull is not completely smooth and rounded on the inside, as it consists of several small bony protrusions and cavities. These same protrusions can sometimes serve as a source of injury. For example, when the head is subject to accelerating–decelerating forces, the soft mass of the brain may be thrown against these ridges and become torn and contused in consequence. Nevertheless, the skull serves as the first line of defense against traumatic brain injury.

SKULL INJURIES

If struck by a blunt object, a flattening of the skull with stress oscillating outward laterally results—like a rock hitting a pool of water. If sufficient pressure is applied, the skull will fracture. Usually the break occurs at the site of impact.

Skull fractures are of three types: depressed, linear, and basilar. Basilar fractures are

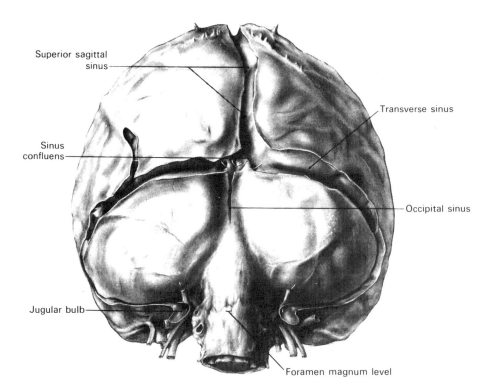

FIGURE 50. Posterior superior view of the dura surrounding the brain. Reproduced, by permission, from *Neuroanatomy*, 2nd Ed., by F. A. Mettler, 1948, C. V. Mosby Company, St. Louis, MO.

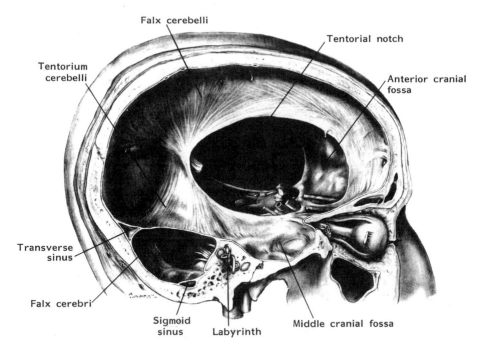

Falx cerebelli

Tentorial notch

Tentorium
cerebelli

Anterior cranial
fossa

Transverse
sinus

Falx cerebri

Sigmoid
sinus   Labyrinth

Middle cranial fossa

FIGURE 51. Parasagittal (lateral) view with brain removed depicting the dura and its compartments. Reproduced, by permission, from *Neuroanatomy*, 2nd Ed., by F. A. Mettler, 1948, C. V. Mosby Company, St. Louis, MO.

relatively uncommon whereas approximately 75% are linear, the remainder being depressed. In general, head injuries are also considered as either closed or open if accompanied by scalp laceration and/or if the fracture extends into the sinuses or middle ear.

Basilar Fractures

Basilar fractures often extend into the base of the skull and are difficult to detect unless quite severe. However, existence of a basal skull fracture may be indicated by cranial nerve damage or hormonal–endocrine abnormalities (such as from damage to the pituitary). Fractures near the sella tursica (at the base of the skull) may tear the stalk of the pituitary; diabetes, impotence, and reduced libido may result.

In some instances, these fractures may extend in an anterior, posterior, or lateral direction. If they extend in an anterolateral direction, tearing of the olfactory, optic, oculomotor, trochlear, first and second branches of the trigeminal, and the facial and auditory nerves may occur, disrupting olfaction, vision, eye movements, and/or causing unilateral facial paralysis and hearing loss. If extending laterally, they may damage the mastoid bone and tympanic membrane of the inner ear, resulting in dizziness and in disturbances involving equilibrium, as well as a loss of hearing. Basilar fractures are sometimes associated with tearing of the dura as well as cerebrospinal (CSF) leakage. Hence, a variety of related complications may occur including infection (Figs. 57 and 58).

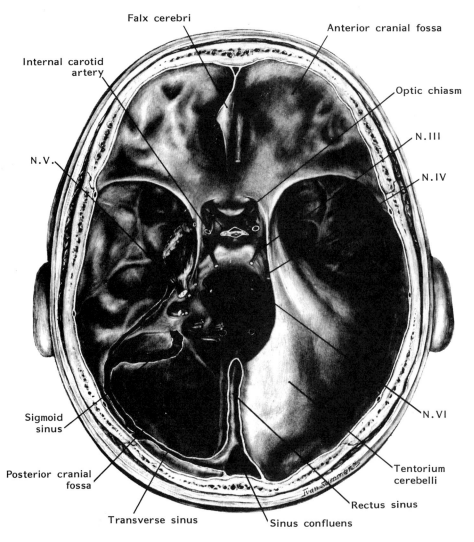

Falx cerebri

Anterior cranial fossa

Internal carotid artery

Optic chiasm

N.III

N.V.

N.IV

Sigmoid sinus

N.VI

Posterior cranial fossa

Tentorium cerebelli

Rectus sinus

Transverse sinus

Sinus confluens

FIGURE 52. View from the base of the skull of the dura mater. The tentorium and falx cerebri have been removed and/or cut away. Reproduced, by permission, from *Neuroanatomy,* 2nd Ed., by F. A. Mettler, 1948, C. V. Mosby Company, St. Louis, MO.

Depressed Fractures

Usually with depressed factures, part of the skull will shatter into several fragments, which are driven downward toward the brain. If the dura is torn, the brain is often lacerated as well. Moreover, if the dura has been torn, the patient becomes vulnerable to infection, particularly because pieces of hair or other debris may be driven into the cranial vault. This in turn will later give rise to a host of symptoms including the possible development of meningitis (Jennett & Teasdale, 1981).

Frequently, but not always, the meningeal artery may be torn, and intracerebral,

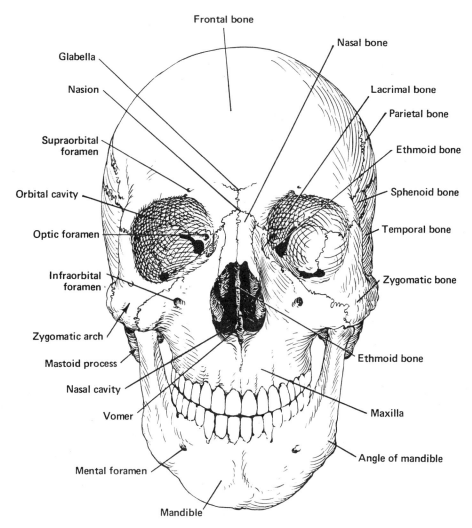

FIGURE 53. Anterior (frontal) view of human skull. Reproduced, with permission, from *Correlative neuroanatomy,* 20th Ed., by J. DeGroot & J. G. Chusid, copyright Appleton & Lange, E. Norwalk, CT, 1988.

extracerebral, or epidural hematomas may develop. Laceration and contusions are usually found beneath the broken bone fragments, and subdural hematomas may develop on the contralateral side (Bakay *et al.*, 1980). If not accompanied by a laceration of the scalp, depressed fractures are described as closed.

In some cases, particularly if bone fragments have been driven into the brain and/or with development of hematomas, patients develop focal neurological signs, depending on which part of the brain has been compromised. Approximately 50% of those who suffer a depressed skull fracture do not lose consciousness (Bakay *et al.*, 1980; Jennett & Teasdale, 1981). In many instances, the dura is spared and there is no gross evidence of

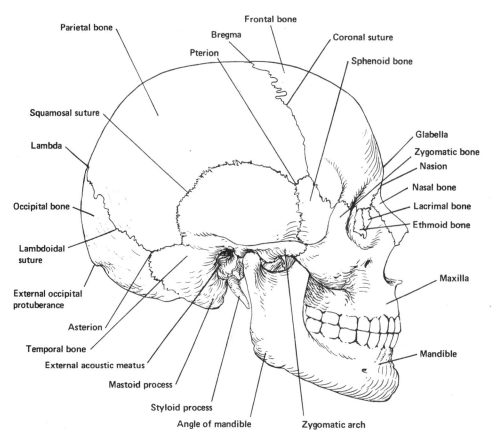

FIGURE 54. Lateral view of the skull. Reproduced, with permission, from *Correlative neuroanatomy,* 20th Ed., by J. DeGroot & J. G. Chusid, copyright Appleton & Lange, E. Norwalk, CT, 1988.

neurological compromise. This does not mean, however, that the brain has not been injured.

Linear Fractures

When the head is struck, an inward deformation of the skull usually results immediately beneath the site of impact, whereas the surrounding area is bent outward. In some instances, the skull shatters (i.e., depressed fracture), whereas in most cases, it will crack. Linear fractures are of two types: longitudinal and transverse.

Like depressed fractures, patients may or may not lose consciousness. However, it has been reported that patients with linear fractures who retain consciousness are 400 times more likely to develop a mass lesion (e.g., hematoma) as compared with comatose patients who are 20 times more likely to develop intracranial hemorrhage (Jennett & Teasdale, 1981).

The most common sites of linear fractures involve the temporal and parietal bones. Indeed, the temporal portion of the skull may fracture following trauma to any portion of the cranium.

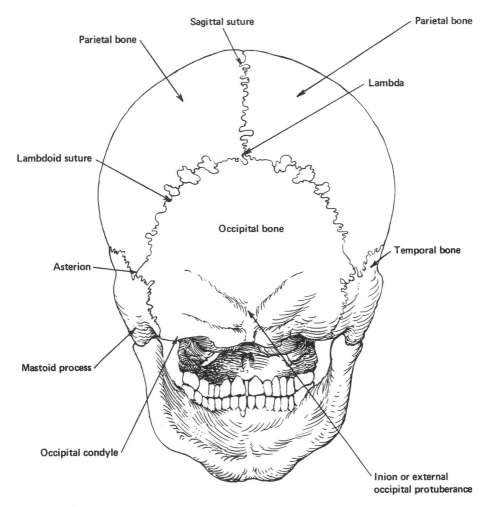

FIGURE 55. Posterior view of the skull. Reproduced, with permission, from *Correlative neuroanatomy,* 20th Ed., by J. DeGroot & J. G. Chusid, copyright Appleton & Lange, E. Norwalk, CT, 1988.

Hearing Loss, Tinnitus, and Vertigo

Linear fractures involving the temporal–parietal bones may damage the auditory meatus, auditory tube, and eardrum, causing hearing loss, tinnitus, disorders of equilibrium and vertigo.

Facial Paralysis

In some instances, longitudinal fractures may damage the cochlear nucleus and cause injuries to the seventh and fifth cranial nerves, which pass through this area before innervating the skin and muscles of the face. When these nerves are crushed or damaged, a unilateral facial paralysis and loss of sensation result. Transverse fractures can also cause stretching of the seventh and eighth nerves and may damage the vestibular and

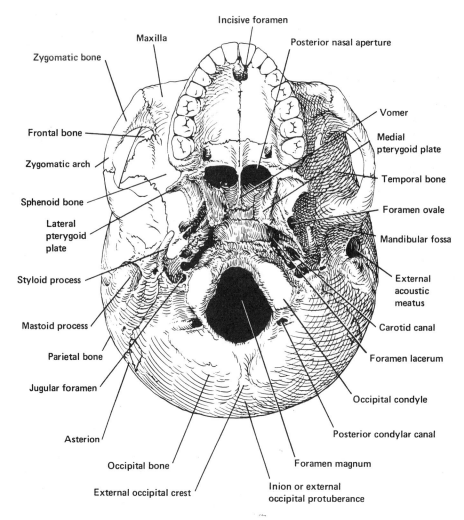

FIGURE 56. The base of the skull. Reproduced, with permission, from *Correlative neuroanatomy*, 20th Ed., by J. DeGroot & J. G. Chusid, copyright Appleton & Lange, E. Norwalk, CT, 1988.

cochlear portions of the labyrinth. Thus, facial paralysis and hearing-related abnormalities may also occur.

Anosmia

Anosmia (loss of the sense of smell) and an apparent loss of taste (loss of aromatic flavor perception) are frequent sequelae of head injury, especially following injuries to the face and fractures involving the back of the head or frontal bone. Anosmia is caused by damage to the olfactory nerve, usually in the vicinity of the cribriform plate.

The cribriform plate is a wafer-thin sheet of perforated bone through which the olfactory nerves pass on their journey from the nasal mucosa to the olfactory bulbs. Because this thin sheet of bone is perforated, it is predisposed to fracture during head trauma, regardless of where the patient was struck. This may cause the olfactory nerves to shear off, resulting in a permanent loss of smell, known as anosmia. Patients are unable to detect even markedly unpleasant odors. If odors can be detected, the olfactory nerve is intact (Fig. 59).

If the shearing is unilateral, the loss of smell will not be recognized by the patient. It is only with complete bilateral shearing that patients begin to complain, usually noting that they have suffered a loss of the ability to taste.

With damage to the olfactory nerve and cribriform plate, sometimes a laceration or rupture of the meninges may also result. If there is meningeal rupture, CSF will leak into the nose. Frequently, the only symptom is what appears to be a continually "running nose." In some instances, CSF has gushed into the patient's nose when he has coughed or sneezed—well after the injury. Therefore, if a patient has a runny nose, loss of smell, but no cold or allergy, and has had a head injury, a CSF fistula secondary to meningeal rupture and cribriform plate fracture should be considered. If this is suspected, the patient should be referred immediately to a neurosurgeon. Sometimes a secondary consequence of a rupture that goes untreated is bacterial infection, which can develop into meningitis.

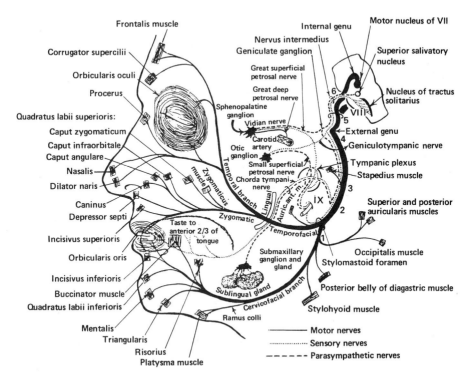

FIGURE 57. The distribution of the seventh (facial) nerve. Reproduced, with permission, from *Correlative neuroanatomy,* 20th Ed., by J. DeGroot & J. G. Chusid, copyright Appleton & Lange, E. Norwalk, CT, 1988.

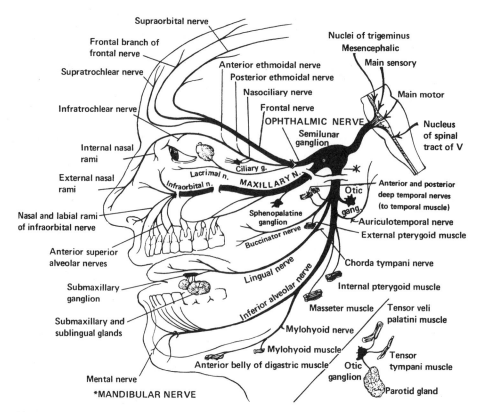

FIGURE 58. The distribution of the fifth (trigeminal) nerve. Reproduced, with permission, from *Correlative neuroanatomy,* 20th Ed., by J. DeGroot & J. G. Chusid, copyright Appleton & Lange, E. Norwalk, CT, 1988.

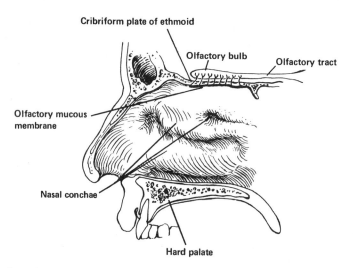

FIGURE 59. Lateral view of the nose and olfactory nerve. Reproduced, with permission, from *Correlative neuroanatomy,* 20th Ed., by J. DeGroot & J. G. Chusid, copyright Appleton & Lange, E. Norwalk, CT, 1988.

Blindness

Fractures near the sphenoid bone (which juts out beneath and below the frontal bone within the skull) may result in laceration of the optic nerve. When this occurs the patient becomes immediately and permanently blind. The pupil becomes permanently dilated and is unreactive to light, although consensual reflexes are maintained.

HEMATOMAS

Following a head injury, with or without skull fracture, the arteries and veins running above, below, or through the meningeal membranes may be stretched, broken, pierced, or ruptured. This results in blood loss and in the development of a blood clot, a hematoma. There are various types of hematomas. Some form below the dura, i.e., intradural hematoma, whereas others develop between the skull and the meninges and are referred to as extradural. Both are caused by bleeding inside the skull and the formation of a clot. The clot in turn acts to compress the brain. Extradural hematomas are often secondary to a skull fracture and laceration of the meningeal arteries below the site of primary impact.

Intradural Hematomas

There are several subtypes of intradural hematoma; epidural, subdural, and intracerebral. All can occur and develop either immediately at the time of primary insult or slowly, with symptoms delayed until days, weeks, or even months after the original head injury. Hematomas develop in 30–55% of those with severe head injuries, but they occur with mild injuries as well.

Intracerebral hematomas are not very common. They are usually secondary to ruptured aneurysms, gunshot or stab wounds, and lacerations from depressed skull fractures. Epidural hematomas are also not very common, as they tend to occur in fewer than 10% of all patients with severe head injury. Most are secondary to fractures of the temporal–parietal area and to laceration of the middle meningeal artery. They are frequently quite slow to develop, appearing hours or even days after the injury (Nikas, 1987).

In most cases, a patient will be struck and will lose consciousness for a brief time period. Upon waking, they seem lucid, but then, as the hematoma develops, they begin to complain increasingly of headache, irritability, confusion. As the hematoma increases in size, compressing and damaging the brain, the patient's symptoms become more severe, and consciousness again may be lost. If the hematoma is not evacuated, the patient is likely to die (Gallagher & Browder, 1968).

Subdural hematomas are the most common of all and are associated with a very poor prognosis. These hematomas develop following damage to the various veins that crisscross the subdural space. This results in the development of a pool of blood over the surface of the entire brain. Patients may deteriorate slowly or rapidly and become markedly depressed or even stuporous as the hematoma enlarges and increasingly compresses the brain (Bucci, Phillips, & McGillicuddy, 1986). In slowly developing undetected cases, patients may complain continually of headache and develop alterations in personality as well as changes in level of consciousness. Eventually, they may develop hemiparesis, language disorders, and other focal signs. Mortality has ranged from 30–70%—even when removal of the hematoma is attempted (Nikas, 1987).

Unfortunately, CT scan (Cooper, Maravilla, Moody, *et al.*, 1979) and, in particular, MRI (Snow, Zimmerman, Gandy, 1986) are not very useful in detecting the initial development of subdural hematomas, even when associated with hemorrhage. The physician should bear in mind that although an initial CT scan may have failed to detect any abnormalities, if the patient's condition subsequently deteriorates, the possibility of hematoma should be entertained.

Acute and chronic subdural hematoma may be unilateral or bilateral with an onset latency period of days or weeks. There may be headache, drowsiness, confusion, and disturbances in consciousness, all of which worsen progressively. Focal or lateralizing signs are less prominent. In the chronic condition, the traumatic etiology may not be clear or may seem very minor (e.g., striking the head against a branch of a tree), particularly among older patients. Headaches, giddiness, and slowness in thinking, may not develop until weeks after the initial injury and may give the initial impression of a vascular lesion, tumor, or drug intoxication.

HERNIATION

Hematomas are potentially life-threatening and can cause extensive brain injury (even when initially brain damage seemed minimal). This is because of the effects of compression as well as secondary increases in intracranial pressure (ICP).

The brain and skull are very tightly fitted, and there is little room for expansion. Thus, when blood leaks into or around the brain, something has to give and make room. Because the skull is rigid and relatively inflexible, pressure is thus exerted on the soft tissue of the brain, which in turn becomes compressed. Because of the compression, the brain will shift within the cranial vault, press up and/or beneath the various dural tentorial compartments, or even become forced down into the foramen magnum at the base of the skull, compressing the brainstem—which leads to death. These latter conditions are referred to collectively as herniations. Not all herniations are secondary to hematoma and many arise from tumors, stroke, or a combination of factors.

Falx, Cerebellar, and Temporal Lobe Herniations

The skull is subdivided into compartments through the dura. Because of its compartmental arrangement, pressure may be high in one region of the brain and less so in yet another. Nevertheless, force will be exerted from a high-pressure region into a low-pressure zone, causing displacement of the brain. The brain is sometimes displaced over or under the dura, causing tearing and further compression effects. Nevertheless, depending on where the brain is displaced, various types of herniation and subsequent brain damage may result. These include subfalcial, tonsillar, and temporal lobe/tentorial herniations.

Subfalcial Herniation

Subfalcial herniation may occur secondary to frontal or parietal hematomas. With increased pressure in these areas, the frontal–parietal areas tend to herniate medially under the falx cerebri, which separates the two hemispheres. With subfalcial herniation, the medial part of one frontal or parietal lobe is pushed under the falx, damaging not only these regions but the cingulate gyrus as well.

Tonsillar/Cerebellar Herniation

Pressure developing from a mass lesion tends to displace the brain and in particular the cerebellum in a downward direction. This also results in brainstem compression as the cerebellum is forced down in the foramen magnum. This leads to respiratory and vasomotor abnormalities, and eventually loss of consciousness. With increasing expansion, respiratory arrest and death result. This form of herniation can also occur secondary to an expanding frontotemporal lobe hematoma.

Tentorial/Temporal Lobe Herniation

Tentorial/temporal lobe herniation is caused by swelling and pressure acting on the medial uncal region of the temporal lobe. As pressure develops, the temporal lobe is forced into the tentorial opening, within which sits the midbrain. Consequently, the midbrain, diencephalon, and subthalamic regions are pressed against the opposite edge of the tentorial opening. Usually the oculomotor nerve becomes compressed, causing ptosis, pupil dilation, and loss of eye movement.

As pressure continues to develop, the midbrain and diencephalon are shoved down into the posterior fossa compressing the brainstem. Because of interference with the reticular activating system, patients begin to experience rapid changes in conscious-awareness; become stuporous; descend into somnolence, to semicoma, to coma; and develop irregular respiration, hemiplegia (due to compression of descending motor tracts), and/or decerebrate rigidity (i.e., extension of the extremities), until finally respiration is arrested and the patient dies. In part, this is a consequence of disconnection of the brainstem from upper cortical centers and can also occur with subfalcial or cerebellar herniation. Even in less severe cases, there may be infarction (i.e., stroke) within these regions secondary to compression of the blood vessels surrounding these various subcortical centers. In these instances, death is also a likely sequela.

CONTUSIONS

Following a blow to the head, the skull will bend inward and sometimes strike the brain, causing a contusion directly below the site of impact, i.e., a coup injury. This is because the brain, being more fluid, moves more slowly than the skull in response to force. However, except in cases of depressed skull fracture, contusions are not commonly found beneath the site of impact (Adams, Graham, & Scott, 1980). Indeed, damage can be widespread or localized to the contralateral half of the brain.

The force of the impact will usually force the brain to shift and/or bounce against and strike the inner bony prominences of the opposite half of the skull (i.e., contrecoup injury) as well as the falx cerebri and tentorium. This results in contusions to the neocortical surface, particularly along the temporal and frontal lobes. Indeed, contusions and bruises are usually found in the orbital frontal regions and anterior and lateral temporal lobes bilaterally as well as along the convexity, regardless of where the skull was struck (Adams et al., 1980). Frequently, the medial portions of the brain, including the corpus callosum, may also be traumatized due to rotational forces such that they bump and slide against the falx and/or tentorium. By contrast, contusions are rarely encountered along the occipital lobe, even when the back of the head has been struck.

In general, contusion may consist of multiple hemorrhages that develop immediately upon impact along the crests of the various cerebral gyri. Contusional hemorrhages may increase in size during the first few hours after injury, extending from the superficial layers of the neocortex into the white matter. Edema is usually a secondary consequence. Thus, widespread damage, varying in severity, is a likely consequence of head injury.

Necrosis

When the brain has been contused, severely compressed, or subjected to rotational shearing forces, axons are often severed and cells crushed. This results in cell death (necrosis) within the first 24 hours after injury—a process that may continue for up to 1 week. After a few months, these cells are reabsorbed, leaving behind glial scars and small cavities in the cortex and white matter. These scars can in turn become a source of abnormal activity and may cause the development of seizures.

Consciousness

When consciousness is not lost following a head injury, it is frequently erroneously assumed that the brain was not damaged. However, a patient may in fact suffer from extensive contusions and lacerations throughout the brain, even with no loss of consciousness (Bakay, Glasauer, & Alker, 1980; Teasdale & Mendelow, 1980). Moreover, there may be complete memory for the accident with no anterograde or retrograde amnesia.

COUP AND CONTRECOUP CONTUSIONS

In some instances, it has been postulated that because of the differential movement of the brain, both coup or contrecoup lesions can result. Coup contusions are caused by the slapping effect of the skull hitting the brain. Tissue is damaged directly below the point of impact. Generally the head is stationary at the time of the injury. Contrecoup contusions are usually associated with translational linear acceleration injuries and the free movement of the head. Translational (linear) acceleration of the brain occurs at the moment of impact and/or as there is a rapid linear acceleration in the motion of the head, such as if thrown from a car. This causes the brain to bounce against and strike the rough bony protusions on the opposite side of the skull.

Contrecavitation. As pertaining to coup and contrecoup lesions, rapid increases in acceleration sometimes cause the development of increased ICP at the trauma point and decreased (contrecoup) pressure at the opposite side of the cerebrum. In addition to the brain striking the opposite side of the skull, this decreased pressure at the contrecoup site can cause the development of cavitation bubbles, which, upon bursting or collapsing, cause local tissue damage, i.e., a contrecoup lesion (Bakay *et al.*, 1980). Contusions are sometimes associated with this type of injury (Unterharnscheidt & Sellier, 1966).

Differential Effects of Impact Site

The development of coup and/or contrecoup lesions is also dependent on what part of the skull was initially impacted. That is, an impact to certain regions of the skull seems to result commonly in coup lesion, whereas other zones struck give rise to coup and contrecoup damage. For example, impact at the occipital region often forces the brain to move in an anterior direction, causing a contrecoup lesion to the frontal lobe (Bakay *et al.*, 1980; Lindgren, 1966). Indeed, although there is some evidence of considerable movement of the parietal–occipital region, regardless of the impact site (see Bakay, Glasauner & Alker, 1980, for review), direct blows to the occiput seldom cause occipital damage.

By contrast, impact to the front of the skull almost always results in frontal lobe (coup) injuries. However, in about 50% of cases, both coup and contrecoup lesions result. Temporal impacts also create contrecoup lesions. If struck from the top of the head, contrecoup contusions frequently develop in the corpus callosum and the orbital frontal lobes due to the downward force of the blow (Bakay *et al.*, 1980).

Caveats

Not all investigators accept the notion of contrecoup damage, however. Indeed, the fact that the frontal and temporal regions are most severely affected regardless of impact site argues against the notion of contrecoup injuries (Ommaya, Grubb, & Naumann, 1971), as do the findings that when there is a skull fracture, contusions are maximal on the side of impact (Adams *et al.*, 1980). Rather, it has been postulated that much of the damage that occurs secondary to impact or nonimpact (including coup and contrecoup) injuries is secondary to the effects of rotational acceleration and shearing forces.

ROTATION AND SHEARING FORCES

In certain types of head injuries, such as those involving a great deal of force and movement, the brain will swirl, rotate, oscillate, and slosh around inside the skull in a rotary fashion (Pudenz & Shelden, 1946). This can occur at the moment of impact or if the head is suddenly subjected to rapid changes in motion (such as when the patient is airborne after being thrown through the windshield of their car, as opposed to receiving a blow to the head when stationary). Indeed, rotational damage may occur even when the head has not been struck but can result from rapid skull movement alone, e.g., whiplash, severe and repeated shaking, or extreme motion of the head and neck (Unterharnscheidt & Sellier, 1966). This is in contrast to linear acceleration injuries, which are not usually associated with this differential swirling movement of the brain.

Nevertheless, as the brain swirls about, the neocortical surface becomes contused, sliced, and sheared by the bony protrusions (e.g., the sphenoid wing) within the cranium, and hemorrhages will develop over the surface of the cerebrum. The frontal–temporal regions are at particular risk for these types of injuries.

Brainstem and Subcortical Lesions

However, rotational acceleration and decelerations injuries can create extensive sub-cortical and brainstem damage as well. For example, the cerebral hemispheres, brainstem, and different parts of the brain will actually move in somewhat different directions as well as at different speeds, causing widespread stretching, straining, and snapping of axons running throughout the white matter, including the corpus callosum (Adams *et al.*, 1981; Gennarelli, 1986; Zimmerman, Bilianiuk, & Gennarelli, 1978). Indeed, because these strains are not uniform but affect various parts of the cerebrum differently, such that one part of the brain is moving in one direction while another portion is sliding at a somewhat different angle, certain regions can literally snap and break loose.

For example, when subject to severe rotational forces, there is sometimes tearing at the pontine–medullary junctions (where the brainstem meets the midbrain), such that the brainstem is partly torn loose and disconnected from the rest of the brain (Hardman, 1979; Jennett & Plum, 1972). Because the cerebral hemispheres sit atop the thin brainstem, torque in the pontine–midbrain junction can result, thereby disconnecting these lower from higher regions. When this occurs, consciousness is lost, and the patient either dies or remains in a prolonged coma.

In addition to contusions, rotational injuries are associated with venous tears, arterial shearing stresses, and hemorrhagic lesions in the midline region and throughout the brain. Nevertheless, the degree and type of damage that occurs are dependent on the speed and direction at which the head moves (Gennarelli, 1986).

DIFFUSE AXONAL INJURY

Independent of actual impact (Gennarelli, Spielman, & Lanfitt, 1982), when the brain is subject to severe rotational and acceleration/deceleration forces, there can result severe diffuse microscopic damage and profound shearing and stretching of axons throughout the brain and brainstem as well as focal lesions in the corpus callosum. Axons are literally torn in half because of the twisting strains placed on them. This condition is referred to as diffuse axonal injury (DAI).

When axons are severed or stretched, the capacity to transmit electrochemical impulses and thus transmit information is attenuated. If severe, a permanent loss of functional capability can result, accompanied by an immediate and prolonged loss of consciousness. Conditions that give rise to DAI are also associated with brainstem damage and to decorticate and/or decerebrate posturing. When this occurs, many patients, if they survive, end up in a vegetative state. Most will die, however (Gennarelli *et al.*, 1982; Gennarelli, Thibault, Adams, Graham, *et al.*, 1982). If less severe there may be a temporary inability to function due to strains involving the axonal membrane (Gennarelli, 1986).

In general, DAI takes the form of axonal retraction balls in those who die within days, microglial scars in those who live days to weeks, as well as degeneration of the fiber tracts among those who survive longer time periods, e.g., months (Adams, Graham, Murray, & Scott, 1981). That is, a few days after an injury in which axons and nerve fibers have been torn, often the nerve cell dies and the glial cellular reactions around these damaged, dying, and dead cells creates microglial scars. Often these scars become epileptogenic.

Moreover, because of this diffuse damage, various widespread regions of the brain are no longer able to function or intercommunicate, i.e., disconnection. Because of this, patients with DAI who have lost consciousness, yet who continue to live, tend not to regain consciousness but remain in a prolonged coma (Adams *et al.*, 1981; Gennarelli *et al.*, 1982). Interestingly, this condition occurs more frequently among those who do not suffer skull fractures.

HYPOXIA AND BLOOD FLOW

The energy required to run the brain is produced through the oxidative metabolism of glucose. Indeed, the brain's need for these substances is quite substantial, as it uses almost 20% of the body's oxygen supply (which the brain is unable to store), and consumes more than 25% of total body glucose. The source for both is the vascular system.

Reduction in oxygen and glucose create disturbances involving neuronal functioning, including seizures and/or a temporary cessation of brain activity—even if the deprivation is transient. If prolonged, the consequence is neuronal death. Reduction in the brain's oxygen supply is referred to as hypoxia.

In general, mild degrees of hypoxia are associated with blurring of vision or difficulty seeing in the dark, whereas moderate degrees produce loss of vision, nausea, coma, and amnesia. If prolonged, severe permanent neuronal damage, coma, and death result. This is a serious concern, as 50–70% of those with severe head trauma are hypoxic following injury (Klauber, Marshall, Toole, *et al.*, 1985).

Characteristically, following head trauma there is an immediate and global reduction in cardiac output and blood flow for a few seconds, which in turn results in oxygen deprivation. This is followed by a transient hypertension and then a prolonged hypotension (Crockard, Iannotti, & Kang, 1982). The overall consequences are reductions in arterial blood perfusion and thus hypoxia throughout the brain, as well as decreased blood flow within the damaged tissue. Metabolism is disrupted and energy failure results. In addition, the blood and oxygen supply in the brain can be reduced or diverted following chest injury, scalp laceration, or fractures involving the limbs.

Unfortunately, a vicious circle of deteriorative feedback can be produced by these conditions, further reducing supply of blood and oxygen in the brain. For example, hypoxia induces vasodilation and constriction of the blood vessels, a condition that result in intracranial hypertension. This creates an overall increase in ICP. When ICP increases, the brain and blood vessels become compressed (due to displacement pressure), further reducing blood and oxygen flow within the brain and to the damaged tissue. This causes the development of ischemia and focal cerebral edema (Jennett & Teasdale, 1981; Miller, 1985), all of which in turn add to displacement pressures (herniation).

Respiratory Distress

With severe head injury many patients may also suffer from transient disturbances involving respiration and apnea (Miller, 1985), i.e., a decrease in respiratory rate. With decreased respiration, there is decreased reoxygenation of the blood, all of which favor the development of hypotension and hypoxia (Staller, 1987).

With respiratory distress, hypotension, and hypoxia, pulmonary hypoperfusion and an increase in blood platelets in the capillaries result. Unfortunately, the increased number of blood platelets actually act to obstruct the blood vessels, thus further reducing blood flow. This has been referred to as neurogenic pulmonary edema. Onset is often delayed and may occur 48 hours after injury. However, arterial hypotension may be an immediate sequela if there has been blood loss from a scalp laceration or other injury (Miller *et al.*, 1981).

Vascular Trauma

Frequently, particularly with severe head injuries, the vascular system may be traumatized because of shearing and stretching of the blood vessels. Moreover, the blow itself or the action of rotational forces can cause vascular spasms in the carotid arteries as well as in the anterior and middle cerebral arteries (Bakay *et al.*, 1980). Although vasospasm can temporarily increase cerebral blood flow, it also increases the likelihood of stroke and/or blockage of the small arteries due to the breaking off of tiny plaques and other debris lining the large vessel walls. (See Chapter 9, Stroke and Cerebrovascular Disease.)

Myocardial Trauma

Head trauma can also result in secondary cardiovascular abnormalities, including myocardial damage. For example, if the brainstem medulla has been compromised, there may be abnormal activation of the vagus nerve, which influences heart rate, the result being atrial fibrillations—a condition that in turn can result in stroke (chapter 9).

Moreover, if the head-injured patient has suffered a chest injury, the heart may be bruised and injured (i.e., myocardial contusion). In these instances, the heart is unable to contract adequately. This leads to reduced output and hypotension—all of which can lead to respiratory distress and hypoxic conditions (Staller, 1987).

Chest Trauma

It is important to note that even with a minor head injury, if there is an injury to the chest (i.e., a pneumothorax, hemothorax), hypoxia may be produced as a result of inadequate ventilation of air. For example, pulmonary edema or lung shunting reduces the ability of the lungs to transport oxygen to the blood (systemic hypoxia). This results in brain damage, even if cerebral blood circulation is normal.

Summary

A variety of conditions associated with head injury can conspire to produce widespread hypoxia and disturbances involving cerebral metabolism. Neuronal death, independent of impact or rotational acceleration–deceleration forces, is the long-term consequence, even in mild cases. A patient with a minor head injury may suffer graver disturbances than someone who has sustained a more serious injury, if bones have been broken or if the chest has been injured.

COMA AND CONSCIOUSNESS

Reticular Damage and Immediate Cessation of Consciousness

In general, the loss of consciousness following a brain injury is often attributed to abnormalities involving the reticular formation of the brainstem. Indeed, destruction of the brainstem reticular formation invariably induces states of prolonged unconsciousness and unresponsiveness, accompanied by a slow synchronized electroencephalogram (EEG) and frequently irreversible coma; i.e., the remainder of the brain cannot be activated. However, damage need not be severe or extensive, as even small lesions in the brainstem, midbrain, and thalamus can induce a protracted loss of consciousness.

Hematomas and Hemorrhage

Frequently, brainstem, midbrain, and thalamic damage are secondary to acceleration rotational forces and/or develops as a consequence of intracranial hemorrhage, ischemia, compression, and herniation. However, these effects of trauma may also be slow to develop. That is, a small artery or capillary may be damaged resulting in a slow and gradual loss of blood (e.g., epidural hemorrhage), in which case patients will lose consciousness some time after the injury. These conditions are also associated with temporal–parietal fractures and laceration of the middle meningeal artery and vein.

Nevertheless, in these latter instances, the patient may seem normal for some time after the accident. However, as blood continues to leak and the brain becomes increasingly compressed, within a few hours or even days the patient begins to complain of headache, drowsiness, and confusion. With increasing blood loss, the patient may suddenly experience seizures, hemiparesis, and eventually loss of consciousness. If blood loss continues, there is a great threat of temporal lobe herniation and eventual crushing of the midbrain. These disturbances are life-threatening and require surgical intervention and identification of the bleeding vessel.

Loss of consciousness some time after the injury is not always attributable to the development of hemorrhage. In some instances, pain and emotional upset give rise to a vasopressor syncopal attack. Following the injury, the patient may walk about the room, seemingly returning to normal, and then turn pale and fall unconscious to the ground. By contrast, those who develop a hemorrhage or other disturbance lose consciousness at the time of injury but regain it after a few moments or minutes, only to fall back into unconsciousness later.

Levels of Consciousness

In general, the ability to obey simple commands is often considered indicative of the return of consciousness. However, patients may fade in and out of consciousness and/or display fluctuating levels of awareness. That is, the patient may appear confused, stuporous, or delerious.

Stupor

In stupor, the patient is unresponsive and can only be aroused by intense, loud, or painful stimulation. The patient may open their eyes and in some cases make some type of verbal response only when vigrously stimulated.

Confusion

In confusion, the patient has difficulty thinking in a coherent fashion and cannot carry out two-step or complex commands. Speech may consist of just a few words. These patients seem unaware of what is happening around them and cannot grasp their immediate situation or the circumstances surrounding their condition. As such, they are disoriented as to time and place.

Delirium

This condition can be secondary to toxic disturbances as well as cerebral contusion. The patient is disoriented and shows fear and irritability, overreactivity, and faulty perception of sensory stimuli sometimes accompanied by visual hallucinations.

Coma

One need not actually suffer a severe head trauma in order to sustain significant damage to the brain. Nor is loss of consciousness at the time of injury a prerequisite. In some cases, patients may experience a severe injury to the skull (e.g., depressed fracture) yet suffer only mild brain damage. Another patient may seem to have sustained a mild skull injury and later demonstrate moderate to severe cognitive loss.

Nevertheless, it does appear that when a patient has lost consciousness, the longer the period of unconsciousness, the more widespread and debilitating the injury and the loss of cognitive capability, including memory functioning. However, as pertaining to mild head traumas, particularly in cases in which consciousness was not lost, there simply have not been enough studies conducted by trained neuropsychologists to properly delineate the full potential ramifications of these injuries.

The Glasgow Coma Scale

Two general indicators of severity are length of unconsciousness and extent of memory loss, both retrograde and anterograde (i.e., post-traumatic amnesia) from the time of injury. One major advance in this regard was the development of the Glasgow Coma Scale (GCS) (Teasdale & Jennett, 1974). The GCS in effect provides standardized criteria for the assessment and description of head injury severity. Subsequently, tremendous interrater reliability has been found in the use of this scale.

The GCS is composed of three major categories: eye opening, motor response, and verbal response. The patients rating (or score) is based on his degree of ability to respond or react to various stimuli. If there is no response, the patient receives a score of 1. Thus, the minimum score possible is 3.

Eye opening: If the patient opens his eyes spontaneously, he receives a score of 4. If he opens them only in response to speech and pain, he receives a score of 3, if only in reaction to pain, the score is 2.

Motor response: If the patient can motorically respond to and obey commands adequately, his score is 6. If his reaction is more limited and he is capable of responding only to pain in a generalized, albeit localized, manner (e.g., attempting to brush away the source), his score is 5. If he can only withdraw a limb in response to pain, the score is 4. Responses limited to abnormal flexion (decorticate) are given a score of 3 whereas abnormal extensions (decerebrate) in response to pain receive a score of 2.

Verbal response: If the patient is oriented to time, person, and place, the score received is 5. Confused spontaneous verbalizations yield a score of 4. Inappropriate verbalizations (yelling, swearing) are given a rating of 3, and incomprehensible verbalizations limited, for example, to moaning, are scored 2.

Severity

A patient in a vegetative coma who is completely unresponsive would receive a score of 3, whereas a patient who is fully responsive and alert would receive a score of 15. A patient who speaks inappropriate words and opens his eyes and motorically withdraws only in response to painful stimuli would have a score of 9. In general, a GCS score of 8 or less is indicative of a severe head injury, 9–12 is considered moderate, and 13–15 is rated mild.

MORTALITY

Mortality and GCS

On the basis of a review of a number of reports, it appears that patients with a GCS score of 8 or less have a mortality rate of approximately 40% (35–50%) and that as the scores decrease, death rate increases. For example, those with a score of 3–5 have a mortality rate of approximately 60%, whereas patients with a coma score of 6 or 7 aged 30–50 have about a 50–50 chance of living or dying (see Nikas, 1987*a*, for a review of the literature).

There is also a significantly high mortality rate for patients who remain in a coma for 6 hr or more (Jennett, Teasdale, Galbraith, *et al.*, 1977). Indeed, in one study, of 700 such cases who were still alive 6 months after their injury, one half of this group died over the course of the next 6 months, i.e., within 1 year of injury.

In addition, the longer the coma, the worse the prospects for rehabilitation and the greater the long-term disability (Najenson *et al.*, 1974). Similarly, among children, intellectual deficits and academic difficulties become more severe as coma length increases (Brink, Garrett, Hale, Woo Sam, & Nickel, *et al.*, 1970).

Mortality and Age

Mortality as well as severity are also a function of age. Children suffer a lower risk of mortality from head injury as compared with adults (Berger, Pitts, Lovely, *et al.*, 1985; Luerssen, Klauber, & Marshall, 1988). However, very young children and infants have a mortality rate that is higher than that of older children (Humphreys, 1983; Raimondi & Hirschauer, 1984).

In general, however, the mortality rate increases with age. For example, those over age 40 with severe injuries have a death rate of up to 70%, whereas the mortality rate for those below age 40 is 23% (Nikas, 1987). Specifically, it has been estimated that for each year over age 35, the odds of death increase by 3.6% and decrease by the same amount for each year under 35 (Teasdale, Skene, Spiegelhater, & Murray, 1982).

Mortality and Motor Functioning

The death rate is also inversely correlated with residual motor functioning. That is, the mortality rate increases as motor function deteriorates. Disturbances in motor function are often indicative of widespread cortical or brainstem damage. Prognosis is particularly poor among those who show posturing or flaccidity of the muscles (Nikas, 1987*a*).

General Complications

Complications affecting recovery and leading to mortality most commonly include hypoxia, hypotension, seizures, infections (e.g., meningitis, abscess), and unrecognized mass lesions (Nikas, 1987*b*). Indeed, many patients talk and show some alertness after injury but die as a result of later development of hypoxia and associated complications (Rose, Valtonin, & Jennett, 1977).

Most patients who die when first seen, however, are in a state of shock with subnormal blood pressure, hypothermia, fast pulse, and pale-moist skin. If this state persists along with deep coma, widely dilated pupils, no eye movements, flaccid limbs, and irregular or rapid respiration, death usually follows. Therefore, these are all grave prognostic signs.

At autopsy, there is usually evidence of cerebral contusion, focal swelling, hemorrhage, and necrosis. Some of these patients, do not die, however, but persist in a state of profound disability.

VEGETATIVE STATES

Some patients will remain in a coma for months or even years and never regain consciousness. Others, although having suffered profound and very severe brain injuries, open their eyes after a few weeks or months and seemingly recover from their sleeplike coma, yet never truly regain consciousness; i.e., recognizable mental and purposeful motor functioning never reappears. These patients are in a persistent vegetative state (Jennett & Plum, 1972). Often such individuals demonstrate an absence of cortical functioning, although the lesion may be in the brainstem. In most cases, the brainstem is actually well preserved, with the hemispheres and subcortical white matter most severely affected (Berrol, 1986).

According to Jennett & Plum (1972), after a few weeks, these patients may open their eyes, first in response to pain, and later spontaneously. They may grimace, flex the limbs, or blink to threats or to loud sounds and may make roving movements of the eyes. Sometimes they seemingly follow objects and may fixate on a physician or family member. This usually gives a family member or an inexperienced physician the erroneous impression of cognition.

Nevertheless, among those in a vegetative state, there is wakefulness without awareness. The patient remains inattentive and never speaks or gives any consistent sign indicating cognition or awareness of inner need. The limbs are often extended in a posture called decerebrate rigidity (i.e., arms and legs extended with the feet and hands inwardly rotated). However, after a few weeks or months, this condition may wear off. Sometimes fragments of coordinated movements look purposeful, such as scratching or movement toward a noxious stimulus. Patients may swallow food and water and may chew and grind their teeth for long periods. Grunting and groaning may also be provoked although most of the time these patients are silent (see also Berrol, 1986). In this regard, however, their behavior is little different from that of an "anencephalic monster," i.e., a child born with only a brainstem.

It has been argued that the term "persistent" should not be applied until at least 1 year has elapsed since injury (Berrol, 1986). This is because some patients may actually improve from the vegetative state to one of severe disability, e.g., those with traumatic versus hypoxic damage. However, the longer the patient is in a persistent vegetative state, the less potential there is for any realistic change.

MEMORY

When the brain has been traumatized, the ability to process information or retain, store, and recall ongoing events may be seriously altered and disturbed—even following a mild head injury and/or when consciousness has not been lost (e.g., see Yarnell & Lynch, 1970). The patient may suffer from a brief or prolonged period of amnesia. If consciousness is merely altered (i.e., the patient is dazed), the amnesia may be only for the events that occurred at the moment of impact and for a few seconds thereafter.

Usually following a significant head injury, there is a period of amnesia for events that occurred just before and just after the injury. However, because the brain may remain dysfunctional for some time even after the return of consciousness, memory functioning and new learning remain deficient for a long time. Indeed, following the recovery of consciousness, patients may be unable to recall anything that occurred for days, weeks, or even months after their injury. This condition has been referred to as post-traumatic (anterograde) amnesia (Russell, 1971).

Frequently the amnesia includes events that occurred well before the moment of impact as well, i.e., retrograde amnesia. Retrograde amnesia may extend for seconds, minutes, hours, days, months, or even years, depending on the severity of the injury (Blomert & Sisler, 1974). In part, this is a consequence of damage to the hippocampus within the temporal lobe as well as frontal lobe injuries, which disrupt attentional functioning. It has been suggested that the length of both retrograde and anterograde amnesia may be used as indicants of the severity of the injury. The longer the memory lapse, the more severe the injury.

Retrograde Amnesia

Retrograde amnesia (RA) is measured by determining the last series of consecutive events recalled prior to impact. Patients may show islands of memory, hence the need to determine continuous memory. RA is not necessarily a permanent condition; slowly, memory for various events may return, usually the older memories returning before more recent experiences. This has been referred to as a shrinking retrograde amnesia. However, the shrinkage is not complete, as events occurring seconds or minutes before the trauma are permanently forgotten (Schacter & Crovitz, 1977).

Not all patients show a shrinking RA (Sisler & Penner, 1975). In fact, there is some possibility that although memory for some events well in the past may have returned, the return (or shrinkage) is not complete. Rather, only islands of events are recalled. As pointed out by Squire, Slater, and Chace (1975), "questions about the remote past tend to sample a greater time interval and tend to be more general than questions about the recent past" (p.77). That is, recent events become telescoped such that lapses are more apparent. Therefore, rather than shrinkage, it is probable that only islands of memory have returned. With these caveats in mind, it is apparent that true RA is difficult to assess and probably should not be used as an indicant of the severity of brain injury, except in the most general of terms.

Post-Traumatic/Anterograde Amnesia

Many patients who suffer brief or extended period of coma or unconsciousness experience protracted periods of disorientation and confusion upon recovery (Levin *et al.*, 1982). Indeed, frequently there is a period of complete amnesia for continuously occurring events for some time after the return of consciousness (Russell, 1971). Although consciousness returns, since the brain is impaired, information processing and thus memory remain faulty for a variable length of time, depending on the severity as well as the location of the injury. This has been referred to as post-traumatic amnesia (PTA). Nevertheless, PTA is not caused by an inability to register information, for immediate recall may be intact, whereas short- and long-term memory remain compromised (Yarnell & Lynch, 1970). Although patients are responsive and may interact somewhat appropriately with their environment, they may continue to have difficulty consolidating and transferring information from immediate- to short- to longer-term memory.

Post-traumatic anterograde amnesia has long been considered a useful method for determining the severity of the brain injury (Russell, 1971). According to Russell (1971), mild injuries are associated with PTA of less than 1 hr. PTA of 1–24 hr is associated with moderate injuries, 1–7 days of PTA suggest moderate to severe injuries, and PTA over 7 days is associated with severe injuries.

In attempting to calculate PTA, it is important to bear in mind that the first appearance of normal memory does not indicate the end of the amnesia period. That is, although ostensibly normal, it may be temporary and followed by another period of PTA.

Thus, PTA is determined by the return of continuous memory. PTA seems to correlate well with severity of the trauma and the degree of cognitive impairment during the first 3 months following injury—at least for moderate and severe injuries. Beyond 3 months postinjury, these correlations become increasingly weak, except among those with profound injuries and long periods of PTA, in which case correlations remain constant for many years (Dailey, 1956; Wowern, 1966). In these instances, however, patients are so severely disabled that estimates of severity based on PTA are completely superfluous.

Some investigators have also argued that the duration of PTA is related to the development of subsequent impairment in memory functioning (Russell, 1971). For example, patients with coma lasting at least 1 day, a GCS of 8 or less, and PTA of 2 or more weeks continue to have significant memory problems for up to 1 year after injury (Dikman, Tempkin, McLean, Wyler, & Machamer, 1987). However, these relationships are largely dependent on how one measures memory and are also a function of which brain regions may have been damaged.

There is some evidence, however, that PTA is somewhat correlated with the extent of RA. For example, among patients with PTA exceeding 7 days, RA is less than 30 min in more than 50% of patients (Russell, 1971). If PTA is less than 1 hr, RA is often less than 1 min (Bromlert & Sisler, 1974).

Caveats

It seems that regardless of the nature and severity of the initial trauma, abnormalities involving memory are the most frequently reported disturbances following a head injury. Moreover, although memory functioning may improve, depending on which part of the brain has been compromised, it may remain abnormal and never completely recover, even after 10–20 years have elapsed (Brooks, 1972; Smith, 1974; see also Schacter & Crovitz, 1977, for review). This is not entirely surprising, given the fact that the frontal and especially the temporal lobes are particularly vulnerable to the effects of hypoxia, herniation, hematomas, and contusions.

Because of this, PTA and the period in which one is rendered unconscious should only be used as a general indicant of brain injury severity, for what appears to be a mild injury to one part of the brain may in fact yield more severe long-term consequences than what appears to be a more significant injury involving yet a different portion of the cerebrum. For example, a patient may suffer a brief loss of consciousness and a PTA of less than 20 min following a mild head injury involving the anterior–inferior temporal lobes, yet continue to suffer disturbances involving attention, motivational functioning, and verbal and/or visual memory for years. In this regard, one cannot with any sense of assurance make blanket statements that those with mild versus moderate head injuries (based on PTA estimates) will subsequently suffer less severe memory or cognitive impairment.

Moreover, when we consider the numerous intervening variables (e.g., hypoxia, a slowly developing hematoma, chest injury) that may add to the severity of what appears initially to be an inconsequential head injury, too heavy a reliance on PTA and length of coma in determining severity will certainly result in an erroneous diagnosis. Therefore, rather than relying on PTA estimates or on the period in which the patient has lost consciousness, one must examine the patient in question adequately in order to arrive at a true measure of his or her capability as well as the possible extent and severity of the injury. Thus, in general, PTA and time unconscious are probably only applicable in regard to those with moderate and severe injuries and do not offer adequate estimates for large numbers of patients with what appears to be a mild injury.

PERSONALITY AND EMOTIONAL ALTERATIONS

Emotional and personality disturbances secondary to head injury are often more debilitating and disruptive than any residual cognitive or physical impairment. They are also the most resistant to treatment. This is because the emotional and personality changes are frequently a direct consequence of the brain injury, and no one can talk (or counsel) a patient out of a damaged brain. That is, just as a patient may become aphasic following an injury to Wernicke's area, the patient may become emotionally abnormal secondary to injuries involving those portions of their brain that govern personality and emotion. Indeed, with severe injuries, a considerable number of patients may in fact develop what appear to be psychotic features, including schizophrenic-like psychosis, hysteria, euphoria, manic-excitement, and indifference (reviewed in Chapters 1–4) due to damage involving the limbic system, the frontal lobes, the temporal lobes, or the right parietal area.

A more common sequela is depression and anxiety. Indeed, many patients seem anxious and depressed, stay depressed for long periods, and tend to become socially withdrawn (Dikmen & Reitan, 1976; Fordyce, Roueche, & Prigatano, 1983). In many instances, disturbances such as depression are reactive and therefore secondary to a realistic appraisal of the patient's injury. Nevertheless, marked alterations in personality and emotional functioning occur even in those with little or no physical handicap (Bond, 1979).

Delayed Development of Emotional Changes

In some cases, emotional and personality disturbances may intensify over time (Fordyce et al., 1983; Oddy, Coughlan, Tyerman, & Jenkins, 1985) with the maximal amount of change noted during the first 3 months following injury (Brooks & McKinlay, 1983). The deterioration is often unrelated to the severity of the initial injury or the degree of neuropsychological impairment (Fordyce et al., 1983).

Sometimes the delay in the development of emotional problems corresponds to the period in which the patient has reached a high level of recovery (Brooks & McKinlay, 1983). Therefore, this may be the result of a greater or developing awareness of their disability as well as difficulties with social interaction and adjustment. Indeed, common complaints include feelings of worthlessness, uselessness, loneliness, and boredom (Lezak, 1987). Frequently, however, patients have a unrealistic appraisal of their condition (Tobias, Puria, & Sheridan, 1982) and in fact will actively deny or refuse to acknowledge the extent of their deficits.

Family Stress

Alterations in personality also place severe strains on relatives and close friends—more so in fact than subsequent physical limitations (Thomsen, 1974; Jennett, 1975;

Rosin, 1977). Often family members have considerable difficulty tolerating or accepting the personality changes, and frequently there is much denial, guilt, and disengagement, and sometimes rejection (Rosin, 1977; Tobias *et al.*, 1982). There is frequently a perception that the head-injured family member is no longer the same person, particularly in that behaviorally they may seem drastically different (e.g., impulsive, amotivated). Because they seem different, these patients are easier to reject, since the person being rejected is a stranger. Family members may treat the patient differently, and spouses may in fact refuse to continue their marriages, depending on the nature of the change. For example, patients who develop sexual preoccupations are four times more likely to become separated or divorced (Dikmen & Reitan, 1976).

Premorbid Personality

Patients who develop psychiatric abnormalities after head injury sometimes have premorbid indications of instability and other problems (Lishman, 1978). But this is not always the case (Rimel, Giordani, Barth, Boll, & Jane, 1981; Barth, Macciocchi, Giordani, Rimel, Jane, & Boll, 1983). Personality changes may be completely opposite to what was observed premorbidly (Tobias *et al.*, 1982), particularly among those with frontal and temporal lobe injuries (Joseph, 1986a). (See Chapter 4, The Frontal Lobes.)

For example, one young man who was described as being very kind, courteous, law abiding, and gentle, following a frontal head injury subsequently raped and savagely beat several women. Other examples of behavior change include mania and hysteria, even among formerly quite conservative and reserved people (Joseph, 1986a, 1988; see also Chapters 1 and 4).

Moreover, children commonly develop behavioral patterns quite inconsistent with those observed premorbidly. For example, an older child may begin to act like a younger child or an infant, such that he seems to have regressed. Common behavioral changes among children include enuresis, impulsiveness, hyperactivity, short attention span, destructive and agressive behavior, and temper tantrums (Brink *et al.*, 1970). Nevertheless, the development of neurosis and even psychoses may occur even after a mild head injury with little or no loss of consciousness (Bennett, 1969).

RECOVERY

Severe injuries to the brain are generally associated with profound disturbances involving all aspects of sensory, motor, cognitive, intellectual, and social–emotional functioning. However, there is no general rule as to which functions may be the most seriously compromised, as this is determined by which parts of the brain have been most seriously damaged. Nevertheless, in comparing large groups of moderately and severely injured patients, certain generalizations may be made regarding recovery.

For example, sensory, motor, and language skills tend to show the greater degree of recovery, whereas writing skills, math ability, memory, attention, intelligence, and social–emotional difficulties persist longer and tend to exert more devastating effects (Dikmen & Reitan, 1976; Jennett, Snoek, Bond, & Brooks, 1981; Miller & Stern, 1965; Najenson Groswasser, Mendelson, & Hackett, 1980; Najenson, Mendelson, Schechter, David, Mintz, & Groswasser, 1974; Tobias, 1982; Weddell, Oddy & Jenkins, 1980). In general, the bulk of motor and speech recovery takes place within 3–6 months of injury (Bond, 1979; Brooks, 1975), and the recovery of speech parallels the recovery of motor functioning (Brink *et al.*, 1970). Recovery of learning, memory, and constructional skills appears to proceed at a slower rate compared with other skills (Brooks & Aughton, 1979), and attention and memory show the least recovery (Dikmen & Reitan, 1976).

Intellect

A number of studies purport that even with severe injuries, intellect may return to normal. These impressions are based on repeated administration of various measures over time and do not account for practice effects. Nor is premorbid IQ taken into account. Finally, as noted with frontal injuries, although the patient may have an average or even superior IQ, this does not mean that the patient can use their intelligence effectively.

Employment

Only approximately one third of all patients with severe closed head injuries, even with extensive rehabilitation, return to gainful employment (Weddell, Oddy, & Jenkins, 1980). Those with personality and emotional problems tend to have the most difficulty (Prigatano, Fordyce, Zeiner, Roueche, Pepping, & Wood, 1984). Perhaps this will change as more is learned about the brain and methods of enhancing recovery.

Age

In general, the outlook for recovery is grim among persons over age 45 who suffered prolonged unconsciousness (Najenson *et al.*, 1974). In fact, the rate of severe disability becomes greater in older persons, i.e., as age increases, there is an exponential increase in the number of patients who fail to make meaningful gains (Carlsson, von Essen, & Lofgren, 1968; Teasdale, Skene, Spiegelhater, & Murry, 1982).

Pediatric patients with severe head injuries have a higher percentage of good outcome compared with adults and a significantly lower mortality rate as well (Alberico, Ward, Choi, Marmarou, & Young, 1987). At 1 year postinjury, the ratio was 2 : 1 in good outcome in comparing children with adults. However, children below the age of 4 seem to be more vulnerable than their older counterparts (Alberico *et al.*, 1987). Indeed, some functions are more impaired after early versus late lesions (see Schnieder, 1979, for review); in some cases, the recovery of some functions occurs at the expense of those that originally were not compromised (Joseph, 1982, 1986*b*).

There is also some suggestion that long-term intellectual deficits are more pronounced among younger children than among older children (i.e., adolescents), even among those whose duration of coma was shorter than that of those of the older groups (Brink *et al.*, 1970). This is consistent with other findings suggesting that very young children are more susceptible than older individuals to the more debilitating effects of severe head injury, including a higher mortality rate and the development of epilepsy.

Nevertheless, in general, children and young adults have better prospects for recovery and rehabilitation than do older individuals (Tobias *et al.*, 1982), which indicates that the aged brain has a reduced potential for recovery.

Recovery over Time

It has long been known that recovery is greatest over the course of the first 3 months after injury and that considerable recovery may continue during the first year (Dikmen & Reitan, 1976). Significant recovery also continues, albeit at a reduced rate, well beyond the first year for simple as well as complex abilities (Brink *et al.*, 1970; Dikmen, Reitan, & Temkin, 1983), even among those who suffered prolonged periods of unconsciousness (Najenson *et al.*, 1980).

Severe Injuries and Recovery

Nevertheless, the longer the coma and the more severe the injury, the greater the long-term disabilities and the worse the prospects for rehabilitation among children and adults (Brink *et al.*, 1970; Najenson *et al.*, 1974, 1980). Indeed, those with severe injuries often remain severely disabled, as only a small minority of patients may progress from severe to moderate disability, or from vegetative conditions to severe disability (Rosin, 1977). Moreover, the potential for severely head-injured patients to return to a socially and vocationally functional life is severely limited (Tobias, Puria, & Sheridan, 1982). Indeed, those with severe injuries seem to have "little potential for improvement over and beyond some very basic functional levels that they may reach fairly rapidly" (Dikmen *et al.*, 1983, p. 337). Some patients with severe injury may in fact deteriorate after having recovered to some degree (Brooks & Aughton, 1979).

EPILEPSY

When the brain has been damaged, neurons die and are replaced by glial scars. Sometimes these scars generate abnormal activity and/or disrupt neural activity in neighboring tissue, a phenomenon described as kindling. Kindling is the induction of epileptiform potentials in neighboring brain areas (see Nobels & Prince, 1978; Pedley, 1978). This results in an expanding lesion. However, not all glial scars are epileptic. Nevertheless, certain regions of the brain are more susceptible to developing epileptic activity than others, the anterior and mesial temporal lobe, for example.

Patients at highest risk of immediately developing epilepsy are those with temporal lobe damage, focal neurological signs (e.g., hemiparasis), intracranial hematomas, depressed skull fractures, and penetrating head injuries, as well as those with closed head injuries with PTA exceeding 24 hr (Jennett & Teasdale, 1981); 25–50% of those with penetrating injuries develop epilepsy, and 10% will suffer an epileptic seizure and develop epilepsy within 1 week of the injury, most experiencing their first attack within 24 hr (Jennett *et al.*, 1974). Among those with nondepressed skull fracture, the incidence of epilepsy is much lower, 7–13% (Jennett, 1973; Jennett *et al.*, 1974; Najenson *et al.*, 1980). In general, 20% of those with severe injuries developed epilepsy (Najenson *et al.*, 1980), and children are more likely to develop epilepsy than are adults (Jennett & Teasdale, 1981).

Post-traumatic seizures tend to decrease in frequency as the years pass, and 10–30% of patients may cease to have seizures altogether, particularly if their first seizure occurred within 1 year after injury. Those who develop seizures 1 or more years following head trauma may in fact suffer increasing episodes unless their condition is properly controlled by medication. Alcoholism has an adverse effect on these conditions, and seizures may be precipitated after a bout of hard drinking. Among women, seizures may occur more frequently around the time of menstruation.

CONCUSSION AND MILD HEAD INJURIES

Although various definitions for what constitutes a mild head injury have been offered, one loses a considerable degree of predictive ability in attempting to apply them. Moreover, what appears to be mild frequently may be quite serious. Indeed, some patients will die from a mild injury. By contrast, often the aftereffects are quite insignificant. Frequently, it is also assumed that one must lose consciousness in order for brain damage to occur. However, there is considerable evidence to indicate otherwise.

In general, the period that encompasses mild head injury for many investigators includes PTA and a loss of consciousness for up to 1 hr. However, based on the patients I have personally examined, it is my impression that a loss of consciousness for up to 20 min can be quite serious, regardless of the extent of PTA.

Concussion

Although a patient may suffer a concussion and memory loss without losing consciousness (Yarnell & Lynch, 1970), concussion is characterized by a brief period of unconsciousness followed by an immediate return of consciousness. There are usually no focal neurological signs, and the loss of consciousness is usually attributable to mechanical forces, such as a blow to the head. As the magnitude of the applied force is increased, the severity of the concussion increases.

Often immediately after an insult to the head, the patient will drop motionless to the ground, and there may be an arrest of respiration and an eventual drop in blood pressure (following rise at impact); death can occur from respiratory arrest. Vital signs usually return, even if the patient is unconscious, within a few seconds. Once respiration returns, the patient may begin to move about in a restless random fashion and may speak, usually unintelligibly. The patient may become abusive and irritable and may shout and resist contact (Russell, 1971).

Mild and Classic Concussion

As described in detail by Gennarelli (1986), there are two broad categories of concussion as well as distinct subtypes. These include mild concussion, in which there is no loss of consciousness, and classic concussion, which involves a short period of coma.

Mild Concussion

Mild concussion consists of several subtypes. Focal concussion is caused by involvement of a localized region of the cerebral cortex. For example, transient left-sided weakness may be due to right motor involvement, whereas the patient who "sees stars" may have received an occipital injury (Gennarelli, 1986). A diffuse concussion results in transient confusion and disorientation. Either of these concussive injuries may or may not be accompanied by amnesia.

With greater impact, although the patient does not lose consciousness, he may be confused and disoriented and may continue to interact motorically with his environment (Yarnell & Lynch, 1970). That is, he may walk around and even speak to others. However, although immediate recall is intact, he later becomes amnesic for the event as well as for the events leading up to the injury, i.e., anterograde and retrograde amnesia. The anterograde and retrograde amnesia may extend forward and backward in time for up to 20 min, even without loss of consciousness (Yarnell & Lynch, 1970). When this occurs, it is evident that the patient has suffered a significant insult to the brain.

Classic Concussion

Classic concussion is accompanied by a brief loss of consciousness at the instant of injury and is almost always associated with post traumatic amnesia. However, according to Gennarelli (1986), a patient with a classic concussion may remain unconscious for as long as 6 hr. If longer than 6 hr, the patient has probably suffered diffuse axonal injuries such that large-scale regions of the cerebrum have become partially disconnected.

In general, a mild (classic) concussion is associated with amnesia of less than ½ hr, a moderate concussion with amnesia of 1–24 hr, and severe concussion with amnesia of 24 hr or more (Tubbs & Potter, 1970). Nevertheless, although the concussion may be considered mild, the accompanying brain damage may be minimal, moderate, or in a few rare cases severe.

In cases of classic concussion, immediately following the injury, the patient develops apnea, hypertension, bradycardia, cardiac arrhythmias, and neurological disturbances such as decerebrate posturing and pupilary dilation. Thus, the patient may seem temporarily paralyzed. Often, upon regaining consciousness, the patients will vomit and complain of headache. Even in mild cases, temporary alterations in the permeability of the blood–brain barrier (BBB) and damage involving the neuronal mitochondria can result (Bakay, Glasauer, & Alker, 1980).

Mild Head Injury

A mild head injury is usually indicated by a GCS score of 13–15, no CT or radiological abnormalities, and a loss of consciousness for less than 20 min (some authorities include those with unconsciousness lasting up to 1 hr, (e.g., Dikmen et al., 1986). This has also been referred to as cerebral concussion, and patients need not have lost consciousness at the time of injury (Dikmen et al., 1983).

Although described as mild, these injuries can be quite serious and involve various degrees of permanent brain damage. For example, 1–5% of those with mild head injuries may demonstrate focal neurological deficits (Coloban, Dacey, Alves, Rimel, & Jane, 1986; Rimel et al., 1981). In addition, 2–3% of those with mild injuries deteriorate after initially appearing alert and responsive (Dacey, Alves, Rimel, et al., 1986; Fischer, Carlson, & Perry, 1981). Moreover, 3% of those with mild head injury will develop increased ICP and life-threatening hematomas that must be removed (Dacey et al., 1986).

Indeed, approximately 1 out 100 individuals with mild head injury die (Luerssen *et al.*, 1988).

Brainstem Abnormalities

It has been suggested that sheer strain secondary to mild acceleration–deceleration injuries causes tearing of axons, followed by degeneration of the neural tracts in the brainstem. Brainstem axonal degeneration has been experimentally demonstrated in monkeys with mild acceleration–deceleration-induced injuries (Jane, Rimel, Pobereskin, Tyson, Stewart, & Genarelli, 1982), and among humans over 40% of those with "mild" head injuries may demonstate abnormal brainstem-evoked potentials (Rowe & Carlson, 1980). Similarly, those who have died from other causes demonstrate microscopic neuronal damage, microglial scars, and fiber degeneration within the brainstem and cerebral hemispheres—even among those who received what were considered "trivial" injuries (Oppenheimer, 1968; Strich, 1969).

DAI and Contusions

Diffuse axonal injuries (DAI) have been noted among those suffering brief period of unconscious (Teasdale & Mendelow, 1984). Moreover, contusions within the anterior temporal regions and frontal lobes have been found among those with mild nonimpact concussions due to acceleration/deceleration injuries (Adams, Graham, & Scott, 1981).

Neuropsychological Deficits

Patients who have sustained mild head injuries have been repeatedly shown to suffer a variety of neuropsychological, psychosocial, and emotional impairments even in the absence of gross or focal neurological deficits (Barth *et al.*, 1983; Dikmen, McLean, & Temkin, 1986; Gronwall & Wrightson, 1974; Rimel *et al.*, 1981). These include pervasive neurobehavioral impairments involving attention, memory, and rate of information processing (Levin, Mattis, Ruff, *et al.*, 1987). Patients may suffer word-finding and expressive speech difficulties, reduced reaction time, perceptual–spatial disorders, and abnormalities involving abstract reasoning abilities. Moreover, although generalized recovery is often noted within 3 months of injury, memory disturbances often remain and may in fact persist for years (Lidvall, Linderoth, & Norlin, 1974; Jennett, 1978).

In some studies, it has been reported that 3 months after a mild injury, a significant number of patients continue to demonstrate visual–spatial abnormalities, memory disorders, reduced ability to concentrate, and persistent headaches, and as many as 34% of those with mild injuries may be unemployed at this time (Barth, Macciocchi, Giordani, Rimel, Jane, & Boll, 1983; Rimel *et al.*, 1981). Interestingly, these deficits are in no manner correlated with length of unconsciousness, PTA, or lawsuits; in one study, only 6 of more than 400 patients were involved in litigation. Hence, purposeful malingering is not likely among most of these cases.

Premorbid Influences

It is noteworthy that recovery appears to be dependent on previous mental abilities (Dikmen & Reitan, 1976) such that the debilitating effects of mild head injury appear to affect patients with minimal educational backgrounds more so than those with initially higher levels of functioning and education. This may be because these patients have "bad brains" to begin with and/or are less able to compensate for cognitive disturbances secondary to brain injury because of their more limited capabilities. That is, those with higher-level abilities have more to draw from and to fall back on. Of course, they also have more to lose.

POSTCONCUSSION SYNDROME

Frequently, a few days or even weeks or months after a mild (versus severe or moderate) trauma to the head, patients begin to complain of cognitive disturbances (Alves, Coloban, O'Leary, Rimel, & Jane, 1986), even when consciousness has not been lost. Symptoms are often nonspecific and are hard to quantify or objectively document. In general, these are referred to as postconcussive disorders. Indeed, about 50% of those who suffer mild head injuries (Alves *et al.*, 1986) are at risk of developing postconcussion symptoms (PCS). PCS is manifested somewhat differently for adults versus children.

Among adults, complaints regarding PCS may include persistent headaches, transient dizziness, nausea, impaired memory and attention, irritability, depression, anxiety, easy fatiguability, nystagmus, as well as inner ear disturbances such as vertigo, tinnitus, and hearing loss (Elia, 1972; Levin, High, Goethe, *et al.*, 1987; Lishman, 1973; Ommaya, Fass, & Yarnell, 1968; Toglia, Rosenberg, & Ronis, 1970). Headache, dizziness, memory problems, weakness, nausea, and tinnitus are often the most common complaints, even at 12 months following injury (Alves *et al.*, 1986). Other symptoms may include hyperacoutism, photophobia, decreased judgment, loss of libido, and difficulty with self-restraint and inhibition.

By contrast, children often may become withdrawn, antisocial, and aggressive and may develop enuresis, as well as sleep disturbances (Dillon *et al.*, 1961). Moreover, it has also been reported that some individuals, children in particular, develop transient migrainelike attacks following even minimal injuries, when consciousness was not necessarily lost (Haas & Lourie, 1988). These attacks include blurred, tunnel, and/or partial or complete loss of vision; paresthesias; dysphasia; confusion; agitation; headache; drowsiness, and vomiting—all of which come on like spells, particularly soon after the injury (Haas & Lourie, 1988). It has been suggested that this is due to traumatic spasm of the larger cerebral arteries.

In general, postconcussion symptoms are variable in degree and duration (Symonds, 1962), although frequently they may persist for long periods, from months to years or sometimes indefinitely (Dikmen & Reitan, 1976; Merskey & Woodforde, 1972; Symonds, 1962). Nevertheless, even when PCS begins to wane, it is sometimes followed by a long period of depression (Merskey & Woodforde, 1972).

Emotional Sequelae

Many patients with PCS in fact develop a variety of emotional and personality difficulties that seem to be triggered by the experience of having had an injury (Bennett, 1969). Patients may seem to be extremely anxious, fearful, depressed, and/or preoccupied with the details surrounding the accident (Bennett, 1969; Merskey & Woodforde,

1972) and remain (albeit periodically and transiently) upset for long periods. Others may appear intolerant of noise, emotional excitement, and crowds and may complain of tenseness, restlessness, an inability to concentrate, and feelings of nervousness and fatigue. Many patients with this syndrome also seem unable to tolerate the effects of alcohol. The emotional disturbances may persist for months or years but usually lessen as time passes.

It has been argued, and frequently it is suspected that PCS has in fact no objective basis and represents an exacerbation of premorbid personality characteristics or is motivated by a desire for financial compensation (Miller, 1961). Undoubtedly, this is true in a few cases. Nevertheless, often most of these patients are not even involved in litigation (Barth *et al.*, 1983; Merskey & Woodforde, 1972; Rimel *et al.*, 1981). Moreover, sometimes the actual deficit is greater than the patient realizes (Waddell & Gronwall, 1984).

Cerebral Blood Flow

Neuronal damage involving the brainstem and cerebral hemispheres as well as significant decrease in cerebral blood flow have been demonstrated among patients with mild and trivial head injuries (Taylor & Bell, 1966). In fact, many of these same patients were without PCS complaints and demonstrated normal circulation during the first 12 hr after their injuries and then within a period of 3 days developed postconcussive symptoms and decreased cerebral blood circulation that lasted weeks or months. It has been suggested that this may be secondary to vasomotor abnormalities caused by brainstem (medullary) impairment (Taylor & Bell, 1966).

Attention and Information Processing

It has also been shown that patients with PCS and mild head injury are unable to process information at a normal rate (Gronwall & Wrigthson, 1974) and tend to become overwhelmed. Frequently, however, patients do not complain about this until days or weeks later, as this does not become apparent to them until they return to work and discover that they are having problems. They may find that tasks that require attention to a number of details and that were formerly performed quite easily now seem difficult and beyond their capacity. The patient says that he cannot concentrate (Gronwall & Wrigthson, 1974).

Presumably, many of the postconcussion symptoms are secondary to shearing forces associated with the acceleration/deceleration nature of their injuries as well as torque and other forces exerted on the brainstem. Indeed, following whiplash, patients may develop PCS, including vestibular symptoms and dizziness (Ommaya *et al.*, 1968; Toglia *et al.*, 1970).

Whiplash and Blood Flow

In whiplash, the head is like a ball at the end of a whip; rapid or extreme rotations or extensions of the head may cause decreased blood flow by compressing the vertebral arteries that supply the brainstem, cerebellum, occipital lobe, and hippocampal region of the temporal lobe (Toole, 1984). (See Chapter 9, Stroke and Cerebrovascular Disease.) This leads to symptomatic vestibular insufficiency and other brainstem responses (feelings of giddiness, lightheadnesss, loss of balance) and can exert disrupting effects on memory and visual functioning. If the patient is suffering from atherosclerosis or abnormalities involving the cervical vertebrae (e.g., cervical osteoarthritis), the overall effects can become exacerbated even further (Toole, 1984).

Similarly, as is well known, the internal carotid artery is also very vulnerable to trauma, particularly in the neck, where it is exposed. Rapid extensions and rotations as well as karatelike blows can tear and dissect the artery, resulting in obstruction.

In general, tall people suffer whiplash more often than do shorter people, and those riding in the front of an automobile are 50% more likely than are those in the rear of the car to sustain such an injury (Elia, 1972). Slow-speed crashes carry a greater chance of whiplash injury than do high-speed incidents (see Elia, 1972, for review) presumably because passengers become tense in realization of the impending accident. Acceleration/deceleration injuries are most likely to affect the brainstem, and temporal and frontal lobe. In fact, there is some suggestion that frontal injuries are more likely to give rise to postconcussional disturbances (Rabavilas & Scarpalezos, 198). However, brainstem and temporal lobe abnormalities are obviously contributory.

Vertigo, Hearing Loss, and Tinnitus

Damage to the inner ear is frequently associated with the development of vertigo, dizziness, and tinnitus. The temporal bone (which contains the auditory meatus) is often subject to injury, including fracture regardless of where the head was initially struck. Therefore, the presence of vertigo and tinnitus following a head injury suggests a concussion of the inner ear (Elia, 1972).

Some patients also complain of hearing loss or even unilateral deafness. In some cases, this deficit is secondary to an injury to the tympanic membrane, external auditory canal, or the inner skin of the ear: the injury results in some bleeding, with the potential development of dried blood clots (and cerumen) in the auditory canal, subsequently plugging the ear and reducing auditory acuity by impeding sound transmission. In addition, in cases of temporal bone fracture, CSF may escape into the ear, temporarily disrupting functioning (Fig. 60). Other patients complain of increased sound sensitivity. It has been proposed that this is secondary to rotational acceleration forces that stretch and cause traction of the stapedius muscle, which is attached to the vestibule and stapes of the ear.

Diploplia and Photophobia

It has been proposed that visual problems such as diplopia may occur secondary to traction of the eye muscles. However, if the oculomotor nerve is injured in any manner, this too may cause diplopia and may also contribute to the development of nystagmus (Elia, 1972). In these cases, nystagmus usually resolves over time.

Photophobia and excessive sensitivity to light may also be secondary to occulomotor traction. Interestingly, it has been demonstrated that many such patients who have sustained minor head injury are consequently more sensitive than they realize (Waddell & Gronwall, 1984); some demonstrate a hypersensitivitiy to both sound and light when, in fact, this was not a complaint.

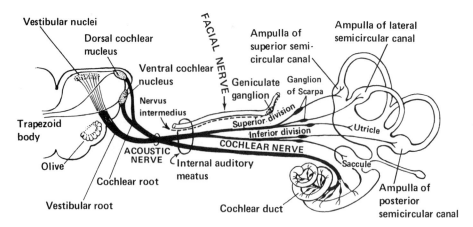

FIGURE 60. Distribution of the acoustic nerve as it projects from the ear to the brainstem. From *Correlative neuroanatomy,* 20th Ed., by J. DeGroot & J. G. Chusid, 1988. Courtesy of Appleton & Lange, E. Norwalk, CT.

PCS and Severe Head Injury

It has been noted repeatedly that those with mild injuries complain of PCS more than those with severe injuries (Levin *et al.,* 1987). This in turn has led to the unfounded suspicion that these disturbances have no objective basis. However, in some cases, as patients recover and progress from severe to moderate or moderate to mild degrees of disability, they begin to make these same complaints. Moreover, there is some possibility that the greater degree of cognitive and personality disorganization among those with severe injuries lessens their ability to appreciate and complain of these disturbances (i.e., lack of insight, decreased motivation). In this regard, patients with severe brain injuries often do not become depressed until after they have demonstrated considerable recovery (Merskey & Woodforde, 1972).

PREMORBID CHARACTERISTICS

In taking histories from my various patients, I was soon impressed with the number of people who seemed to have done rather poorly in school before having suffered the head injury. Moreover, many had already suffered one or more previous head traumas. On the basis of my records, approximately 30% of more than 350 such patients fell within these two categories. Indeed, other researchers have found that as many as 50% of head-injured patients have a history of poor premorbid academic performance, including learning disabilities, school dropout, multiple failed subjects, as well as social difficulties (Fahy, Irving, & Miller, 1967; Fuld & Fisher, 1977; J. F. Haas, Cope, & Hall, 1987). In fact, children who do poorly in school are at increased risk of sustaining a head injury as a teenager or adult (J. F. Haas *et al.,* 1987). As suggested by J. F. Haas *et al.* (1987), this relationship may be attributable to poor attention span, distractability, limited frustration tolerance, poor judgment, impulsivity, difficulty anticipating consequences, perceptual–

motor abnormalities, and other problems, all of which make these individuals more susceptible to being involved in an automobile accident later in life.

The finding that many head-injured and even spine-injured patients (Morris, Roth, & Davidoff, 1986) have also suffered previous cerebral traumas has led some investigators to suggest that these people have a life-style that seems to predispose them to violence and injuries to the cranium (Tobias *et al.*, 1982). However, it is also possible that once a person has sustained a head injury, subsequent decreases in overall functional efficiency make them less likely to avoid situations in which a second (or third) injury may occur.

Life-style and premorbid social–emotional stability are in fact important contributors to the possibility of suffering a head trauma. For example, chronic alcoholics are especially suspectible to cerebral injury (Bennett, 1969). It has also been reported that many head-injured patients suffered a bout of depression or other emotional disturbances (e.g., fight with a girlfriend) immediately before their injury (Tobias *et al.*, 1982). Overall, those most at risk of suffering a head injury at some point in time are young males with a history of learning disability, alcohol abuse, social–emotional difficulties, and previous head trauma.

REFERENCES

Adams, J. H., Graham, D. I., Murray, L. S., & Scott, G. (1981). Diffuse axonal injury due to nonmissile head injury in humans: An analysis of 45 cases. *Annals of Neurology, 12,* 557–563.

Adams, J. H., Graham, D. I., Scott, G. (1980). Brain damage in fatal non-missile head injury. *Journal of Clinical Pathology, 33,* 1132–1145.

Alberico, A. M., Ward, J. D. Choi, S. C., Marmarou, A., & Young, H. F. (1987). Outcome after severe head injury. *Journal of Neurosurgery, 67,* 648–656.

Alves, W. M., Coloban, A. R. T., O'Leary, T. J., Rimel, R. W., & Jane, J. A. (1986). Understanding posttraumatic symptoms after minor head injury. *Journal of Head Trauma Rehabilitation, 1,* 1–12.

Bakay, L., Glasauer, F. E., & Alker, G. J. (1980). *Head injury.* Boston: Little, Brown.

Barth, J. T., Macciocchi, S. N., Giordani, B., Rimel, R., Jane, J. A., & Boll, T. J. (1983). Neuropsychological sequelae of minor head injury. *Neurosurgery, 13,* 529–533.

Bennett, A. E. (1969). Psychiatric and neurologic problems in head injury with medicolegal implications. *Diseases of the Nervous System, 30,* 314–318.

Berger, M. S., Pitts, L. H., Lovely, M., *et al.* (1985). Outcome from severe head injury in children and adolescents. *Journal of Neurosurgery, 62,* 194–199.

Berrol, S. (1986). Evolution and the persistent vegetative state. *Head Trauma Rehabilitation, 1,* 7–13.

Bromlert, D. M., & Sisler, G. C. (1974). The measurement of retrograde post-traumatic amnesia. *Canadian Psychiatric Association Journal, 19,* 185–192.

Bond, M. R. (1976). Assessment of the psychosocial outcome of severe head injury. *Acta Neurochirurgica, 34,* 57–70.

Bond, M. R. (1979). The states of recovery from severe head injury with special reference to late outcome. *International Rehabilitation Medicine, 1,* 155–159.

Brink, J. D., Garrett, A. L., Hale, W. R., Woo Sam, R. A., & Nickel, M. G. (1970). Recovery of motor and intellectual function in children sustaining severe head injuries. *Developmental Medicine and Child Neurology, 12,* 565–571.

Brooks, D. N., & Aughton, M. E. (1979). Cognitive recovery during the first year after severe blunt head injury. *International Rehabilitation Medicine, 1,* 166–172.

Brooks, D. N., & McKinlay, W. (1983). Personality and behavioural change after severe blunt head injury—A relative's view. *Journal of Neurology, Neurosurgery and Psychiatry, 46,* 336–344.

Bucci, M. N., Phillips, T. W., & McGillicuddy, J. E. (1986). Delayed epidural hemorrhage in hypotensive multiple trauma patients. *Neurosurgery, 19,* 65–68.

Carlsson, C. A., von Essen, C., & Lofgren, J. (1968). Factors affecting the clinical course of patients with severe head injuries. *Journal of Neurosurgery, 29,* 242–251.

Coloban, A. R. T., Dacey, R. G., Alves, W., Rimel, R. W., & Jane, J. A. (1986). Neurologic and neurosurgical implications of mild head injury. *Journal of Head Trauma Rehabilitation, 1,* 13–21.

Cooper, P. R., Maravilla, K., Moody, S., *et al.,* (1979). Serial computerized tomographic scanning and the prognosis of severe head injury. *Neurosurgery, 5,* 566–569.

Crockard, A., Iannotti, F., & Kang, J. (1982). Posttraumatic edema in the gerbil. In R. G. Grossman & P. L. Gildenberg (Eds.), *Head injury: Basic clinical aspects.* New York: Raven Press.

Dacey, R. G., Alves, W. M., Rimel, R. W., *et al.* (1986). Neurosurgical complications after apparently minor head injury. *Journal of Neurosurgery, 65,* 203–210.

Dailey, C. A. (1956). Psychological findings five years after head injury. *Journal of Clinical Psychology, 12,* 349–353.

Dikmen, S., McLean, A., & Temkin, N. (1986). Neuropsychological and psychosocial consequences of minor head injury. *Journal of Neurology, Neurosurgery and Psychiatry, 49,* 1227–1232.

Dikmen, S., & Reitan, R. M. (1976). Psychological deficits and recovery of functions after head injury. *Transactions of the American Neurological Assoication, 101,* 72–79.

Dikmen, S., & Reitan, R. M., & Temkin, N. R. (1983). Neuropsychological recovery in head injury. *Archives of Neurology, 40,* 333–338.

Dikmen, S., Temkin, N., McLean, A., Wyler, A., & Machamer, J. (1987). Memory and head injury severity. *Journal of Neurology, Neurosurgery and Psychiatry, 50,* 1613–1618.

Dillon, H., & Leopold, R. L. (1961). Children and the post-concussion syndrome. *Journal of the American Medical Association, 14,* 175–186.

Elia, J. C. (1972). The postconcussion syndrome. *Industrial Medicine, 41,* 23–31.

Fahy, T. J., Irving, M. H., & Miller, P. (1967). Severe head injuries. *Lancet, 2,* 475–478.

Fischer, R. P., Carlson, J., & Perry, J. F. (1981). Postconcussive hospital observation of alert patients in a primary trauma center. *Journal of Trauma, 21,* 920–924.

Fordyce, D. J., Roueche, J. R., & Prigatano, G. P. (1983). Enhanced emotional reactions in chronic head trauma patients. *Journal of Neurology, Neurosurgery and Psychiatry, 46,* 620–624.

Fuld, P. A., & Fisher, P. (1977). Recovery of intellectual ability after closed head injury, *Developmental Medicine and Child Neurology, 19,* 495–502.

Gallagher, J. B., & Browder, E. F. (1968). Extradural hematoma. *Journal of Neurosurgery, 8,* 434–437.

Gennarelli, T. A. (1986). Mechanisms of pathophysiology of cerebral concussion. *Journal of Head Trauma Rehabilitation, 1,* 23–29.

Gennarelli, T. A., Spielman, G. M., Lanfitt, T. W., *et al.,* (1982). Influence of the type of intracranial lesion on outcome from severe head injury. *Journal of Neurosurgery, 56,* 26–32.

Gennarelli, T. A., Thibault, L. E., Adams, H., *et al.* (1982). Diffuse axonal injury and traumatic coma in the primate. *Annals of Neurology, 12,* 564–574.

Gronwall, D. (1976). Performance changes during recovery from closed head injury. *Proceedings of the Australian Association of Neurologists, 13,* 143–147.

Gronwall, D., & Wrightson, P. (1974). Delayed recovery of intellectual function after minor head injury. *Lancet, 2,* 607–609.

Haas, D. C., & Lourie, H. (1988). Trauma-triggered migraine: An explanation for common neurological attacks after mild head injury. *Journal of Neurosurgery, 68,* 181–188.

Haas, J. F., Cope, D. N., & Hall, K. (1987). Premorbid prevalence of poor academic performance in severe head injury. *Journal of Neurology, Neurosurgery and Psychiatry, 50,* 52–56.

Hardman, J. M. (1979). The pathology of traumatic brain injuries. In R. A. Thompson & J. R. Green (Eds.), *Advances in neurology* (Vol. 22). New York: Raven Press.

Humphreyes, R. P. (1983). Outcome of severe head injury in children. In A. J. Raimondi (Ed.), *Concepts in pediatric neurosurgery* (Vol. 3). Basel: Karger.

Jane, J. A., Rimel, R. W., Pobereskin, L. H., *et al.* (1982). Outcome and pathology of head injury. In R. G. Granman & P. L. Gildenburg (Eds.), *Head injury: Basic and clinical aspects.* New York: Raven Press.

Jennett, B. (1975). Scale, scope and philosophy of the clinical problem. In R. Porter & D. W. Fitzsimons (Eds.), *Outcome of severe damage to the central nervous system.* (Ciba). Amsterdam: North-Holland.

Jennett, B. (1978). The problem of mild head injury. *Practitioner, 221,* 77–82.

Jennett, B., & Plum, F. (1972). Persistent vegetative states after brain damage. *Lancet, 1,* 734–737.

Jennett, B., Miller, J. D., & Braakman, R. (1974). Epilepsy after nonmissile depressed skull fracture. *Journal of Neurosurgery, 41,* 208–216.

Jennett, B., Snoek, J., Bond, M. R., & Brooks, N. (1981). Disability after severe head injury. *Journal of Neurology, Neurosurgery and Psychiatry, 44,* 285–293.

Jennett, B., & Teasdale, G. (1977). Aspects of coma after severe head injury. *Lancet, 1,* 878–881.

Jennett, B., & Teasdale, G. (1981). *Management of head injuries.* Philadelphia: F. A. Davis.

Jennett, B., Teasdale, G., Galbraith, S., *et al.* (1977). Severe head injuries in three countries. *Journal of Neurology, Neurosurgery and Psychiatry, 40,* 291–298.

Joseph, R. (1982). The neuropsychology of development: Hemispheric laterality, limbic language, and the origin of thought. *Journal of Clinical Psychology, 38,* 4–33.

Joseph, R. (1988*a*). Confabulation and delusional denial: Frontal lobe and lateralized influences. *Journal of Clinical Psychology, 42,* 507–519.

Joseph, R. (1986*b*). Reversal of cerebral dominance for language and emotion in a corpus callosotomy patient. *Journal of Neurology, Neurosurgery and Psychiatry, 49,* 628–634.

Joseph, R. (1988). The right cerebral hemisphere: Neuropsychiatry, neuropsychology, neurodynamics. *Journal of Clinical Psychology, 44,* 630–674.

Klauber, M. R., Marshall, L. F., Toole, B. M., *et al.* (1985). Cause of decline in head-injury mortality rate in San Diego County, California. *Journal of Neurosurgery, 62,* 528–531.

Levin, H. S., Benton, A. L., & Grossman, R. G. (1982). *Neurobehavioral consequences of closed head injury.* New York: Oxford University Press.

Levin, H. S., High, W. M., Goethe, K. E., *et al.* (1987). The neurobehavioral rating scale: Assessment of the behavioural sequelae of head injury by the clinician. *Journal of Neurology, Neurosurgery and Psychiatry, 50,* 183–193.

Levin, H. S., Mattis, S., Ruff, R. M., *et al.* (1987). Neurobehavioral outcome following minor head injury. *Journal of Neurosurgery, 66,* 234–243.

Lezak, M. D. (1987). Relationships between personality disorders, social disturbances and physical disability following traumatic brain injury. *Journal of Head Trauma Rehabilitation, 2,* 57–69.

Lidvall, H., Linderoth, B., & Norlin, B. (1974). Causes of the post concussional syndrome. *Acta Neurologica Scandinavica, 56,* 1–87.

Lindgren, S. O. (1966). Experimental studies on mechanical effects in head injury. *Acta Scandinavica, 132,* 1–87.

Lishman, W. A. (1973). The psychiatric sequelae of head injury. A review. *Psychological Medicine, 3,* 304–322.

Lishman, W. A. (1978). The psychiatric sequela of head injuries. *Journal of the Irish Medical Association, 71,* 306–314.

Luerssen, T. G., Klauber, M. R., & Marshall, L. F. (1988). Outcome from head injury related to patient's age. *Journal of Neurosurgery, 68,* 409–416.

Merskey, H., & Woodforde, J. M. (1972). Psychiatric sequelae of minor head injury. *Brain, 95,* 521–528.

Miller, E. (1979). The long term consequence of head injury. *British Journal of Social and Clinical Psychology, 18,* 87–98.

Miller, H. (1961). Accident neurosis. *British Medical Journal, 1,* 919–925, 992–998.

Miller, H., & Stern, G. (1965). The long term prognosis of severe head injuries. *Lancet, 1,* 225–227.

Miller, J. D. (1985). Head injury and brain ischaemia—Implication for therapy. *British Journal of Anesthesiology, 57,* 120–129.

Miller, J. D., Butterworth, J. F., Gudeman, S. K., *et al.* (1981). Further experience in the management of severe head injury. *Journal of Neurosurgery, 54,* 289–299.

Morris, J., Roth, E., Davidoff, G. (1986). Mild closed head injury and cognitive deficits in spinal-cord-injured patients. *Journal of Head Trauma Rehabilitation, 1,* 31–42.

Najenson, T., Groswasser, Z., Mendelson, L., & Hackett, P. (1980). Rehabilitation outcome of brain damaged patients after severe head injury. *International Rehabilitation Medicine, 2,* 17–22.

Najenson, T., Mendelson, L., Schechter, I., *et al.* (1974). Rehabilitation after severe head injury. *Scandinavian Journal of Rehabilitative Medicine, 6,* 5–14.

Nikas, D. L. (1987*a*). Prognostic indicators in patients with severe head injury. *Critical Care Nursing Quarterly, 10,* 25–34.

Nikas, D. L. (1987*b*). Critical aspects of head trauma. *Critical Care Nursing Quarterly, 10,* 19–44.

Noebels, J. L. & Prince, D. A. (1978). Development of focal seizures in cerebral cortex: Role of axons terminal bursting. *Journal of Neurophysiology, 41,* 1267–1281.

Oddy, M., Coughlan, T., Tyerman, A., & Jenkins, D. (1985). Social adjustment after closed head injury. *Journal of Neurology, Neurosurgery and Psychiatry, 48,* 564–568.

Ommaya, A. K., Fass, F., & Yarnell, P. (1968). Whiplash injury and brain damage: An experimental study. *Journal of the American Medical Association, 204,* 285–289.

Ommaya, A. K., Grubb, R. L., & Naumann, R. A. (1971). Coup and contrecoup injury. *Journal of Neurosurgery, 35,* 503–516.

Oppenheimer, D. R. (1968). Microscopic brain lesions after trauma. *Journal of Neurology, Neurosurgery and Psychiatry, 31,* 299–306.

Pedley, T. A. (1978). The pathophysioogy of focal epilepsy: Neurophysiological considerations. *Annals of Neurology, 3,* 2–9.

Prigatano, G., Fordyce, D. J., Zeiner, H., *et al.* (1984). Neuropsychological rehabilitation after closed head injury in young adults. *Journal of Neurology, Neurosurgery and Psychiatry, 47,* 505–513.

Pudenz, R. H., & Shelden, C. H. (1946). The lucite calvarium—A method for direct observation of the brain. II. *Journal of Neurosurgery, 3,* 487–505.

Rabavilas, A. D., & Scarpalezos, S. (1981). The post-traumatic syndrome. Some considerations related to psychiatric prevention. *Bibliotheca Psychiatrica, 160,* 73–77.

Raimondi, A. J., & Hirschauer, J. (1984). Head injury in the infant and toddler. *Childs Brain, 11,* 344–351.

Rimel, R. W., Giordani, B., Barth, J. T., Boll, T. J., & Jane, J. A. (1981). Disability caused by minor head injury. *Neurosurgery, 9,* 221–228.

Rose, J., Valtonen, S., & Jennett, B. (1977). Avoidable factors contributing to death after head injury. *British Medical Journal, 2,* 615–618.

Rosin, A. J. (1977). Reactions of families of brain-injured patients who remain in a vegetative state. *Scandinavian Journal of Rehabilitative Medicine, 9,* 1–5.

Rowe, M. J., & Carlson, C. (1980). Brainstem auditory evoked potentials in post-concussion dizziness. *Archives of Neurology, 37,* 679–683.

Russell, W. R. (1971). *The traumatic amnesias.* London: Oxford University Press.

Schacter, D. L., & Crovitz, H. F. (1977). Memory function after closed head injury: A review of the quantitative research. *Cortex, 13,* 150–176.

Schneider, G. E. (1979). Is it really better to havfe your brain lesion early? A revision of the "Kennard principle." *Neuropsychologia, 17,* 557–583.

Sisler, G., & Penner, H. (1975). Amnesia following severe head injury. *Canadian Psychiatric Association Journal, 20,* 333–336.

Smith, E. (1974). Influence of site of impact on cognitive impairment persisting long after severe closed head injury. *Journal of Neurology, Neurosurgery and Psychiatry, 37,* 719–726.

Snow, R. B., Zimmerman, R. D., Gandy, S. E., (1986). Comparison of magnetic resonance imaging and computed tomography in the evaluation of head injury. *Journal of Neurosurgery, 18,* 45–52.

Squire, L. R., Slater, P. C., & Chace, P. M. (1975). Retrograde amnesia. *Science, 187,* 77–79.

Strich, S. J. (1961). Shearing of nerve fibers as a cause of brain damage due to head injury. *Lancet, 2,* 443–448.

Symonds, C. (1962). Concussion and its sequelae. *Lancet, 1,* 1–5.

Staller, A. G. (1987). Systemic effects of severe head trauma. *Critical Care Nursing Quarterly, 10,* 58–68.

Taylor, A. R., & Bell, T. K. (1966). Slowing of cerebral circulation after concussional head injury. *Lancet, 2,* 178–180.

Teasdale, G., Mendelow, D. (1984). Pathophysiology of head injuries. In N. Brooks (Ed.), *Closed head injury.* New York: Oxford University Press.

Teasdale, G., Skene, A., Spiegelhater, D., & Murry, L. (1982). Age, severity, and outcome of head injury. In R. G. Grossman & P. L. Gidenberg (Eds.), *Head injury: Basic and clinical aspects.* New York: Raven Press.

Thomsen, I. (1974). The patient with severe head injury and his family. *Scandinavian Journal of Rehabilitative Medicine, 6,* 180–183.

Tobias, J. S., Puria, K. B., & Sheridan, J. (1982). Rehabilitation of the severely brain-injured. *Scandinavian Journal of Rehabilitative Medicine, 14,* 83–88.

Toglia, J. U., Rosenberg, P. E., & Ronis, M. L. (1970). Post traumatic dizziness. *Archives of Otolaryngology, 92,* 7–13.

Toole, J. F. (1984). *Cerebrovascular disease*. New York: Raven Press.

Tubbs, O. N., & Potter, J. M. (1970). Early post concussion headache. *Lancet, 2,* 128–129.

Unterharnscheidt, F., & Sellier, K. (1966). Mechanisms and pathomorphology of closed head injury. In W. F. Caveness & A. E. Walker (Eds.), *Head injury*. Philadelphia: J. B. Lippincott.

Waddell, P. A., & Gronwall, D. M. A. (1984). Sensitivity to light and sound following minor head injury. *Acta Neurologica Scandinavica, 69,* 270–278.

Weddell, R., Oddy, M., & Jenkins, D. (1980). Social adjustment after rehabilitation. *Psychological Medicine, 10,* 257–263.

Wowern, Von F. (1966). Post traumatic amnesia and confusion as an index of severity in head injury. *Acta Neurologica Scandinavica, 42,* 373–378.

Yarnell, P. R., & Lynch, S. (1970). Retrograde memory immediately after concussion. *Lancet, 1,* 863–864.

Zimmerman, R. A., Bilianiuk, L. T., & Gennarelli, T. A. (1978). Computerized tomography of shearing injuries of the cerebral white matter. *Radiology, 127,* 393–396.

Stroke and Cerebrovascular Disease

CEREBRAL INFARCTION

When the brain is not adequately perfused with blood and is deprived of oxygen, glucose, and other nutrients, a variety of neurological, neuropsychiatric, and neuropsychological abnormalities may result, depending on how long and which portions of the cerebrum are involved. As is well known, the complete deprivation of blood for longer than 3 min produces neuronal, glial, and vascular necrosis and irreversible brain damage; i.e., cerebral infarction (stroke) and ischemic necrosis. If blood flow is reduced for a shorter period, transient neurological abnormalities may occur.

Frequently a cerebral infarct and the neurological symptoms that accompany it may develop quite abruptly and within a matter of seconds. However, the full symptomatic development of an infarct can be more prolonged, taking perhaps minutes, hours, or days; this is known as stroke in evolution.

Specifically, cerebral infarction is characterized by lack of oxygen, nutrients, and/or the impaired removal of metabolic products—conditions that result in the death of neurons, glia, and the vasculature. Moreover, when cells die, their membranes burst, releasing lipids, fatty acids, and other substances that can produce systemic and local effects that magnify damage in surrounding zones.

Cerebral infarction or stroke is often secondary to cerebrovascular disease and vascular abnormalities involving either the heart or blood vessels, or both. This condition includes atherosclerosis, occlusion of the cerebral arteries by thrombus or embolus, or rupture of a vessel that causes hemorrhage. Other major risk factors for stroke include diabetes mellitus, atrial fibrillation, transient ischemic attacks (TIAs), left ventricular hypertrophy, congestive heart failure, and coronary heart disease (Toole, 1984; Wolf, Kannel, & Verter, 1983). Diseases or damage involving the heart, including myocardial infarction, are leading contributors to stroke.

FUNCTIONAL ANATOMY OF THE HEART AND ARTERIAL DISTRIBUTION

The heart is a four-chambered muscular organ, about the size of a man's fist, that lies predominantly to the left of the body's midline. The upper two chambers are referred to as the atria (or auricles), and the lower chambers are the ventricles. In general, blood flows from the atria to the ventricles (when the atria valves contract) and from the right and left ventricles, respectively, into the pulmonary artery and aorta (when the ventricular valves contract).

Oxygenation

From the pulmonary artery, blood is shunted to the lungs, where carbon dioxide is removed and oxygen replaced. This oxygenated blood is then transmitted to the left atrium by the pulmonary veins. From the left atrium, blood is transported to the left ventricle, which pumps the oxygenated blood through the aorta.

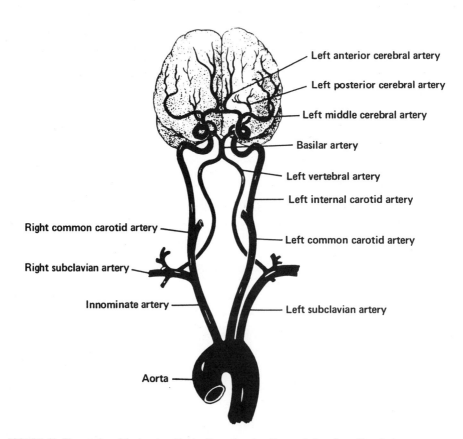

FIGURE 61. The arteries of the heart and brain. Reproduced, with permission, from *Correlative neuroanatomy,* 20th Ed., by J. DeGroot & J. G. Chusid, copyright Appleton & Lange, E. Norwalk, CT, 1988.

Arterial Cerebral Pathways

It is through the aorta that blood is transmitted directly to the brain. Thus, clots or other debris cast off from the heart commonly affect cerebral integrity. Specifically, the aorta gives rise to the left common carotid and brachiocephalic artery. The brachiocephalic artery bifurcates into the right common carotid and right subclavian arteries. Each common carotid divides into the external and internal carotid arteries. The subclavian arteries give rise to the vertebral arteries.

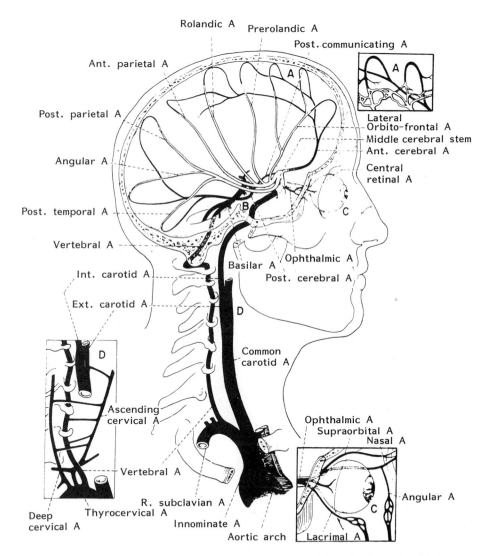

FIGURE 62. The distribution of arteries from the heart to the right side of the brain. The arteries of the heart and brain. Reproduced, with permission, from *Correlative neuroanatomy,* 20th Ed., by J. DeGroot & J. G. Chusid, copyright Appleton & Lange, E. Norwalk, CT, 1988.

Thus, the brain is actually nourished by two separate systems of vasculature: the carotid and the vertebral. The carotid system supplies the frontal and parietal lobe, all but the inferior–posterior third of the temporal lobe, the hypothalamus, basal ganglia, and the eyes. The vertebral system nourishes the posterior temporal lobe, the occipital lobe, the upper part of the spinal cord, the brainstem, midbrain, thalamus, cerebellum, and inner ear. Abnormalities involving either of these circulatory systems can result in widespread, albeit characteristic, disturbances (Figs. 61 and 62).

THE BLOOD SUPPLY OF THE BRAIN

The Carotid System

The internal carotid artery gives rise to four major arterial branches: the middle cerebral, anterior cerebral, ophthalamic, and anterior choroidal arteries (Figs. 63–65).

Middle Cerebral Artery

The middle cerebral artery is a direct extension of the internal cartoid and receives almost 80% of the blood passing through this arterial system. As a major recipient of the carotid blood supply, it is often the most commonly affected part of the vasculature when

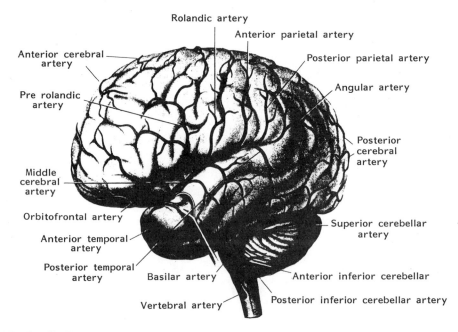

FIGURE 63. The principal arteries on the lateral surface of the cerebrum and cerebellum. From *Human neuroanatomy* by R. C. Truex & M. B. Carpenter, 1969. Courtesy of The Williams & Wilkins Co., Baltimore, MD.

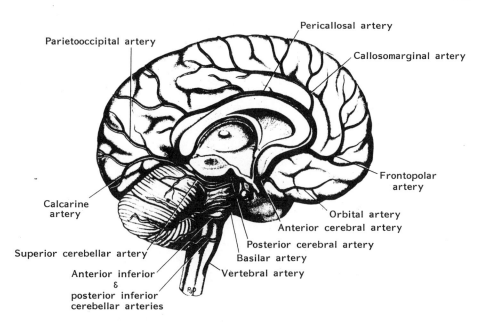

FIGURE 64. The principal arteries of the brainstem, cerebellum and medial surface of the cerebrum. From *Human neuroanatomy* by R. C. Truex & M. B. Carpenter, 1969. Courtesy of The Williams & Wilkins Co., Baltimore, MD.

debris are cast off from the heart and vessel walls. Through its branches, this artery supplies the lateral part of the cerebral hemispheres, including the neocortex and white matter of the lateral/inferior convexity of the frontal lobes, the motor areas, primary and association somesthetic areas, the inferior parietal lobule, and the superior portion of temporal lobe and insula. Its penetrating branches supply the putamen, portions of the caudate and globus pallidus, posterior limb of the internal capsule, and corona radiata.

Anterior Cerebral Artery

Through its branches, the anterior cerebral artery supplies the orbital frontal lobes, all but the most posterior portion of the medial walls of the cerebral hemispheres, and the anterior four fifths of the corpus callosum. In this regard, it might better be referred to as the anterior medial–orbital artery.

Ophthalmic Artery

The ophthalmic artery is the first large branch given off by the internal carotid. The ophthalmic artery supplies and nourishes the eye and the orbit as well as some skin on the forehead. The ophthalmic artery also gives off branches that feed the posterior limb of the internal capsule, the thalamus, the wall of the third ventricle, and portions of the optic chiasm.

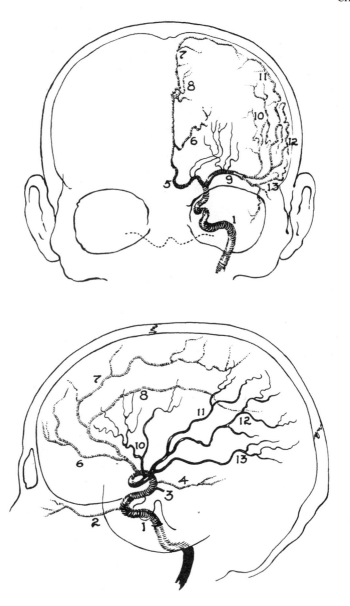

1. Internal carotid artery.
2. Ophthalmic artery.
3. Posterior communicating artery.
4. Anterior choroidal artery.
5. Anterior cerebral artery.
6. Frontopolar artery.
7. Callosomarginal artery.

8. Pericallosal artery.
9. Middle cerebral artery.
10. Ascending frontoparietal artery.
11. Posterior parietal artery.
12. Angular artery.
13. Posterior temporal artery.

FIGURE 65. The distribution of the internal carotid artery. From *Correlative neuroanatomy,* 20th Ed., by J. DeGroot and J. G. Chusid, 1988. Courtesy of Appleton & Lange, E. Norwalk, CT; based on a figure from ''Intracranial Angiography'' by List, Burge, & Hodges, 1945, *Radiology, 45,* p. 1.

Anterior Choroidal Artery

The anterior choroidal artery arises from the lateral side of the internal carotid. It supplies the medial portion of the globus pallidus and Ammons horn and parts of the internal capsule. In general, the terminal arterial branches of the anterior, middle, and posterior cerebral arteries (which is part of the vertebral system) interconnect over the surface of the brain such that there is some overlap in distribution.

The Vertebral System

Through its branches, the vertebral system supplies the brainstem, cerebellum, and the occipital and inferior temporal lobes. Specifically, the vertebral arteries unite to form the basilar artery, and the basilar artery gives rise to the cerebellar and posterior cerebral arteries.

Vertebral Arteries

Each vertebral artery arises from the right and left subclavian and ascends to the medulla, where they unite to form the basilar artery at the caudal base of the pons. The vertebral arteries are the chief arteries of the medulla; they supply the lower three fourths of the pyramids, the medial lemniscus, the restiform body, and the posterior–inferior cerebellum.

Basilar Artery

The basilar artery supplies the pons and gives rise to the inferior and superior cerebellar arteries, which nourish the cerebellum. As the basilar artery ascends, it bifurcates into the two posterior cerebral arteries.

Posterior Cerebral Artery

The major trunks of the posterior cerebral artery irrigate the hippocampus, medial portion of the temporal lobes, occipital lobes, including areas 17, 18, 19, and the splenium of the corpus callosum. Through its deep penetrating branches, it also feeds the thalamus, subthalamic nuclei, substantia nigra, midbrain, pineal body, and posterior hippocampus (Figs. 66 and 67).

CEREBROVASCULAR DISEASE

Arteries

By definition, an artery (with the exception of the pulmonary artery) is a vessel that carries oxygenated blood away from the heart to other parts of the body. Small arteries are referred to as arterioles. Capillaries are microscopic vessels that transport blood from the arterioles to venules. Venules carry blood to veins. In general, the capillary density is

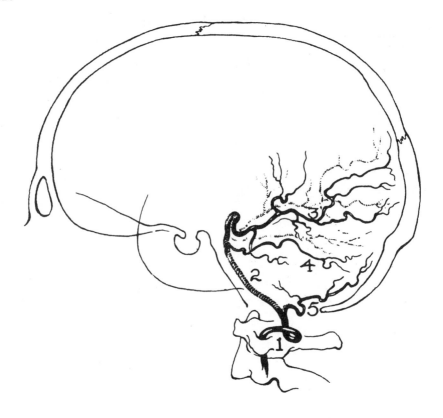

1. Vertebral artery.   4. Superior cerebellar artery.
2. Basilar artery.   5. Posterior inferior cerebellar artery.
3. Posterior cerebral artery.

FIGURE 66. The distribution of the vertebral-basilar arteries. From *Correlative neuroanatomy,* 20th Ed., by J. DeGroot & J. G. Chusid, 1988. Courtesy of Appleton & Lange, E. Norwalk, CT; based on a figure from ''Intracranial Angiography'' by List, Burge, & Hodges, 1945; *Radiology, 45,* p. 1.

greater in the gray matter than in white matter, and the gray matter receives about five times as much blood and seven times as much oxygen as the white matter.

Arteries consist of an outer coat of tough fibrous tissue, an inner lining of endothelium, and a smooth inner coat of muscle that acts to constrict and dilate the vessel. Any alteration in the smoothness of this muscular coat can give rise to the development of blood clots and thrombi. Most rough spots are secondary to atherosclerosis. Atherosclerosis is a major risk factor for stroke. If an artery is severed, it has the capacity to regenerate.

ATHEROSCLEROSIS

Atherosclerosis is a noninflammatory degenerative disease that can result in arterial abnormalities throughout the body. These include roughening of the blood vessel intima;

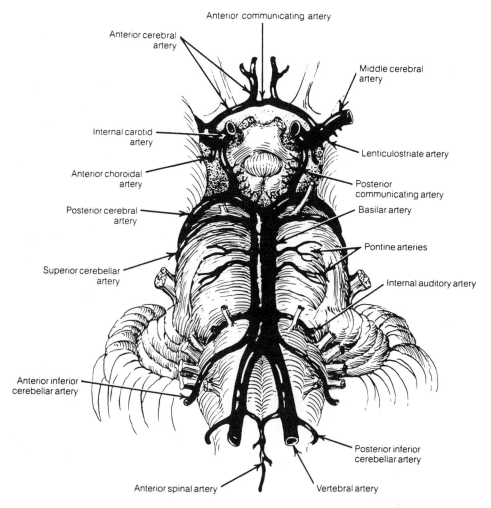

FIGURE 67. The base of the brain. The circle of Willis and the principal arteries of the brain. Reproduced, with permission, from *Correlative Neuroanatomy,* 20th Ed., by J. DeGroot & J. G. Chusid, copyright Appleton & Lange, E. Norwalk, CT, 1988.

elongation and stiffening of the artery, which may cause it to kink and buckle (which in turn reduces blood flow and pressure); reductions in the caliber or dissection or tearing of the lumen; obstruction or occlusion of the lumen with possible diversion of flow through collateral channels; focal dilations; and plaque formation.

Atherosclerosis exerts its effects indirectly on the brain by decreasing perfusion pressure and reducing flow through the tissues supplied by the various blood vessels. This is accomplished by promoting the development of thrombi and emboli (fibrin, platelets, or cholesterol crystals), which in turn increasingly occlude the arterial lumen. The metabolic demands of many areas of the brain can thus become partially deprived of oxygen and glucose.

Thrombi

Clot Formation

Atherosclerotic development usually begins early in life, exerting its initial roughening effects at the bifurcation of the various blood vessels. Endothelial cells lining the blood vessel begin to die, ulceration occurs, and blood platelets, lipids, and cholesterol begin to be deposited in the arterial intima, forming a mound of tissue. Indeed, within a matter of seconds, blood platelets will begin to adhere to any portion of a vessel that is not perfectly smooth and contains rough spots (e.g., a patchlike accumulation of lipid or cholesterol). When this occurs, the adhering blood platelets will rupture, triggering the formation of thrombin and insoluble fibrin proteins: thromboplastin. These thrombin proteins act to create clots.

Specifically, these fibrin proteins resemble weblike threads that are tangled together. These tangles act like nets, trapping more blood cells and other debris, which then clot together. Once started, the clot tends to grow as more and more platelets are enmeshed and rupture, thereby releasing more thromboplastin fibrin proteins. Furthermore, the plaques that narrow the lumen may serve as a nidus upon which even more thrombi come to adhere and from which emboli may be dislodged. These elevated fibrous plaques (thrombi) invariably grow larger and may even become vascularized. A complicated lesion is thus formed.

Obstructive Influences

As the clot grows, blood flow is reduced, leading to the accumulation of even more thromboplastin; these deposits create turbulence or eddy currents, further damaging the smooth endothelium of the artery as well as reducing resilience.

As the clot grows and thrombi increase in thickness, the lumen becomes progressively smaller, resulting in arterial dilation. By reducing the resilience and the diameter of the large arteries, atherosclerosis can induce systolic hypertension. Thus, the driving force of the blood against vessel walls is increased, leading to further roughening and plaque formation. Atherosclerosis is thus an insidious process.

When the lumen of the artery is narrowed by about 50%, pressure in the proximal segment increases, whereas distal to the clot pressure begins to fall. With 70% reduction, flow is significantly decreased and neurological functioning may be altered. Typically, however, patients remain asymptomatic until there is a sudden reduction in blood flow or thrombi or emboli are thrown off, creating a complete obstruction. However, if the core of the plaque becomes necrotic and calcifies, the surface may disintegrate, exposing the weakened underlying surface of the vessel. When this occurs, the vessel may rupture and hemorrhage.

Obstruction of the artery due to atherosclerosis may produce disastrous neurological consequences or may be associated with no symptoms whatsoever. The outcome depends on (1) the configuration of the arterial tree with which the patient was born; (2) the segment of artery involved; (3) the rapidity of obstruction development; (4) the presence or absence of collateral vessels; (5) associated diseases such as hypertension; and (6) triggering mechanisms, such as a sudden blow or turn of the head.

Susceptible Arteries

There is a tendency for atheromatous plaques to form at branching and curves of cerebral arteries—most frequently, the internal carotid artery and carotid sinus; the vertebral arteries and their junction, which forms the basilar; the main bifurcation of the middle cerebral artery; the posterior cerebral arteries as they wind around the midbrain; and in the anterior cerebral arteries as they curve over the corpus callosum (Adams & Victor, 1981; Toole, 1984).

Atherosclerosis seldom exists in either the coronary of cerebral artery system without the other being involved as well—it occurs in both (Toole, 1984). When the heart is involved, this can lead to myocardial infarction, mural thrombi may be cast off that then flow directly to the lungs and brain. Atherosclerotic heart disease can also cause cardiac dysrhythmias or decreases in cardiac output—possibly to such a degree that cerebrovascular insufficiency results.

Risk Factors

Risk factors for cerebrovascular and carotid atherosclerosis include hypertension, increased age, diabetes mellitus, and cigarette smoking, age and hypertension being the most important (see Crouse, Toole, McKinney, *et al.*, 1987; Wolf, 1985). In general, the onset of atherosclerotic disease is usually in childhood and remains silent, growing slowly for 20 or 30 years before becoming symptomatic. It appears to reach its peak incidence between the ages of 50–70 years; men are twice as likely as women to suffer.

CEREBRAL ISCHEMIA

When emboli, thrombi, and/or atherosclerosis reduce perfusion of brain tissue below a critical level, ischemia occurs and the patient suffers a cerebral infarct. Cerebral infarction and ischemia are caused by insufficiency of the oxygen and blood supply. Ischemia leads to hypoxia and impaired delivery of glucose as well as a failure to remove metabolites and waste, such as lactic acid and carbon dioxide. As infarction evolves, local edema results, which may cause an increase in tissue pressure and further reduce tissue perfusion by compressing capillaries, thereby enlarging the infarction. The severity and extent of the neurological deficit are increased even further.

During ischemic attacks, there is usually reduced blood flow extending far beyond the infarct borders. This further reduces neuronal activity such that transient, as well as permanent, neurological deterioration occurs. This transient blood flow reduction is produced by metabolic changes, compression of the local vasculature, and temporary cessation of neural activity, due to disconnection. Initially, this condition may make the functional effects of the stroke appear more pervasive and profound. Nevertheless, blood flow is still sufficient in these border areas to keep the tissues alive (Torvik & Svindland, 1986). Thus, as the ischemia subsides and blood flow is increased to these depressed areas, there appears to be a considerable degree of recovery.

Most infarcts are sharply delineated. Nevertheless, surrounding the area of ischemia is a concentric zone of hyperemia caused by a local loss of autoregulatory capacity and vasomotor paralysis; that is, increased flow to the immediately surrounding area acts to divert blood from other areas of the brain as well as from the ischemic zone, thereby increasing ischemic damage to this area (Toole, 1984). This loss of autoregulation is most evident during the acute phase of cerebral infarction. As the infarction evolves, there is local edema and swelling, causing increased tissue pressure which further reduces tissue perfusion by compressing capillaries. The infarction is enlarged even further. The pathological effects of ischemia and reduced blood flow may be massive, if, for example, the internal carotid or middle cerebral artery is obstructed. The effects may be minute if impaired circulation is limited to the smaller arteries and arterioles.

With moderate or massive infarction, even if quite focal, regions within the opposite hemisphere also exhibit similar but less extensive changes due perhaps to local reflexia, increased intracranial pressure (ICP), or the spillage and spread of vasoactive chemicals that affect the entire brain (Toole, 1984). Moreover, infarction of one hemisphere may cause so much swelling that it leads to symptoms of increased ICP. When pressure increases blood flow decreases. Blood flow tends toward normal in those who recover but remains slow throughout the affected hemisphere in those who do poorly.

Risk Factors

Risk factors for ischemic stroke include older age, male sex, hypertension, TIAs, hypertensive heart disease, coronary heart disease, congestive heart failure, and diabetes mellitus (Davis, Dambrosia, Schoenberg, *et al.,* 1987).

THROMBOSIS

When a thrombotic clot enlarges sufficiently, the patient suffers a cerebral infarct, i.e., thrombosis. A thrombosis is caused by a thrombus—a clot produced by coagulated blood (thromboplastic: a protein that forms clots). Thrombotic strokes often occur during periods of prolonged inactivity or sleep, such that the symptoms are present upon arising in the morning. As these patients attempt to swing out of bed or a chair, they find that they are weak on one side, that they cannot speak, or that some other deficit has developed.

Thrombotic strokes develop gradually. Symptoms and signs usually progress in a stepwise fashion, sometimes taking 2–4 days to develop fully. Patients deteriorate, improve slightly, then deteriorate further, a process referred to as stroke in evolution. This stepwise evolution is due to edema and alterations in blood flow and metabolism as thrombotic particles continually form and break off. Stabilization with improvement begins after 7–14 days after stroke onset (Baxter, 1984). The size of the infarct in part is dependent on the presence and integrity of collateral vessels. If collateral circulatory channels are not in existence, occlusion exerts drastic effects and the infarct is quite large.

Warning signs include headache and/or previous transient neurological symptoms or a TIAs. When TIAs precede a stroke, they almost always stamp the process as thrombotic (Toole, 1984; Adams & Victor, 1981). The most common cause of thrombotic stroke is arteriosclerosis. Thrombosis follows clotting of the blood at a site at which its flow is impeded by a sclerotic plaque, usually in the bifurcations of the carotids. Complete occlusion of the carotids is always the consequence of thrombosis (Toole, 1984).

EMBOLISM

In contrast to thrombosis, which is caused by a localized buildup, emboli are free particles that become lodged within a vessel, causing occlusion. Like thrombosis, embolic strokes create an ischemic cerebral infarct. Unlike thrombosis, however, embolitic strokes are often followed later by hemorrhage. Both thrombotic and cerebral embolic strokes occur most commonly among older persons. By contrast, among younger age groups, embolism is the most frequent culprit.

An embolism may be composed of thrombotic particles that have broken off from a clot, air bubbles, masses of bacteria, or blood clots. They may also consist of cholesterol crystals thrown off from atheromatous plaques situated in the vertebrobasilar and carotid arteries; pieces of tumor cells from the lung, stomach, or kidney that subsequently take root in the brain after drifting in the bloodstream; and fat globules released into the bloodstream after trauma to the marrow of the long bones. Oral contraceptives among women can give rise to the develoment of embolism, and an association among those with mitral valve prolapse has been noted (Jackson, 1986; Toole, 1984).

Cardiac Embolic Origins

Cerebral emboli may develop when there is plaque buildup on the cardiac or carotid valves. It may also result from mitral stenosis, atrial fibrillation, aortic valve calcification, fragments of left atria or ventricular thrombus, mitral value polyps, myocardial infarction, or vegetations of infective endocarditis. Heart disease, mitral stenosis, and atrial fibrillation are thus major risk factors for cerebral embolism. Chronic atrial fibrillation in particular carries a high risk of stroke (Petersen & Godtfredsen, 1986; Wolf, Kannel, McGee, Meeks, *et al.,* 1983), the clot coming from a paralyzed atrium. When the embolus is infected, meningitis or abscess may develop. Indeed, an estimated 90% of emboli from the heart end up in the brain. Thus, embolic stroke is often a sign of systemic heart disease.

The Carotid and Left Middle Cerebral Artery

In general, emboli expelled from the heart and the left ventricle are carried into the brachiocephalic artery and then to the left common carotid. From the left carotid, emboli are transmitted and occlude the arteries supplying the left cerebral hemisphere. Thus, the left side of the brain is a common destination of emboli originating in the heart. When emboli are repeatedly freed into the blood stream, they tend to lodge in the same artery, usually the middle cerebral. This is because the middle cerebral artery is a direct extension of the internal cartoid and receives almost 80% of the blood. Thus, most emboli end up within the middle cerebral system. Embolic cerebral strokes tend to produce focal effects such as an expressive aphasia, a monoplegia, or receptive aphasia. Global effects are less common.

Vertebrobasilar Artery

Emboli entering the vertebrobasilar system produce deep coma and total paralysis. Indeed, a 1-mm speck lodged in an artery of the brainstem can cause catastrophic neurological consequences (Toole, 1984). Embolic infarction of the undersurface of the cerebellum (via the cerebellar arteries) may cause fatal brainstem compression. If it enters the posterior cerebral artery, it may produce either a unilateral or bilateral homonymous hemianopia or severe memory loss.

Onset

After lodgment of an embolus, the vessel usually goes into spasm; thrombosis may occur. Embolic strokes characteristically begin suddenly, often while the patient is awake and active. There is usually no warning, and the effects of the infarction reach its peak almost immediately. Cerebral embolization will be major if the embolus is large or temporary if the fragment is small. Smaller fragments have a greater likelihood of disintegrating. Not infrequently, an extensive deficit from embolism reverses itself dramatically within a few hours or a day or two. In many cases, the first episode will be followed by another, frequently with severe damage. Early anticoagulant therapy should be emphasized, as it is important in the prevention of embolic stroke recurrence (Lodder & van der Lugt, 1983; Koller, 1982).

Embolic Hemorrhage

Approximately 65% of patients with a cerebral embolic stroke develop hemorrhagic infarction. Conversely, fewer than 20% of those with thrombosis will develop hemorrhage (Ott, Zamani, Kleefield & Funkenstein, 1986). Similarly, approximately 50% of all hemorrhagic infarcts are associated with embolic strokes (Fisher & Adams, 1951; R. G. Hart & Easton, 1986). Thus, embolic strokes have a special propensity for hemorrhagic transformation, and hemorrhagic infarction nearly always indicates embolism.

Blood vessels affected by embolism characteristically hemorrhage within 12–48 hr (Cerebral Embolism Study Group, 1984; Hart & Easton, 1986). However, it may take several days to develop (Laureno, Shields, & Narayan, 1987). Hemorrhagic transformation occurs when the embolus disintegrates and/or migrates distally, permitting reperfusion of the damaged vessel (Fisher & Adams, 1951; Jorgenson & Torvic, 1969). That is, when a vessel is occluded, it is damaged and weakened, and both the brain and the involved portion of the vessel may become necrotic. When the weakened portion of a previously occluded vessel is subsequently reexposed to the full force of arterial pressure, it ruptures and hemorrhages.

Embolic hemorrhages are frequently asymptomatic (Hakim, Ryder-Cooke, & Melanson, 1983; Ott *et al.*, 1986) and benign, as the tissue involved has already been damaged. However, if the hemorrhage is secondary to anticoagulant therapy, the bleeding may be more profuse and cause significant neurological deterioration and even death (Hart & Easton, 1986).

TRANSIENT ISCHEMIC ATTACKS

Transient ischemic attacks are caused by a brief and temporary reduction in blood flow to a focal region within the brain. They are accompanied by transitory and focal neurological disturbances, which seem to resolve both immediately and completely with no apparent residual effects. The most frequent cause of TIAs is atherosclerosis and microembolization of platelet aggregates from ulcerated atherosclerotic plaques within the carotids or from the cardiac valves. These conditions act to reduce blood flow. Other causes include vascular spasm, aggregations of cholesterol crystals, fibrin and/or blood platelets that temporarily occlude a vessel, or a combination of these factors.

Transient ischemic attacks are related to the microcirculation, in which small irritants such as an embolus can lead to blockage. However, they can involve any cerebral or cerebellar artery. They may last a few seconds or up to 12–24 hr. Most last 2–15 min (Toole, 1984). The symptoms are transient, because the occluding embolus almost immediately disintegrates, allowing for the immediate reestablishment of blood flow and functional recovery.

Transient ischemic attacks that last less than 60 min are different from those of longer duration. The shorter TIAs are caused by emboli that travel from one artery to another, whereas the longer TIAs are caused by emboli passed by the heart (Toole, 1984). Thus, artery-to-artery emboli tend to be smaller and to disintegrate more quickly, whereas those from the heart tend to be larger and/or greater in number. Some patients may experience only a single episode of TIA in a lifetime, whereas others may have as many as 20 attacks in a single day. In most patients, there are fewer than one or two TIAs per week (Toole, 1984).

Weakness or numbness of a single finger may be the only manifestation of a TIA. However, a person may suffer a TIA and not be conscious of it, or the manifestation may be a disturbance in memory or speech and word finding or brief confusion. With these types of disturbances, patients and their families ignore, fail to notice, or attribute little significance to these attacks, as they are transient.

In some instances, the TIA may take the form of temporary blindness, like a shade being pulled over the eye. It is when the patient becomes aware that there is a loss of vision, or a loss of strength in the hand or foot, that rapidly progresses to involve the entire extremity that they become alarmed. TIAs can occur within any region of the cerebral vasculature. Some investigators, however, have classified them as either ophthalmic, hemispheric, or vertebrobasilar.

Hemispheric TIAs

In hemispheric attacks, ischemia occurs foremost in the distal territory of the middle cerebral artery, producing weakness or numbness in the opposite hand and arm, but different combinations may occur; such as in the face and lips, hand and foot, or fingers alone. In ocular attacks, transient monocular blindness occurs and is described as a shade falling smoothly over the visual field until the eye is blind. The attack clears smoothly and uniformly.

Vertebrobasilar TIAs

If the TIA occurs in the vertebrobasilar system, there may be dizziness, diplopia, dysarthria, bifacial numbness, and weakness or numbness involving part or parts of the body, or even both body halves (due to the involvement of diverse regions of the brainstem and thalamus supplied by the vertebrobasilar system). Other symptoms may include, in order of frequency, headache, staggering, veering to one side, sensation of crosseyed-ness, dark or blurred or tunnel vision, partial or complete blindness, pupillary changes, and paralysis of gaze (Toole, 1984). In basilar artery disease, each side of the body may be affected alternately. There is good evidence that TIAs may be abolished by anti-coagulant drugs.

TIA and Stroke

As many as 40% of patients with TIAs subsequently suffer brain infarction, most occurring within the first 6 months of the initial episode (Wolf et al., 1983). Stroke may occur after the first or second TIA or only after hundreds have occurred over a period of weeks or months. However, the greatest risk of stroke following TIA is within the first year, and in particular the first 30 days; 20% occurring during the first month and 50% within a year (Wolf et al., 1983).

When TIAs precede a stroke, however, they almost always stamp the process as thrombotic (atherosclerotic thrombosis). Nevertheless, it is noteworthy that although thrombotic strokes are said to occur predominantly at night, most infarctions occur be-tween 6 AM and 6 PM(Van Der Windt & Van Gijn, 1988).

Risk Factors

Risk factors include cigarette smoking, previous history of stroke or TIA, ischemic heart disease, and diabetes. (Howard, Toole, Frye-Pierson, & Hinshelwood, 1987). How-ever, as the number of risk factors increases, the prognosis for recovery following stroke declines.

LACUNAR STROKES

The term lacune is associated with the development of small holes in the subcortical tissue, often secondary to the occlusion of a deep single perforating artery (Fisher, 1969). The most common type is attributable to an occlusion via macrophage plaques. Approx-imately 20% of all infarcts are lacunar (Kunitz, Gross, Heyman, et al., 1984). However, the incidence increases with age. In lacunar strokes, there is usually no impairment of consciousness or higher cognitive functioning. However, if the lesion involves the inter-nal capsule, there may be motor disturbances, including paralysis or facial or arm weak-ness. If involving the thalamus, sensory sensation over various body parts may be attenu-ated. The incidence of fatality is very low. Nevertheless, more than one third of affected patients may be seriously impaired as long as 1 year post-stroke (Bamford et al., 1987). Usually, since the stroke is so tiny, the computed tomography (CT) scan is negative.

MULTI-INFARCT DEMENTIA

In some instances, patients will repeatedly suffer small strokes over a number of years. At first these strokes seem asymptomatic or have only mild consequences. However, with repeated incidences, patients (or family members) may notice that their memory is not as good as before, that they are having difficulty concentrating, that they are sometimes confused, and that they have increased word-finding difficulty, as well as other linguistic problems. Personality and emotional changes may be subtle at first as well.

Essentially, as the lesion expands, as a result of repeated, albeit small strokes, the patient gradually deteriorates, until finally what was a series of minor deficits is "suddenly" a major alteration in personality functioning and intellectual capability. Frequently these persons and family members erroneously describe the onset as sudden, as they tended to ignore the stepwise progression of increasing severity. Careful questioning will reveal that the patient's symptoms had been progressing over time.

In addition, patients with multi-infarct dementia have been reported to have bilateral patchily reduced blood flow in the gray matter, particularly within the distribution of the middle cerebral artery (Yamaguchi, Meyer, Yamamoto, et al., 1980). The reductions are related to the degree of dementia severity (Kitagawa, Meyer, Tachibana, et al., 1984; Meyer, Rogers, Judd, Mortel, & Sims, 1988). In general, the pattern of reduction is suggestive of widespread and diffuse cerebral ischemia or infarction; the regions involved include the thalamus and the frontal and temporal lobes. Nevertheless, patients with multi-infarct dementia are frequently misdiagnosed as suffering from Alzheimer's disease.

HEART DISEASE, MYOCARDIAL INFARCTION, AND CARDIAC SURGERY

Ischemia and Heart Disease

The delivery of oxygen to the brain depends on the vascular, pulmonary, and cardiac system; the flow characteristics of the blood; and the quality and quantity of the hemoglobin molecules and the binding of oxygen to those molecules (Grotta, Manner, Pettigrew, & Yatsu, 1986). Abnormalities involving red blood cell structure or concentration are frequent causes of cerebrovascular abnormalities (Grotta et al., 1986) and can create conditions that promote coronary heart disease and abnormal clotting, hence reduced blood flow.

Coronary heart disease, even when asymptomatic, is a major underlying contributor to the development of regional decreases in cerebral blood flow, cerebral infarction, and ischemia (Di Pasquale, Andreoli, Pinelli, et al., 1986). In many cases, patients suffer cerebral deterioration even in the absence of stroke. In fact, I have examined a considerable number of patients who, when questioned, note that their memory or other cognitive disturbances began soon following a heart attack or major surgery.

Myocardial Infarction

During a myocardial infarct, blood pressure, cerebral blood flow, and metabolism fall by as much as 50% (Toole, 1984). Cerebrovascular insufficiency and cerebral infarction are a likely consequence. With cardiac arrest, blood pressure and blood flow cease, and widespread cerebral ischemic damage results. Myocardial infarction is a major contributor to stroke. When myocardial infarction occurs, thrombi are cast off from the heart and supporting vessels into the blood and carried to the cerebral vasculature, causing occlusion. In fact, following a heart attack, embolic events may continue for up to 1 month, with the patient suffering a series of small or major cerebral infarctions. This is because during the healing process, mural thrombi and embolism clots may continually form and break off. If major occlusions occur within the vertebral system, the patient may die. Indeed, myocardial infarction is the leading cause of mortality among patients with stroke (Burke, Callow, O'Donnel, Kelly, & Welch, 1982).

Global Ischemia

Global ischemia is caused by a sudden and complete reduction in arterial pressure such as occurs during myocardial infarction. If it persists for more than a few minutes, widespread damage in the cortex, hippocampus, basal ganglia, brainstem, and cerebellum results. Areas at the junctions between the various vascular territories, i.e., watershed areas, are especially vulnerable.

Valvular Insufficiency

During a heart cycle, the atria and ventricles contract and relax successively; this is the heartbeat. However, if any of these valves loses its ability to close, blood will leak backward, a condition referred to as valvular insufficiency. If the left atrioventricular passageway becomes narrowed (mitral stenosis), blood flow is hindered and circulatory failure results, accompanied by massive cerebral ischemia and neuronal death. The death rate among stroke patients with coronary artery disease has been estimated to be more than 50% (Di Pasquale et al., 1986).

Fibrillation

Atrial fibrillation and tachybradycardia are abnormalities of rhythm and conduction that deprive the brain of adequate perfusion. Moreover, thrombi can be thrown off, becoming a source of emboli and vascular occlusion (Barnett, 1984). The clinical picture may include syncope or severe diffuse hypoxia.

Mitral Valve Prolapse

Mitral valve prolapse is caused by thickening, elongation, altered collagen composition, as well as basic wear and tear of the mitral valve leaflets (Barnett, 1984; Cole, Chan, Hickey, et al., 1984; Jackson, 1986; Lucas & Edwards, 1982). This causes the mitral valves to balloon back (prolapse) into the left atrium during ventricular contraction. This disturbance can in turn disrupt blood flow to the brain and create ischemic conditions. However, thrombi also tend to form on the abnormal mitral valve and thus become thrown off into the blood supply (Barnett, 1984).

The ophthalamic and posterior cerebral arteries seem to be particularly affected, as retinal ischemia as well as transient global amnesia seems to be a frequent consequence

(Jackson, 1986; Wilson, Keeling, Malcolm, *et al.*, 1977). However, the cerebral hemispheres are just as frequently affected (Barnett, 1984; Jackson, 1986). Nevertheless, the risk of stroke, at least among young persons, is rather low. However, mitral valve prolapse is associated with the development of infective endocarditis.

There is also some association with the development of chronic anxiety, agoraphobia, and panic disorders (Klein & Gorman, 1984). The causal nature of this relationship, however, is unclear. Possibly persons who are susceptible to anxiety disorders who also suffer from mitral valve prolapse respond to these symptoms with increased fear and anxiety. That is, mitral valve prolapse exacerbates an already disturbed emotional condition (Jackson, 1986).

Vasospasms

Arteries may spasm when emboli pass and/or occlude an artery, if an aneurysm ruptures, or if a vessel is manipulated or traumatized in some manner (Toole, 1984) such as after a head injury. They have also been known to occur among persons whose arteries tend to be hyperreactive, i.e., young women (Toole, 1984). Spasm may be diffuse or segmental along the artery.

When a spasm occurs, there is a transient stoppage of blood-flow. If prolonged, the patient will suffer ischemic cerebral damage. Moreover, spasm sometimes causes embolic particles to be dislodged from the vessel wall, occluding smaller distal arteries. Cerebral infarction is therefore a likely consequence of spasm.

Murmurs

Murmurs, or bruits, are sometimes produced by changes in the direction of blood flow such as at the bifurcations of the arteries. Frequently they are a consequence of alterations in the wall of the blood vessel, including shrinkage of the luminal diameter. In general, murmurs become audible after the lumen has been reduced by about 50% (Toole, 1984); with increasing stenosis, the volume and pitch become louder and higher. Murmurs are often indicative of atherosclerosis and are most intense over the site of the lesion. However, they may be heard over vessels other than the affected artery. Bruits are graded 1–6, 1 being the mildest and 6 the loudest.

Cardiac Surgery

A few years ago, we were witness to the catastrophic effects of artificial heart surgery and experimental implantation on various human subjects, such as Dr. Barney Clark and others. All these unfortunate patients suffered extremely serious cerebral damage due to repeated and massive strokes. Although not well publicized, the effects of heart transplantation (Hotson & Pedley, 1976; Montero & Martinez, 1986; Schober & Herman, 1973), and even open heart surgery, can create similar disastrous consequences.

For example, a variety of studies have indicated that although motor and other initial impairments secondary to cerebrovascular disease generally improve after open heart surgery, significant deterioration in regard to personality, intellectual, visual–spatial, perceptual, memory, and attentional functioning often results (Aberg & Kihlgren, 1974; Heller, Frank, Kornfled, *et al.,*1974; Gilberstadt & Sako, 1967; Lee, Miller, & Rowe, 1969; Lee, Brady, Rowe, 1971; Raymond, Conklin, Schaeffer, *et al.,* 1984; Shaw, Bates, Cartlidge *et al.,* 1987).

Open heart surgery can also cause and induce stroke (Smith, Treasure, Newman, Joseph, *et al.,* 1986). Frequently, the effects are diffuse rather than focal (Sotaneiemi, Mononen, & Hokkanen, 1986). Cardiac surgery may cause cerebral injury due to reduced blood flow and arterial pressure; macroembolization of fat, air, or other gases; dislodgment of debris from the valves; and the initiation of blood cell and platelet aggregation. (Shaw *et al.,* 1987). In fact, the process of opening the chest cavity via sternal retraction alone can reduce oxygen intake if the brachial plexus is traumatized (Baisden, Greenwald, & Symbas, 1984).

In general, the cerebral effects of heart surgery appear to be age dependent. Children seem to be more resiliant, as the long-term consequences on cerebral functioning are less drastic.

Given the above, and the common knowledge that certain types of heart surgery (e.g., so-called triple bypass) generally seem to have no proven benefit, it may be extremely wise to be cautious before undergoing these procedures. Certainly, to clarify these risks further, there is a need for a series of rigorous neuropsychological studies to be conducted on such patients both pre- and postsurgery. Nevertheless, sometimes central nervous system (CNS) functioning is improved due to the correction of circulatory abnormalities and increased blood flow (Sotaneiemi *et al.,* 1986).

Heart Transplants

A common supposed side effect of heart transplants was personality changes, the explanation being that patients would assume the personality of the donor. In reality, however, many of these patients experienced alterations in mental and personality functioning because they suffered strokes. Based on a review of the few studies conducted, it appears that heart transplantation carries very significant risks in regard to cerebral functional integrity. This is because many of these people have severe vascular disease that is not confined to the heart, such as atherosclerosis and the presence of mural and arterial thrombi. Thus, during the trauma of surgery, debris can be loosened and cast into the blood, and various vessels may go into spasm, creating serious complications involving the brain (Hotson & Pedley, 1976; Montero & Martinez, 1986; Schober & Herman, 1973).

Other primary and secondary consequences of heart transplantion on the brain include vascular lesions due to circulatory collapse, decreased cardiac output and chronic postoperative hypotension, thrombosis, embolism, hemorrhage, as well as hypoxic damage and opportunistic infection due to depressed immune status (Montero & Martinez, 1986). In this regard, it would appear that frequently these patients trade an unhealthy heart for a damaged brain. The 5-year survival rate of heart transplantation is 50% (see Montero & Martinez, 1986, for review).

It is important to note, however, that there is a paucity of neuropsychological research on the effects of heart transplantation on cerebral functional integrity. Perhaps the immediate and long-term effects are not as dismal as this short review suggests.

HEMORRHAGE

Hemorrhage can occur anywhere throughout the brain and may be attributable to a number of factors e.g., head injury, hypertension, rupture of an aneurysm or arteriovenous malformation (AVM), the weakening of a segment of the vasculature secondary to emboli or thrombus, or vessel wall necrosis due to occlusion and ischemia.

Hemorrhages are frequently classified in terms of gross anatomical location: extradural, subdural, subarachnoid, intercerebral/cerebral, and cerebellar. Extradural and subdural hemorrhages are frequently secondary to head injury, whereas subarachnoid, cerebral, and cerebellar hemorrhages are often related to arterial abnormalities. Bleeding from a hemorrhage may be minute and inconsequential or profuse and extensive such that a large pool of blood rapidly develops. In some cases, bleeding may occur at a very slow, albeit continuous, pace, such that the adverse effects are not detected for days.

Subarachnoid Hemorrhage

Subarachnoid hemorrhage results from any condition that causes blood to leak into the subarachnoid space. Massive subarachnoid hemorrhage is usually the result of rupture of an intracranial aneurysm or bleeding from a cerebral angioma. In either case, there is no warning, and the onset is quite sudden and abrupt (Adams & Victor, 1981). If the hemorrhage is severe, it may lead to immediate coma and death. If moderate, the patient may pass into a semistuporous state and/or become confused and irritable. If minor, the patient may complain only of severe headache possibly develop focal deficits after hours or over the course of the first few days or weeks following hemorrhage. Vasospasms and rebleeding are very common during the first 2 weeks.

Subarachnoid hemorrhage carries a mortality of more than 50%, one third of whom will die within the first 24 hours. Only about 25% who survive will make a good recovery (Hijdra, Braakman, van Gijn, Vermeulen, & van Crevel, 1987).

Subarachnoid hemorrhage occurs most often among persons over age 50. When it occurs among younger persons, it is often secondary to congenital vascular abnormalities, including angioma, ruptured aneurysms, or rupture of an AVM on the brain surface (Adams & Victor, 1981; Toole, 1984). Rupture or seepage into the ventricular system may occur, and the cerebrospinal fluid (CSF) is bloody in 90% of cases. Anemic and hemorrhagic infarction may coexist in the same lesion.

Headache and vomiting are immediate common sequelae of hemorrhage (as well as cerebrovascular disease), and most patients will complain of severe backache and neck stiffness in the absence of demonstrable focal signs that develop later (Gorelick, Hier, Caplan, & Langenberg, 1986; Portenoy, Abissi, & Lipton, 1984). Onset is sudden and the intensity is described as severe or violent. These headaches are diffusely distributed over the cranium and/or are localized to the frontoparietal region (Gorelick et al., 1986).

Headaches are usually caused by the pressure effects of escaping blood, which distends, distorts, or stretches pain-sensitive intracranial structures. Pain in or behind the eye is often associated with hemorrhage of posterior communicating-carotid aneurysms (Gorelick *et al.*, 1986).

Cerebral/Intracerebral Hemorrhage

Cerebral hemorrhage is commonly caused by hypertension and associated degenerative changes in the vessel wall of penetrating arteries, making them suceptible to rupture (Kase, 1986). Onset is always sudden. The rupture may be brought on by mental excitement of physical effort or may occur during rest or sleep. The patient usually complains of sudden headache and may vomit and become confused and dazed with progressive impairment of consciousness over several minutes or hours time, except in the mildest of cases. However, it may evolve gradually, taking hours or days to become fully developed, and there may be no warning signs.

After a large hemorrhage, the affected hemisphere becomes larger than the other because of swelling. As the pool of blood increases and begins to clot, surrounding tissues become compressed, the convolutions become flattened, and pressure may be exerted against the opposite half of the brain, causing damage in this region as well. With large hemorrhages, coma and death may ensue due to compression of midline and vital brainstem nuclei (Adams & Victor, 1981). If the patient survives and the clot is not surgically removed, it is eventually absorbed and replaced by a glial scar. In these instances, however, patients are commonly incapacitated to varying degrees. Cerebral hemorrhages occur most often in the vicinity of the internal capsule, corona radiata, frontal lobe, pons, thalamus, and putamen (Adams & Victor, 1981; Kase, 1986).

The neurological deficit is never transitory, good functional recovery being attained by fewer than 40% of survivors, and 30–75% die within 30 days (Adams & Victor, 1981; Fieschi, Carolei, Fiorelli, *et al.*, 1988; Portenoy *et al.*, 1987). Most patients suffer persistent, permanent, and severe neurological abnormalities. Good clinical outcome is related to lower age, size of hemorrhage, the time period during which the patient was unconscious, and high scores on the Glasgow Coma Scale (Portenoy, Lipton, Berger, Lesser, & Lantos, 1987; Toole, 1984).

In more than 60% of cases, intracerebral hemorrhage is related to hypertensive cerebrovascular disease (Mohr, Caplan, Melski, *et al.*, 1978), making the vessels susceptible to rupture. That is, hypertension can induce degenerative changes and may in fact induce the formation of microaneurysms, particularly in the subcortical and perforating arteries (Kase, 1986). However, not all cerebral hemorrhages are caused by hypertension.

HYPERTENSION

Hypertension is a leading cause of vascular hypertrophy, arteriosclerosis, stroke, and hemorrhage. Conversely, approximately 40% of those with arteriosclerosis are hypertensive (Toole, 1984). In some respects, however, hypertension and arteriosclerosis are mutually reinforcing, in that the development of thrombi can act to obstruct blood flow passage, thereby increasing (at least proximal) pressure, whereas vessels damaged by increased pressure are likely to become infiltrated by thrombi.

Specifically, chronic hypertension acts to reduce arterial elasticity by stretching and thickening the walls of the blood vessels, including the capillaries (Garcia, Ben-David, Conger, *et al.*, 1981; Hart, Heistad, & Brody, 1980). It can also potentiate the development of thrombi via pressure-induced erosion or roughening of vessel walls. The space within the vessel through which the blood flows frequently decreases in size. However, in some cases it is actually enlarged.

Chronic hypertension, although associated with increased blood pressure, can actually cause generalized blood flow reductions, particularly in regions served by the middle cerebral artery, i.e., the frontal–parietal and temporal lobes (Rodriguez, Arvigo, Marenco, *et al.*, 1987). One consequence of hypertension is an increased risk of ischemic infarcts; i.e., because the caliber of the lumen becomes fixed and rigid, the ability to dilate and thus compensate for alterations in blood pressure is lost. If there were a decrease in blood pressure, this inability to compensate would result in a significant reduction in blood flow, hence cerebral ischemia.

By contrast, if blood pressure were to increase, this lack of flexibility would predispose the vessels to burst and hemorrhage (Toole, 1984), hence the strong correlation between the incidence of stroke and high blood pressure.

Hypertensive encephalopathy refers to an acute syndrome in which there is an absence of warning signs and a rapid development (minutes to hours) of deficits. Patients often complain of headache, nausea, vomiting, visual disturbances, and confusion. They may develop convulsions, focal neurological signs, and/or lapse into a deepening coma or stuporous state. Onset is often preceded by an extreme and rapid rise in blood pressure and severe hypertension. Autoregulatory responses may become abnormal such that widespread vasospasms occur accompanied by ischemia and/or the rupturing of arterioles and capillaries (Toole, 1984).

ANEURYSMS, AVMs, TUMORS, AMYLOID ANGIOPATHY

Hypertension is only one of many causes of hemorrhage (Brott, Thalinger, & Hertzberg, 1986; Hart & Easton, 1986; Laureno *et al.*, 1987). Hemorrhage may occur secondary to drug use, anticoagulant therapy, medication, AVMs, aneurysms, vessel wall necrosis, brain tumors, and various types of arterial pathology, including small vascular malformations, and cerebral amyloid angiopathy (Adams & Victor, 1981; Kase, 1986; Toole, 1984).

Ischemia and Hemorrhagic Infarcts

Ischemia not only results in the death of brain cells but necrosis of the local vasculature, which is also deprived of metabolic support. These vessel wall ischemic structural alterations make them very suceptible to rupture. Indeed, more than 40% of those with cerebral ischemic infarction will become hemorrhagic within 1–2 weeks (Hornig, Dorndorf, & Agnoli, 1986).

These ischemia-related hemorrhagic infarcts (HI) are not limited to a single vessel, however. Bleeding may be multifocal, particularly if the patient had suffered a large stroke. In part, this is also due to the more extensive edema associated with large strokes. When swelling occurs, not only is brain tissue compressed, but the endothelium of various small vessels is crushed and damaged. When these vessels are compressed, blood flow is prevented, which in turn makes these same vessels and their distal extensions more suceptible to rupture when blood flow is reestablished. (Garcia, Lowry, Briggs, et al., 1983). That is, with blockage of a vessel, the distal part of the vessel may become necrotic. Even with mild degrees of edema, there is compression and subsequent damage to various small vessels surrounding the lesion.

Hemorrhagic infarcts are not usually associated with chronic hypertension (Hart & Easton, 1986). Frequently, however, they are secondary to the reestablishment of blood flow following occlusion. As a result, when anticoagulants are employed to remove the clot, the necrotic vessels rupture and hemorrhage. Thus, anticoagulants can increase the risk of secondary hemorrhagic infarction, particularly when used following large strokes and/or those accompanied by gross neurological disturbances (Cerebral Embolism Study Group, 1983; Hornig et al., 1986).

Aneurysm

Aneurysm, also called saccular or berry aneurysm, take the form of small, thin-walled blisters protruding from the various cerebral arteries. Aneurysms may be single or multiple and are attributed to developmental defects, e.g., a congenital weakness at the junction of two arteries. Often they are located at the bifurcations and branches of various arteries, particularly the internal carotid, the middle cerebral, or the junction of the anterior communicating and anterior cerebral arteries.

Symptoms secondary to aneurysm due to rupture or compression may occur at any age. Before rupture, they are usually asymptomatic. However, as there is a tendency for them to enlarge over time, which in turn makes them more suceptible to rupture, with increasing age there is increasing risk. The peak incidence of rupture is between the ages of 40 and 55 (Adams & Victor, 1981).

Aneurysms may rupture due to sudden increases in blood pressure, while engaged in strenuous activity, during sexual intercourse, or while straining during a bowel movement (Adams & Victor, 1981). One patient I examined suffered a ruptured aneurysm when hyperventilating in his swimming pool.

Occasionally, if large and located near the base of the brain, they may compress the optic nerves, hypothalamus, or pituitary; if within the cavernous sinus, they compress the third, fourth, sixth, or ophthalamic division of the fifth nerve. Thus, a variety of visual, endocrine, and emotional alterations may herald the presence of an aneurysm prior to rupture.

With large aneurysms, when rupture occurs, blood under high pressure may be forced into the subarachnoid space, and the patient may be stricken with an excrutiating generalized headache and/or almost immediately fall unconscious to the ground, or they may suffer a severe headache but remain relatively lucid (Adams & Victor, 1981). If the hemorrhage is confined to the subarachnoid space, there are few or no lateralizing signs and no warning symptoms. In some cases, however, the patient may complain of headache, transitory unilateral weakness, numbness or tingling, or speech disturbance in the days or weeks preceding rupture, due to minor leakage of the aneurysm.

Often those who become unconscious following rupture develop decerebrate rigidity. This is usually due to compression effects, such as herniation, on the brainstem. Persistent deep coma is accompanied by irregular respiration, attacks of extensor rigidity, and finally respiratory arrest and circulatory collapse. In mild cases, consciousness, if lost, may be regained within minutes or hours. However, patients remain drowsy and confused and complain of headache and neck stiffness for several days. Unfortunately, in mild or severe cases, there is a tendency for the hemorrhage to recur (Adams & Victor, 1981).

Cerebral Amyloid Angiopathy

Amyloid angiopathies are associated with the development of microaneurysms and the occlusion of arteries in the superficial layers of the cerebral cortex (Kase, 1986). Following amyloid occlusion, the arteries are often weakened, making them susceptible to rupture. Amyloid angiopathies are often associated with recurrent hemorrhages over a period of months, which in turn may lead to the development of intracerebral hematomas. Sometimes a head trauma can trigger this latter form of hemorrhages.

Arteriovenous Malformations

Arteriovenous malformations (AVMs) consist of a tangle of dilated blood vessels, sometimes referred to as angiomas. This developmental abnormality may become symptomatic at any age, but most commonly between the ages of 20–30. Frequently AVMs form abnormal collateral channels between arteries and veins, thereby bypassing the capillary system. When this occurs, there may be abnormal shunting of blood from the arteries to the veins. As a consequence, underlying brain tissue is not adequately irrigated and may become ischemic, depending on the size of the AVM. AVMs vary in size and tend to be located in the posterior portion of the cerebral hemispheres, near the surface, as well as deep within the brainstem, thalamus, and basal ganglia. Frequently they are multiple and may be found in a variety of separate locations (Toole, 1984). They tend to be more common among males.

Like aneurysms, AVMs are present from birth and can grow larger and more complicated over time. It has been estimated that AVMs can increase in size by 2.8% per year and can become 56% larger over the span of a 20-year period (Mendelow, Erfurth, Grossart, & Macpherson, 1987). As they increase in size, their risk of becoming symptomatic increases, as there is a greater likelihood of collateral shunting.

Arteriovenous malformations are often a cause of intracerebral and subarachnoid hemorrhage (Drake, 1978). When hemorrhage occurs, blood may enter the subarachnoid space, mimicking an aneurysm. However, although the first symptom is usually a hemorrhage, 30% of patients with this disorder may suffer a seizure and 20% experience headaches or focal neurological symptoms.

Small vascular malformations often become symptomatic during the 30s and 40s and occur more often among females (Kase, 1986). These often involve the subcortical white matter of the convexity.

Brain tumors can give rise to hemorrhage in a variety of ways, particularly if the tumor is malignant and is richly vascularized. That is, certain tumors have a tendency to become spontaneously necrotic. When this occurs, their supporting vasculature ruptures. However, tumors are frequently transmitted to the brain via the arterial system, whereas others, such as carcinomas, tend to invade the walls of blood vessels. In either instance, by adhering to or penetrating the walls of the blood vessels, tumors can make them more susceptible to rupture. (See Chapter 10, Cerebral Neoplasms.)

Drug-Induced Hemorrhages

Persons with possible cerebrovascular abnormalities (such as aneurysm, AVM, or even tumor) and who abuse cocaine or amphetamines are at risk of suffering an intracranial hemorrhagic infarct (Golbe & Merkin, 1986; Lichtfeld, Rubin, & Feldman, 1984; Schwartz, & Cohen, 1984; Wojak & Flamm, 1987). Presumably these drug-induced hemorrhages are due to transient increases in blood pressure and/or vasospasm, which in turn act to rupture abnormal vessels.

LOCALIZED HEMORRHAGIC SYMPTOMS

1. *Internal capsule hemorrhage.* A patient who suffers an internal capsular hemorrhage is usually unconscious, has a slow pulse rate, and may exhibit Cheyne–Stokes respiration. The head and eyes deviate to the side of the lesion (due to paralysis), and a divergent squint is common. The corneal reflex is often lost opposite the lesion and may be lost on both sides, if coma is profound. There is also paralysis of the contralateral side of the body and no response to pinprick on paralyzed side. The limbs are extremely hypotonic such that when lifted by the physician they will fall inertly.

2. *Thalamic hemorrhage.* Thalamic hemorrhages also produce a hemiplegia or paresis due to compression of the adjacent internal capsule. Thalamic syndromes include severe sensory loss from both deep and cutaneous (contralateral) receptors as well as transitory hemiparesis. Sensation may return, to be replaced by pain and hyperasthesia. Sensory deficits usually equal or outstrips the motor weakness, and an expressive aphasia may be present if the hemorrhage involves the left thalamus. The eyes may deviate downward, with palsies of vertical and lateral gaze and inequality of pupils with absence of light reaction.

3. *Pontine hemorrhage.* Hemorrhage of the pontine brainstem is usually fatal. Deep coma ensues within a few minutes, and there may be total paralysis, decerebrate rigidity, and pinpoint pupils that do not react to light. The head and eyes are turned toward the side of the hemorrhage, if unilateral. Usually, however, even unilateral brainstem hemorrhages exert bilateral brainstem compression. The eyeballs are usually fixed.

4. *Cerebellar hemorrhage.* Hemorrhage involving the cerebellum usually develops over a period of hours (Adams & Victor, 1981). However, there may be sudden onset with occipital headache, vomiting, inability to stand or walk, and loss of

consciousness. There is a paresis of conjugate lateral gaze to the side of the hemorrhage and forced deviation contralaterally. Pupils are small and unequal but react to light. Also, there may be involuntary closure of one eye, as well as ocular bobbing.

5. *Frontal, parietal, temporal, and occipital hemorrhage.* These hemorrhagic conditions initially give rise to slow or rapidly developing focal syndromes, including headache. However, as the hemorrhage increases in size, syndromes becomes more global with impaired consciousness.

HEMORRHAGES AND STROKES: ARTERIAL SYNDROMES

Internal Carotid Artery Syndromes

Because the cerebral arteries arise from the internal carotid, hemorrhage or occlusion of this artery may be associated with extremely variable as well as widespread symptoms. As the artery becomes increasingly occluded, an occasional patient may complain of hearing a disturbing noise (bruits)—a result of turbulence from stenosis of the carotid artery relayed through the blood supply of the ear.

Stenosis of the internal carotid artery may cause massive infarction involving the anterior two thirds or all of the cerebral hemisphere, including the basal ganglia, and can lead to death in a few days. It usually produces a picture resembling middle cerebral artery occlusion. For example, if the left internal carotid is occluded, the patient may become hemiplegic and globally aphasic. Because occlusion is accompanied by ischemia, the swelling of cerebral tissue may simulate an intracranial neoplasm. If there is massive edema, tentorial herniation and death may ensue.

Since this artery gives rise to the ophthalmic, which nourishes the optic nerve and retina, carotid artery insufficiency may produce transient monocular blindness just prior to stroke onset. Unilateral blindness is the only feature distinguishing the carotid syndrome from that produced by obstruction of the middle cerebral artery.

Nevertheless, since the carotid also gives rise to the middle and anterior cerebral arteries, the most distal parts of the vascular territories of these vessels will suffer, as they are maximally subject to the influences of ischemia; i.e., the most distal portion of any occluded artery is the most severely affected. These zones are also the most vulnerable to TIAs, giving rise to weakness or paresthesias of the arm, and, if extensive, the face and tongue.

In some cases of internal carotid obstruction, the numerous branches of the external carotid (occipital, superficial temporal, and maxillary arteries) can serve as collateral blood-supply channels. In these instances, although occluded, symptoms are mild or nonexistent.

Middle Cerebral Artery Syndromes

The middle cerebral artery through its branches supplies the lateral part of the cerebral hemispheres, including the neocortex and white matter of the lateral/inferior frontal lobes (and motor areas), the superior and inferior parietal regions, and the superior portion of the temporal lobe. Its penetrating branches irrigate the putamen, caudate, globus pallidus, posterior limb of internal capsule, and the corona radiata. Whether caused by trauma, embolus, or atherosclerosis, contralateral hemiplegia is the hallmark of infarction in the territory supplied by this artery (Adams & Victor, 1981).

The classic picture of total occlusion is contralateral hemiplegia, with hemiparesis involving the face and arm more than the leg. Sensory deficits may be severe or mild, with disorders of pain perception, touch, vibration, and position. This includes extinction of pinprick or touch, deficits in two-point discrimination, as well as astereognosis, and perhaps dense sensory loss if the parietal lobe is involved. Visual-field defects consist of a homonymous hemianopsia or inferior quadrantanopia (Fig. 68).

If the left hemisphere is involved, global aphasia is present. However, if the right hemisphere is affected, neglect, denial, indifference, confabulation, and maniclike states may occur, as well as disturbances involving visual–perceptual functioning and the ability to perceive and/or express musical and emotional nonverbal nuances. It is important to note that only a branch of this artery may be obstructed. If the posterior branch of the middle cerebral artery is occluded, the parietal and inferior parietal lobe may be affected. If the left anterior branch is occluded, the patient may develop expressive aphasia.

Anterior Cerebral Artery Syndromes

Through its branches, the anterior cerebral artery supplies the anterior three fourths of the medial surface of the hemispheres, including the medial–orbital frontal lobe, the

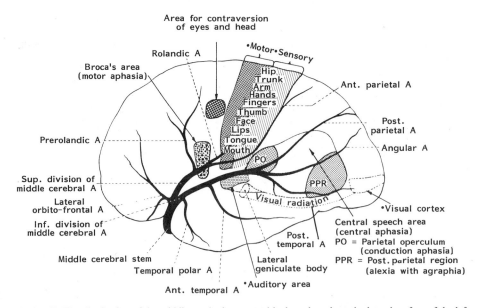

FIGURE 68. The distribution of the middle cerebral artery and its branches along the lateral surface of the left cerebral hemisphere. From *Principles of neurology* by R. D. Adams & M. Victor, 1981. Courtesy of McGraw-Hill, New York.

anterior four fifths of the corpus callosum, and the head of the caudate nucleus and putamen (Fig. 69). Hemorrhage is most often caused by rupture of an aneurysm. With total occlusion or hemorrhage, patients become obtunded and mute; develop grasp, sucking, and snout reflexes, gait apraxia, Gegenhalten, waxy flexibility, and catatonic-like postures; and are incontinent. (For further discussion of orbital and medial symptoms, see Chapter 4.)

Vertebrobasilar Artery Syndromes

Because there may be collateral circulation from the vertebrobasilar system, obstruction of this artery on one side may not produce symptoms. However, if obstruction of the opposite vertebral artery occurs later, disastrous consequences will result. Headache occurs in more than 50% of those with ischemia, beginning as a pounding or throbbing behind the orbit or in the temporal region.

A wide variety of visual and vestibular symptoms also occur when the vertebrobasilar system is compromised, including diplopia, transient blindness, or blurring, and visual hallucinations and illusions. Patients will complain of severe pounding or throbbing headaches (usually localized behind the orbit of the eye or in the temporal region) and will experience episodes of dizziness and vertigo, with or without hearing loss. This is because the auditory and vestibular portions of the ear as well as the brainstem vestibular nuclei are supplied by the vertebrobasilar arterial system. In addition, other brainstem signs include numbness, diplopia, impaired vision in one or both fields, dysarthria, hiccups, and difficulty swallowing.

Lateral Medullary Syndrome

The vertebral arteries are the chief arteries of the medulla; they supply the lower three fourths of the pyramids, the medial lemniscus, the restiform body, and the posterior–

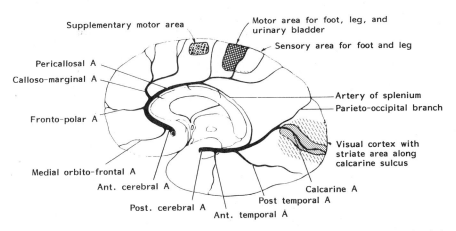

FIGURE 69. The distribution of the anterior cerebral artery along the medial aspect of the right hemisphere. From *Principles of neurology* by R. D. Adams & M. Victor, 1981. Courtesy of McGraw-Hill, New York.

inferior cerebellum (Fig. 70). Rarely does an infarct involve the pyramids or medial lemniscus. Rather, two prominent sites of lesion are the medial, and in particular the lateral, medulla. The classic lateral medullary syndrome is caused by an infarction of a wedge-shaped area of the lateral medulla and inferior surface of the cerebellum. Onset is associated with severe vertigo, and vomiting may occur. Symptoms typically include contralateral impairment of pain and thermal sense; ipsilateral Horner's syndrome (miosis, ptosis, decreased sweating); ipsilateral paralysis of the soft palate, pharynx, and vocal cord (due to involvement of nucleus ambiguous); ninth and tenth nerve dysfunction (hoarseness, dysphagia, ipsilateral paralysis of the palate and vocal cords); loss of balance such that the patient falls to the side ipsilateral to the lesion; loss of taste sensation; and hiccup, nystagmus, and nausea. There may also be dysphagia and pain or paresthesia—a sensation of hot water running over the face. There is some degree of cerebellar deficiency, with nystagmus, hypotonia, and incoordination on the side of the lesion.

Medial Medullary Syndrome

Medial medullary syndrome is a less common consequence of vertebral artery occlusion. Nevertheless, this causes contralateral hemiparesis, ipsilateral paralysis of the tongue due to twelfth nerve involvement near the zone of infarction, and loss of position and vibratory perception with sparing of pain and temperature sensation. Vertical nystagmus implies a lesion at the pontomedullary junction, and a paralysis of gaze suggests a lesion above the medulla (in pons or midbrain).

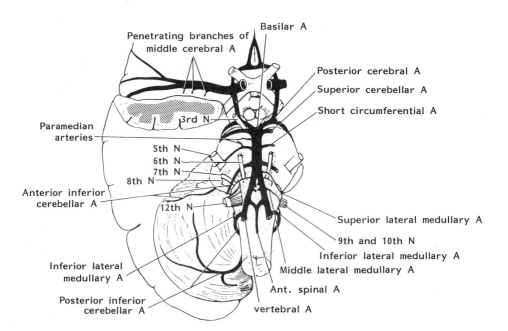

FIGURE 70. The principal blood vessels of the brainstem vertebral–basilar system. From *Principles of neurology* by R. D. Adams & M. Victor, 1981. Courtesy of McGraw-Hill, New York.

Vertebral Artery Trauma

The vertebral arteries are vulnerable to compressions or extremes in extension such as can occur during whiplash (Toole, 1984). Moreover, if the patient suffers from osteoarthritis of the cervical spine, the space through which the vertebral arteries pass may become narrowed, subjecting these arteries to pinching or other stresses with movement of the head. Thus, these patients may be subject to repeated instances of vertebral insufficiency.

Basilar Artery Syndromes

The basilar artery supplies the pons. Infarcts characteristically involve the corticospinal and corticobulbar tracts, cerebellum, cerebellar peduncles, medial/lateral lemniscus, spinothalamic tracts, and third to eighth nerves. The outstanding features of basilar artery infarct are a constellation of cranial nerve signs of both the sensory and motor varieties, cerebellar symptoms, bilateral pyramidal tract signs, ataxia, dysarthria, hemiplegia, and disturbances involving ocular movement and paralysis of gaze. If convergence is preserved, the lesion is in the middle of the inferior pons. If there is no convergence, the lesion is in the superior pons (medial longitudinal fasciculus).

Often patients become comotose because of ischemic compression effects on the reticular formation. Early signs of increasing occlusion or hemorrhage may occur in different combinations: somnolence, visual hallucinations, disorders of ocular movement, delerium, and Korsakoff's amnesic defects (Adams & Victor, 1981).

Medial pontine lesions result in ataxia of the ipsilateral limbs; a contralateral paresis of the face, arm, and leg; and variable sensory loss. If Horner's syndrome is present or if cranial nerves V, VII, or VIII are affected, the lesion is laterally placed. If paralysis of cranial nerves III, IV, VI, or VII or involvement of the pyramidal tract occurs, the lesion is probably medially placed. In general, infarct of the medial pons results (variably) in vertigo; nausea; vomiting; nystagmus; ipsilateral ataxia; ipsilateral Horner's syndrome; paresis of conjugate gaze; contralateral loss of pain; temperature sensation over the face, arm, trunk, and leg; and slurred speech.

Locked-in Syndrome

If occlusion spares the upper brainstem but involves the midpontine level, the locked-in syndrome may occur, in which the patient is alert, conscious of the surroundings, and able to see and hear but is completely paralyzed and unable to communicate, except through eyeblinks. However, because the respiratory, vasomotor, and thermoregulatory centers and pathways are affected, there may be associated abnormalities. Unfortunately, because patients can only interact by means of eyeblinks it is extremely difficult to ascertain just how impaired the patient is.

Posterior Cerebral Artery Syndromes

The posterior cerebral arteries are a branch of the vertebrobasilar system and supply via their own branches the inferomedial temporal and medial occipital regions, including areas 17, 18, and 19 and the posterior hippocampus. By means of deep penetrating branches, the posterior cerebral arteries also supply the thalamus, subthalamic nuclei, substantia nigra, midbrain, and pineal body.

Thalamic infarct or hemorrhage includes severe sensory loss and possible receptive aphasia. However, sensation may return, to be replaced by pain and hyperathesia. Midbrain infarcts includes Weber's syndrome (oculomotor palsy with contralateral hemiplegia), paralysis of vertical gaze, and stupor or coma.

Cortical syndromes include anomia, alexia, apraxia, prosopagnosia (depending on which hemisphere is involved), and related temporal–occipital, parietal–occipital disturbances. Involvement of the optic radiations or infarction of the calcarine cortex causes visual-field impairment, such as scotoma and homonymous hemianopias, particularly of the upper quadrants. With bilateral occlusion, the patient will become cortically blind.

Ischemic lesions in the occipital area may cause variations in the nature and form of visual-field defects experienced by the patient from day to day—occasionally leading to an erroneous diagnosis of hysteria. TIAs in this vicinity are also reflected by fleeting visual-field defects of a hemianopic distribution. Distal occlusion also causes mediotemporal infarction, with hippocampal involvement and memory loss. Transient global amnesia is also sometimes a consequence of transient occlusion of the posterior cerebral arteries.

Cerebellar Artery Syndrome

The cerebellar artery is also a branch of the vertebrobasilar system; it supplies portions of the pons as well as the cerebellum. Deafness and tinnitus may occur with lateral inferior pontine lesions due to occlusion of the anterior–inferior cerebellar artery. Infarction in this area may also cause vertigo, nystagmus, ipsilateral ataxia of limbs, and a contralateral hemiparesis with no sensory defect. With mild lesions, the patient may walk with an unsteady wide-based gait. With more severe lesions, patients may have extreme difficulty walking or even looking to the side of the lesion, although the pupils are normal and reactive to light.

Differential Diagnosis: Carotid versus Vertebral System

The development of deficits such as aphasia, agnosia, apraxia, constructional and manipulospatial deficits, emotional abnormalities and/or delusions indicates a carotid circulatory disturbance. Dizziness, diplopia, ataxia, nystagmus, cranial nerve signs, internuclear ophthalmoplegia, dissociated sensory loss, and/or bilateral abnormalities are hallmarks of a brainstem lesion within the vertebrobasilar territory.

RECOVERY AND MORTALITY

Mortality rates for cerebrovascular disease have declined in the United States over the course of the past 40 years (Gillum, 1986). Nevertheless, the initial death rate for persons in the acute phase and up to 30 days after stroke is about 38%. However, 50% of those who survive this phase die over the course of the next 7 years (Dombovy, Sandok, & Basford, 1986).

The major determinants for short-term mortality are impaired consciousness, leg weakness, and increasing age, with level of consciousness following stroke the single most important predictor of short-term survival (Chambers, Norris, Shurvell, & Hachinski, 1987). The major determinants for long-term mortality are low activity level, advanced age, male sex, heart disease, and hypertension. However, those who suffer hemorrhagic infarcts have a higher mortality rate than do those with infarcts due to other causes (Chambers et al., 1987). Those with right hemisphere damage tend to have poorer outcomes as well as higher mortality rates (see Chapter 1). In particular, right parietal lobule infarcts are associated with very poor outcomes (Valdimaersson, Bergvall, & Samuelson, 1982).

Hyperglycemia and diabetes are also associated with poor neurological recovery and higher short-term mortality, as well as increasing the risk of stroke in general. This is because both diabetes and hyperglycemia accentuate ischemic damage (Pulsinelli, Levy, Sigsbee, Scherer, & Plum, 1983; Woo, Chan, Yu, & Huang, 1988). Hyperglycemia also appears to have a negative effect on energy metabolism due to the generation of severe lactic acidosis (Rehncrona, Rosen, & Siesjo, 1980)—factors that act to retard neuronal recovery.

Some investigators have argued that luxury perfusion and increased cerebral blood flow (CBF) within an infarcted cite is often indicative of a good prognosis, wheras low CBF is a bad prognosis (Olsen et al., 1981). Presumably increased flow acts to nourish damaged tissue. Other studies however, indicate that initial CBF levels are not predictive of clinical outcome (Burke et al., 1986). Apparently, this is because once damage occurs during the initial period of ischemia, these cells cannot be salvaged (Heiss & Rosner, 1983). Thus, blood flow increases only when undamaged neurons return to a functionally active state (Burke et al., 1986) rather than acting to rejuvenate injured tissue. In fact, hyperfusion may endanger neuronal recovery (Mies et al., 1983). By contrast, oxygen metabolism seems to correlate better with clinical status and functional recovery than does blood flow (Wise et al., 1983).

Recovery is often greatest during the first 30 days after stroke (Dombovy et al., 1986; Lind, 1982), but continues up to 6 months in some patients (Wade & Hewer, 1987). It has been estimated that although about 60% of major stroke patients are able to achieve total independence (Wade & Hewer, 1987), only about 10% of initial survivors return to their jobs without gross or obvious disability; 40% demonstate mild disability, 40% are severely disabled, and 10% require institutionalization (Stallones et al., 1972). The 5-year cumulative risk of repeated stroke is about 42% in men and 24% in women (Baxter, 1984).

REFERENCES

Adams, R. D., & Victor, M. (1981). *Principles of neurology.* New York: McGraw-Hill.

Aberg, T., & Kihlgren, M. (1987). Effect of open-heart surgery on intellectual function. *Scandinavian Journal of Thoracic and Cardiovascular Surgery, 15,* 1–63.

Bamford, J., Sandercock, P., Jones, L., & Warlow, C. (1987). The natural history of lucunar infarction. *Stroke, 18,* 545–551.

Baisden, C. E., Greenwald, L. V., & Symbas, P. N. (1984). Occult rib fractures and brachial plexus injury following median sternotomy for open-heart operations. *Annals of Thoracic Surgery, 38,* 192–194.

Barnett, H. J. M. (1984). Cardiac causes of cerebral ischemia. In J. F. Toole (Ed.), *Cerebrovascular disorders* (pp. 174–177). New York: Raven Press.

Baxter, D. (1984). Clinical syndromes associated with stroke. In M. E. Brandstater & J. V. Bamajian (Eds.), *Stroke rehabilitation.* Los Angeles, Williams & Wilkins.

Brott, T., Thalinger, K., & Hertzberg, V. (1986). Hypertension as a risk factor for spontaneous intracerebral hemorrhage. *Stroke, 17,* 1078–1083.

Burke, A. M., Younkin, D., Gordon, J., *et al.* (1986). Changes in cerebral blood flow and recovery from acute stroke. *Stroke, 17,* 173–178.

Burke, P. A., Callow, A. D., O'Donnel, T. F., & Welch, (1982). Prophylactic carotid endarterectomy for asymptomatic bruit. *Archives of Surgery, 117,* 1222–1227.

Cahill, D. W., Knippe, H., & Mosser, J. (1981). Intracranial hemorrhage withampetamine abuse. *Neurology (New York), 31,* 1058–1059.

Calandre, L., Ortega, J. F., & Bermejo, F. (1984). Anti-coagulation and hemorrhagic infraction in cerebral embolism secondary to rheumatic heart disease. *Archives of Neurology, 41,* 1152–1154.

Cerebral Embolism Study Group. (1984). Immediate anticoagulation of embolic stroke. *Stroke, 15,* 779–789.

Chambers, B. R., Norris, J. W., Shurvell, B. L., & Hachinski, V. C. (1987). Prognosis of acute stroke. *Neurology (New York), 37,* 221–225.

Cole, W. G., Chan, D., Hickey, A. J., *et al.* (1984). Collagen composition of normal and myxomatous human mitral valves. *Journal of Biochemistry, 219,* 451–460.

Crouse, J. R., Toole, J. F., McKinney, W. M., *et al.* (1987). Risk factors for extracranial carotid artery atherosclerosis. *Stroke, 18,* 990–996.

Davis, P. H., Dambrosia, J. M., Schoenberg, B. S., *et al.* (1987). *Annals of Neurology, 22,* 319–327.

Di Pasquale, G., Andreoli, A., Pinelli, G., *et al.* (1986). Cerebral ischemia and asymptomatic coronary artery disease: A prospective study of 83 patients. *Stroke, 17,* 1098–1101.

Dombovy, M. L., Sandok, B. A., & Basford, J. B. (1986). Rehabilitation for stroke: A review. *Stroke, 17,* 363–369.

Drake, C. G. (1978). Cerebral arteriovenous malformation: Considerations from an experience with surgical treatment of 166 cases. *Clincal Neurosurgery, 26,* 145–208.

Fieschi, C., Carolei, A., Fiorelli, M., *et al.* (1988). Changing prognosis of primary intracerebral hemorrhage: Results of a clinical and computed tomographic follow up study of 104 patients. *Stroke, 19,* 192–195.

Fisher, C. M. (1969). The arterial lesions underlying lacunes. *Acta Neuropathologica, 12,* 1–15.

Fisher, C. M., & Adams, R. D. (1951). Observations on brain embolism with special reference to the mechanisms of hemorrhage infarction. *Journal of Neuropathology and Experimental Neurology, 10,* 92–93.

Garcia, J. H., Ben-David, E., Conger, K. A. *et al.* (1981). Arterial hypertension injures brain capillaries. *Stroke, 12,* 410–413.

Garcia, J. H., Lowry, S. L., Briggs, L., *et al.* (1983). Brain capillaries expand and rupture in areas of ischemia and reperfusion. In M. Reivich & H. I. Hurtig (Eds.), *Cerebrovascular diseases.* New York, Raven Press.

Gillum, R. F. (1986). Cerebrovascular disease morbidity in the United States, 1970–1983. *Stroke, 17,* 656–661.

Golbe, L. I., & Merkin, M. D. (1986). Cerebral infarction in a user of free-based cocaine (''crack''). *Neurology (New York), 36,* 1602–1604.

Gorelick, P. B., Hier, D. B., Caplan, L. R., & Langenberg, P. (1986). Headache in acute cerebrovascular disease. *Neurology (New York), 36,* 1445–1450.

Grotta, J. C., Manner, C., Pettigrew, C., & Yatsu, F. M. (1986). Red blood cell disorders and stroke. *Stroke, 17,* 811–817.

Hakim, A. M., Ryder-Cooke, A., & Melanson, D. (1983). Sequential computerized tomographic appearance of strokes. *Stroke, 14,* 893–897.

Hart, M., Heistad, D. D., & Brody, M. J. (1980). Effect of chronic hypertension and sympathetic denervation on wall–lumen ratio of cerebral vessels. *Hypertension, 2,* 419–423.

Hart, R. G., & Easton, J. D. (1986). Hemorrhagic infarcts. *Stroke, 17,* 586–589.

Heiss, W-D., & Rosner, G. (1983). Functional recovery of cortical neurons as related to degree and duration of ischemia. *Annals of Neurology, 14,* 294–301.

Heller, S. S., Frank, K. A., Kornfled, D. S., *et al.* (1974). Psychological outcome following open-heart surgery. *Archives of Internal Medicine, 134,* 908–914.

Hijdra, A., Braakman, R., van Gijn, J., Vermeulen, M., & van Crevel, H. (1987). Aneurysmal subarachnoid hemorrhage. *Stroke, 18,* 1061–1067.

Hornig, C. R., Dorndorf, W., & Agnoli, A. L. (1986). Hemorrhagic cerebral infarction—A prospective study. *Stroke, 17,* 179–185.

Hotson, J. R., & Pedley, T. A. (1976). The neurological complications of cardiac transplantation. *Brain, 99,* 673–694.

Howard, G., Toole, J. F., Frye-Pierson, J., & Hinshelwood, L. C. (1987). Factors influencing the survival of 451 transient ischemic attack patients. *Stroke, 18,* 552–557.

Jackson, A. C. (1986). Neurologic disorders associated with mitral valve prolapse. *Canadian Journal of Neurological Science, 13,* 15–20.

Jorgenson, L., & Torvic, A. (1969). Ischaemic cerebrovascular disease in an autopsy series. *Journal of Neurological Science, 9,* 285–320.

Kase, C. S. (1986). Intracerebral hemorrhage: Non-hypertensive causes. *Stroke, 17,* 590–595.

Kitagawa, Y., Meyer, J. S., Rogers, R. L., et al. (1984). Ct-CBF correlations of cognitive deficits in multi-infarct dementia. *Stroke, 15,* 1000–1008.

Klein, D. F., & Gorman, J. M. (1984). Panic disorders and mitral valve prolapse. *Journal of Clinical Psychiatry Monographs, 2,* 14–17.

Koller, R. I. (1982). Recurrent embolic cerebral infarction and anticoagulation. *Neurology (New York), 32,* 283–285.

Kunitz, S. C., Cross, C. R., Heyman, A., et al. (1984). The pilot stroke data bank. *Stroke, 15,* 740–746.

Laureno, R., Shields, R. W., Jr., & Narayan, T. (1987). The diagnosis and management of cerebral embolism and haemorrhagic infarction with sequential computerized cranial tomography. *Brain, 110,* 93–105.

Lee, W. H., Brady, M. P., & Rowe, J. M., et al. (1971). Effects of extracorporeal circulation on behaviour, personality, and brain function. *Annals of Surgery, 173,* 1031–1023.

Lee, W. H., Miller, W., Rowe, J. M., et al. (1969). Effects of extracorporeal circualtion on personality and cerebration. *Annals of Thoracic Surgery, 7,* 562–569.

Lind, K. (1982). A synthesis of studies on stroke rehabilitation. *Journal of Chronic Diseases, 35,* 133–149.

Litchfield, P. J., Rubin, D. M., & Feldman, R. S. (1984). Subarachnoid hemorrhage precipitated by cocaine snorting. *Archives of Neurology, 41,* 223–224.

Lodder, J., & van der Lugt, P. J. M. (1983). Evaluation of the risk of immediate anti-coagulant treatment in patients with embolic strokes of cardiac origin. *Stroke, 14,* 42–46.

Lucas, R. V., & Edwards, J. E. (1982). The floppy mitral valve. *Current Problems in Cardiology, 7,* 1–48.

Mendelow, A. D., Erfurth, A., Grossart, K., & Macpherson, P. (1987). Do cerebral arteriovenous malforamtions increase in size? *Journal of Neurolgoy, Neurosurgery and Psychiatry, 50,* 980–987.

Meyer, J. S., Rogers, R. L., Judd, B. W., Mortel, K. F., & Sims, P. (1988). Cognition and cerebral blood flow fluctuate together in multi-infarct dementia. *Stroke, 19,* 163–169.

Mies, G., Auer, L. M., Ebbardt, G., et al. (1983). D=Flow and neuronal density in tissue surrounding chronic infarction. *Stroke, 14,* 22–27.

Mohr, J. P., Caplan, L. R., Melski, J. W., et al. (1978). The Harvard cooperative registry. *Neurology (New York), 28,* 754–762.

Montero, C. G., & Martinez, A. J. (1986). Neuropathology of heart transplantation: 23 cases. *Neurology (New York) 36,* 1149–1154.

Olsen, T. S., Larsen, B., Kriver, E. E., et al. (1981). Focal cerebral hyperemia in acute stroke. *Stroke, 2,* 598–606.

Ott, B. R., Zamani, A., Kleefield, J., & Funkenstein, H. H. (1986). The clinical spectrum of hemorrhagic infarction. *Stroke, 17,* 630–637.

Petersen, P., & Godtfredsen, J. (1986). Embolic complications in paroxysmal atrial fibrillation. *Stroke, 17,* 622–629.

Portenoy, R. K., Abissi, C. J., & Lipton, R. B. (1984). Headache in cerebrovascular disease. *Stroke, 15,* 1009–1012.

Portenoy, R. K., Lipton, R. B., Berger, A. R., Lesser, M. L., & Lantos, G. (1987). Intracerebral hemorrhage: A model for the prediction of outcome. *Journal of Neurology, Neurosurgery and Psychiatry, 50,* 976–979.

Pulsinelli, W. A., Levy, D. E., Sigsbee, B. Scherer, P., & Plum, F. (1983). Increased damage after ischemic stroke in patients with hyperglycemia with or without established diabetes mellitus. *American Journal of Medicine, 74,* 540–544.

Raymond, M., Conklin, C., Schaeffer, J., et al. (1984). Coping with transient intellectual dysfunction after coronary bypass surgery. *Heart and Lung, 13,* 531–539.

Rehncrona, S., Rosen, I., & Siesjo, B. K. (1980). Excessive cullular acidosis: An important mechanism of neuronal damage in the brain? *Acta Physiologica Scandinavica, 110,* 435–437.

Rodriguez, G., Arvigo, F., Marenco, S., *et al.* (1987). Regional cerebral blood flow in essential hypertension. *Stroke, 18*, 13–20.

Schober, R., & Herman, M. M. (1973). Neuropathology in cardiac transplantation: Survey of 31 cases. *Lancet, 1*, 962–967.

Schwartz, K. A., & Cohen, J. A. (1984). Subarachnoid hemorrhage precipitated by cocaine snorting. *Archives of Neurology, 41*, 705.

Shaw, P. J., Bates, D., Cartlidge, N. E. F., *et al.* (1987). Neurologic and neuropsychological morbidity following major surgery. *Stroke, 18*, 700–707.

Smith, P. L. C., Treasure, T., Newman, S. P., Joseph, P., *et al.* (1986). Cerebral consequences of cardiopulmonary bypass. *Lancet, 1*, 823–825.

Sotaniemi, K. A., Mononen, H., & Hokkanen, T. E. (1986). Long-term cerebral outcome after open-heart surgery. A five year neuropsychological follow-up study. *Stroke, 17*, 410–416.

Stallones, R. A., Dyken, M. L., Fang, H. C. H. *et al.* (1972). Epidemiology for stroke facilities planning. *Stroke, 3*, 360–371.

Roole, J. T. (1984). *Cerebrovascular disorders*. New York: Raven Press.

Torvik, A., & Svindland, A. (1986). Is there a transitional zone between brain infarcts and the surrounding brain? A histological study. *Acta Neurologica Scandinavica, 74*, 365–370.

Valdimaersson, E., Bergvall, U., & Samuelson, K. (1982). Prognostic significance of cerebral computed tomograph results in supratentorial infarction. *Acta Neurologica Scandinavica, 65*, 133–145.

Van Der Windt, C., & Van Gijn, J. (1988). Cerebral infarction does not occur typically at night. *Journal of Neurology, Neurosurgery and Psychiatry, 51*, 109–111.

Wade, D. T., & Hewer, R. L. (1987). Functional abilities after stroke: Measurement, natural history and prognosis. *Journal of Neurology, Neurosurgery and Psychiatry, 50*, 177–182.

Wilson, L. A., Keeling, P. W. N., Malcolm, A. D., *et al.* (1977). Visual complications of mitral leaflet prolapse. *British Medical Journal, 2*, 86–88.

Wise, R. J. S., Bernardi, S., Frackowiack, R. S. J., *et al.* (1983). Serial observations on the pathophysiology of acute stroke. *Brain, 106*, 197–222.

Wojak, J. C., & Flamm, E. S. (1987). Intracranial hemorrhage and cocaine use. *Stroke, 18*, 712–715.

Wolf, P. A. (1985). Risk factors for stroke. *Neurology Clinics, 16*, 359–360.

Wolf, P. A., Kannel, W. B., McGee, D. L., *et al.* (1983). Duration of atrial fibrillation and imminence of stroke: The Framingham Study. *Stroke, 14*, 664–667.

Wolf, P. A., Kannel, W. B., & Verter, J. (1983). Current status of risk factors for stroke. *Neurology Clinics, 1*, 317–343.

Woo, E., chan, Y. W., Yu, Y. L., & Huang, C. Y. (1988). Admission glucose level in relation to mortality and morbidity outcome in 252 stroke patients. *Stroke, 19*, 185–191.

Yamaguchi, F., Meyer, J. S., Yamamoto, M., *et al.* (1980). Non-invasive regional cerebral blood flow measurements in dementia. *Archives of Neurology, 37*, 114–119.

Cerebral Neoplasms

Brain tumors have a number of etiologies and may arise following head injury, infection, metabolic and other systematic diseases, and exposure to toxins and radiation. Some are caused by tumors that developed in other parts of the body that metastasized to the brain. Others are believed to have originated in embryonic cells left in the brain during development. In some cases, tumors are a consequence of embryological timing and migration errors; i.e., if germ layers differentiate too rapidly or if cells migrate to the wrong location, they exert neoplastic influences within their unnatural environment.

Indeed, among children, many tumors are congenital, developing from displaced embryonic cells, dysplasia of developing structures, and the altered development of primitive cells that normally act as precursors to neurons and glia. Most of these tumors tend to occur within the brainstem, cerebellum, and midline structures, including the third ventricle. Among older persons, most tumors are due to dedifferentiation of adult elements.

TUMOR DEVELOPMENT: GENETICS

Tumors are sometimes believed to be caused by a loss of restraint in regard to cellular growth and differentiation such that a malignant progression ensues. For example, oncogenes (J. R. Shapiro, 1986) are genes that are important genetic regulators. The aberrant expression of oncogenes is associated with cancer-causing abnormalities in chromosomal structure (Gilbert, 1983). If these oncogenes becomes abnormal or are inappropriately expressed, they in turn induce malignant cellular formation. Presumably, three groups of chromosomal abnormalities are associated with altered oncogene expression: deletions, duplications, and reciprocal translocations.

Deletions are associated with the removal of the constraints normally exerted on oncogenes, promoting malignant expression through the rapid and abnormal proliferation of cells as well as the possible loss of chromosomes during cell division (Rowley, 1983; Yunis, 1983; J. R. Shapiro, 1986). Deletions are associated with the development of neuroblastomas in children (Gilbert, Feder, Balaban, et al., 1984).

Duplications are associated with the transposition, amplification, and hyperactivation of oncogenes (Alitalo, Schwab, Lin, et al., 1983), such that numerical abnormalties in chromosomal expression result, as well as segregational errors involving the gain of chromosomes during cell division (Shapiro, 1986). Again, this is presumed to be secondary to a loss of regulatory restraint. Thus, if a malignant recessive gene is present, its duplication may result in a malignant overrepresentation, hence the expression of recessive malignant traits. The ability to suppress its expression has been overridden, and a malignant hybrid cell is developed (Shapiro, 1986). Once a primary tumor begins to develop, a series of secondary events contribute to their growth, invasive properties, and metastasis.

ESTABLISHMENT AND GROWTH OF A TUMOR

Vascularization and Necrosis

For a tumor to grow, it must become vascularized. Indeed, it has been suspected that tumors may in fact secrete a substance that potentiates capillary development (Sherbet, 1982). Thus, the initial stages of tumor growth are sometimes associated with local hyperemia. Nevertheless, the blood flow of established tumors is lower and more variable than that of the surrounding normal brain tissue (Blasberg, Groothuis, & Molnar, 1981; Brooks, Beaney, & Thomas, 1986). In fact, tumors have a lower oxygen utilization as well (Ito, Lammerstman, Wise, *et al.*, 1982). Thus, tumors, or at least their centralmost portions, often exist in a state of hypoxia, although what they receive seems adequate for their peripheral proliferation and metabolism. As a consequence, many tumors, particularly those that are rapidly growing, contain central regions of necrosis. This is because, as tumor volume increases, the surface area becomes increasingly inadequate in regard to blood perfusion and the diffusion of nutrients and metablic products, such that, as the periphery proliferates, cells in the center become increasingly deprived of nutrients and undergo death and necrosis (Sherbet, 1982). Subsequently, underlying normal tissue is also destroyed.

Invasion and Decimation

As tumors grow, they increasingly encompass, surround, and destroy neighboring tissue. Invasion also sometimes occurs by the locomotive behavior of individual tumor cells that develop microfilaments. These microfilaments extend into the cytoplasm of surrounding tissue and then infiltrate them.

When a tumor becomes vascularized, its potential to dessiminate is increased because of tumor material escaping into the bloodstream. Capillaries offer little resistance to invading tumors that destroy the endothelium of the vessel walls. Thus, these vessels may also become hemorrhagic.

Once tumor cells enter the bloodstream, they may be carried short or long distances, where they lodge and give rise to secondary growths; i.e., like a thrombus, they will attach to the vessel wall. Moreover, imperfections in the endothelial wall increase the likelihood of adhesion. However, unlike a thrombus or embolus, these tumor cells are able to penetrate the vessel walls so as to form attachments to new host material (Sherbet, 1982).

Interestingly, anticoagulants, including aspirin, have been found to arrest or reduce the development of certain blood vessel-borne tumor cell colonies (Sherbet, 1982). Tumors cells are also transported via the lymphatic system.

Metastasis

It has been estimated that anywhere from 10% to 33% of all cancers located in other body regions will metastasize to the brain (Adams & Victor, 1981; Bloom, 1979; Hirsh, Hansen, Paulson & Vraa-Jensen, 1979; Sherbet, 1982; Williams, 1979). These metastases may be single or multiple. In most cases, the patient has lung cancer, whereas in other instances breast cancer is the culprit (Bloom, 1979; Hirsh et al., 1979; Williams, 1979). These metastases are usually passed via the blood or lymphatic system. However, surgery for tumor often results in the development of cerebral metastases, presumably because of dislodged tumor fragments, which are then carried elsewhere.

Intracranial metastases, or carcinomas, are of three types, those that attach to the skull, those that metastasize to the meninges, and those that infiltrate the brain. Most form in the cerebral hemispheres (60%) and the cerebellum (30%) and seem to develop preferentially along the distribution of the middle cerebral artery (Bloom, 1979). In more than 70% of reported cases, the metastases are multiple and scattered throughout the brain, usually near the surface in the gray and subcortical white matter.

Malignancy

Malignancy refers to the biological ability of a group of cells to become freed of homeostatic controls. When this occurs, they progressively devide, disseminate, invade, and form distant metastases, ultimately killing the host. However, in addition to its infiltrative and proliferative potential, a tumor's malignancy is dependent on its anatomical location, the degree of elevated intracranial pressure (ICP) it induces, the patient's age and neurological status, and its responsiveness to therapy (Salcman & Kaplan, 1986). By contrast, so-called benign tumors are slow growing, generally encapsulated, and localized and have little metastatic potential.

Realistically, however, all tumors have the potential to kill the patient; thus all are potentially malignant (Salcman & Kaplan, 1986; Sherbet, 1982). For example, a so-called benign tumor located in the brainstem or a low-grade astrocytoma located near vital centers may quickly kill the patient. Moreover, a tumor that is recurrent and ineradicable, albeit benign, is just as fatal as a malignant tumor due to the effects of pressure within limited cranial–cerebral space, although they are not considered malignant, rarely metastasize, and may in fact be relatively small. Thus, the grading of a tumor or its malignant versus benign state must be treated with caution (Salcman & Kaplan, 1986).

Tumor Grading

Nevertheless, in determining malignancy, many types of tumors are graded in regard to their cellular architecture, mitotic activity, and in particular their degree of differentiation. Those that are least well differentiated are the most malignant. For example, a tumor that is three fourths differentiated is considered grade 1. If one half of the tumor is differentiated, it is grade 2. If only one fourth of the tumor contains differentiated cells, it is grade 3. Grade 4 tumors are those in which very little or no differentiation is seen. Some investigators have collapsed this point system to three grades, however.

Grade 1 tumors generally do not metastasize, whereas grade 3 and 4 tumors have the greatest degree of potential for forming metastases. Moreover, patients with grade 3 and 4 tumors have the highest and fastest mortality rate. For example, in one study, patients with astrocytomas graded 1–4 had average postoperative survival times of 74, 24, 12, and 7 months, respectively (see Sherbet, 1982, for review).

Some tumors, however, may initially appear to be benign and receive a low grade, whereas as they grow they become progressively less differentiated and more malignant and increase their metastatic potential (Sherbet, 1982). For example, the daughter cells of transformed astrocytes, oligodendrocites, microgliocytes, or ependymocytes tend to become variably dedifferentiated, hence more malignant as the tumor grows and cells divide and proliferate. Thus, what was a benign grade 1 astrocytoma is now a grade 4 glioblastoma multiforme.

Age

There is a bimodal age distribution regarding the development and incidence of brain tumors, as they tend to occur in childhood and then later with increasing risk during the fifth, sixth, and seventh decades, until a decline occurs during the eighth decade of life (Salcman & Kaplan, 1986).

Gliomas, pituitary adenomas, and meningiomas are the most frequently occurring types of brain tumor across all age groups (Salcman & Kaplan, 1986). However, among children, and persons below age 20, ependymomas of the fourth ventricle, pinealomas, cerebellar astroycytomas, and medulloblastomas are the most common. Meningiomas and gliomas are most frequent around 50 years of age.

Extrinsic and Intrinsic Tumors

Most cerebral tumors can be broadly considered either intracerebral (intrinsic) or extracerebral (extrinsic). Extrinsic tumors usually arise from the coverings of the brain and cranial nerves and, although benign, can exert compression on underlying structures. These include meningiomas, acoustic schwannomas, and pituitary adenomas. Intrinsic tumors are often secondary to the dedifferentiation of glia, ependymal cells, and astrocytes. These include ependymomas, various grades of astrocytoma, and oligodendrogliomas, all of which (particularly gliomas) arise from adult elements. These tumors have the capability of becoming increasingly less well differentiated and more malignant. Frequently they involve the lateral portions of the hemispheres or the ventricles.

NEOPLASMS AND SYMPTOMS ASSOCIATED WITH TUMOR FORMATION

Initially, tumor development is associated with localized cerebral displacement, compression, edema, and regional swelling, particularly in the white matter. Because of this, although there are a variety of tumors, the symptoms produced are more dependent on the tumor's rate and location of development rather than the type tumor per se. Their influences are site specific, such that initial localized effects are the most prominent. Hence, the most common modes of onset include progressive focal symptoms (e.g., focal epilepsy, monoplegia, hemiplegia, aphasia, cerebellar deficiency, and symptoms of increased ICP). Most patients also suffer from periodic bifrontal and bioccipital headaches that awaken the patient at night or are present upon waking. Vomiting, mental torpor, unsteady gait, sphincter incontinence, and papilledema are also frequent sequelae.

Nevertheless, as ICP, increases, disturbances of consciousness, cognition, and neurological functioning become progressively widespread. However, generalized symptoms occur late or not at all. Even so, functional disruptions associated with tumor formation are usually slow to appear and develop, taking months or years. The sudden appearance of symptoms is generally indicative of vascular disease. However, in some cases, a silent slow-growing tumor may hemorrhage, in which case the symptoms are of sudden onset.

Fast- versus Slow-Growing Tumors

A tumor may appear, develop, and in fact grow for long periods with hardly any symptoms. This is particularly true of slow-growing tumors, which give the brain time to adjust. Rapidly growing tumors exert more drastic effects. In this regard, a tumor that takes 3 years to reach a size of 5 cm may exert little disruptive influences, whereas a rapidly growing tumor that reaches a size of 2 cm may exert profound consequences, even if localized to the same region. However, tumor location is also of importance, for even tiny tumors of the brainstem may cause death.

Generalized Neoplastic Symptoms

Increased Intracranial Pressure

Because of limitations in the cranial–cerebral space, when tumors (or any mass lesion) form ICP is likely to rise. As ICP increases, disturbances of consciousness, cognition, and neurological functioning become increasingly diffuse and progressively more widespread. This is because the skull is rigid and the development and enlargement of any type of neoplasm or space-occupying mass (such as a hematoma or hemorrhage) occurs at the expense of the brain, which becomes increasingly compressed. Generalized symptoms begin to replace or at least override localized deficits as the tumor enlarges and spreads.

Moreover, a tumor growing in one part of the brain not only will displace underlying brain tissue but can compress local blood vessels as well as decrease the amount of cerebrospinal fluid (CSF) in the ventricles and subarachnoid space. With increased displacement and edema, CSF pressure eventually begins to rise. Compression effects are thereby exerted on midline structures as well as on contralateral brain tissue. If the brain becomes sufficiently swollen and displaced, herniation may result.

Cognitive Abnormalities

As the tumor enlarges and ICP rises, often there is a slight bewilderment, slowness in comprehension, or loss of capacity to sustain continuous mental activity, although specific localized signs of disease are diminished or lacking. There may be a persistent lack of application to the tasks of the day, a slowing of thought processes and reaction time, undue irritability, emotional lability, inertia, faulty insight, forgetfulness, reduced range of mental activity, indifference to common social practices, and the like. There may also be inordinate drowsiness, apathy, or stoicism, becoming more prominent after a few weeks (Adams & Victor, 1981).

With increased tumor development, when questioned a long pause precedes each reply, and the patient may not even bother to reply, as if he did not hear the question. However, responses are more intelligent than one would expect. Much of the drowsiness and general restriction of the mental horizon is related to increased ICP and is unrelated to the site of the lesion.

Headache

The most frequent initial nonlocalizing complaints include headaches, seizures, personality change, weakness, and confusion. Tumor-related headaches are an early symptom and are reported by approximately one third of all patients. Although not usually well localized, they may be bifrontal or located along the vertex of the cranium. Frequently they are moderate to severe in intensity with a deep nonpulsatile quality and are usually quite variable occurring throughout the day as well as nocturnally (Adams & Victor, 198). However, they tend to be worse in the morning when the patient first awakens and may improve if the patient vomits. Tumor-related headaches are often caused by local swelling of tissues and by distortion of blood vessels in and around the tumor.

Vomiting occurs in about one third of all tumor patients and accompanies the headache. Vomiting is not related to the ingestion of food but is sometimes induced by increased ICP and brainstem compression and is found with tumors of the posterior fossa or with low brainstem gliomas.

Seizures

Generalized epileptiform convulsions are a common symptom of tumor and may precede other disturbances by many years. It is the first symptom in 30–50% of all patients, particularly those suffering from astrocytoma, meningioma, or glioblastoma. Indeed, the occurrence of a seizure for the first time during adult years and the existence of a localizing aura almost always suggest tumor. Glioblastoma multiforme, oligodendroglioma, apendymoma, metastatic carcinoma, and primary reticulum cell sarcoma are all associated with the development of seizures. Similarly, tumors of the frontal and temporal lobes frequently trigger seizure activity.

FOCAL SYNDROMES AND NEOPLASMS

Frontal Lobe Tumors

Depending on which quadrant of the frontal lobes are involved, symptoms associated with neoplastic growth can be quite variable. Regardless of location, patients tend to complain of headache even during the early stages of tumor formation. During the later stages, papilledema and frequent vomiting are characteristic—features usually caused by increased ICP.

If the tumor is within the midline region, apathy, mutism, depressive and catatonic-like features with posturing, grasp reflexes, and gegenhalten may be prominent. Some patients are initially misdiagnosed as depressed.

Downward pressure on the olfactory nerve may lead to anosmia on the side of the lesion. Pressure on the corticospinal fibers may led to contralateral weakness that is most marked in face and tongue. If the tumor extends to the medial motor areas, the patient's lower extremity may become paralyzed.

Depressive-like symptoms, disturbances of speech output, as well as some degree of motor impairment are also characteristic of left frontal tumors. By contrast, right frontal tumors may initially give rise to manic and delusional symptoms. (See Chapter 4, The Frontal Lobes.) In general, however, a progressive dementia becomes increasingly apparent, regardless of which quadrant has been most compromised; 50% of all patients with frontal tumors are likely to develop seizures.

Tumors of the motor areas are easy to localize because of the focal convulsions that occur in select body regions. Depending on the extensiveness of the tumor, weakness or paralysis may variably involve the fingers, hand, arm, tongue, face, and trunk. Motor weakness is the result of destruction of corticospinal tract fibers.

Temporal Lobe Tumors

Tumors of temporal lobe can cause receptive and fluent aphasia (if the left temporal region is involved), receptive amusia and agnosia for environmental and emotional sounds (if the right lobe is compromised), and visual-field defects (i.e., a crossed upper quadrant hemianopia with loss greatest in the ipsilateral field). These tumors also cause auditory hallucinations and tinnitus. (See Chapter 7, The Temporal Lobes.) If the inferior regions are involved, there is an increased likelihood of seizures (in more than 50% of all cases), emotional alterations, and disruptions of memory. Like frontal lobe tumors, personality changes may be the most prominent symptom.

Parietal Lobe Tumors

With tumors involving the parietal lobes, sensory disturbances are most prominent. They may also cause sensory jacksonian fits, which consist of paresthesia, tingling, pain, or sensations of electric shock, corresponding to the focus of damage. That is, a patient may feel spasms of shocklike sensations along her leg. Abnormalities involving the spatial and discriminative aspects of sensation may be prominent (e.g., astereognosis), especially of postural sensibility and tactile discrimination, while crude appreciation of pain, heat, and cold is intact. Parietal postcentral tumors are also associated with hypotonia and wasting of the various body parts (parietal wasting).

Occipital Lobe Tumors

Tumors of the occipital lobe are not as common as frontal and temporal neoplasm or parietal tumors. However, visual abnormalities, including blindness if the tumor is situated medially, are common sequelae.

Brainstem Tumors

In 90% of all reported cases, the initial manifestation of a brainstem tumor is a palsy of one or more cranial nerves, most often the sixth and seventh, such that conjugate gaze, gaze deviation, and facial sensation are abnormal. In addition, patients develop hemiparesis, unilateral ataxia of gait, and paraparesis. If the tumor increasingly involves the medulla, the patient may develop uncontrollable hiccups and disturbances of cardiac and respiratory rate. Death is highly likely, as even very small tumors exert drastic effects.

Cerebellar Tumors

The cerebellum is a common site of tumor, especially in childhood. Symptoms are most marked on standing and walking, such that patients tends to fall backward or sometimes forward. Gait is ataxic, and nystagmus may be present if the tumor is laterally placed or absent if localized to the midline. Patients tend to walk with a wide-based gait and have considerable difficulty with balance. Many patients will list to the side of the tumor. Cerebellar tumor growth, via compression, also tends to affect cranial nerves V–XII.

Tumors of the Ventricles: Ependymomas

Ependymomas originate in the dedifferentiation of adult ependymal cells, which line the ventricular walls (Fig. 71). The fourth ventricle is involved about 70% of the time. These tumors usually develop in young adults, and especially children, such that about 40% occur during the first year of life and 75% during the first decade. Presumably, these tumors are benign. However, as they can occlude the ventricles, CSF flow may be impeded and hydrocephalus and increased ICP may result. With increased pressure, there is a danger of herniation and brainstem compression accompanied by paroxysmal headaches, vomiting, difficulty in swallowing, paresthesias of the extremities, abdominal pain, and vertigo. Seizures occur in one third of most cases.

Among infants and young children, initial symptoms include headaches, lethargy, stupor, spastic weakness of the legs, and unsteadyness of gait. In some respects, the symptoms are similar to those of medulloblastoma. The 5-year survival rate is about 50% (Bloom, 1979). Although these tumors form in the walls of the ventricle, they can also grow into the brain. Moreover, they tend to form miniature ventricles, i.e., tubules of cells that are compacted in a radial manner, like spokes in a wheel, such that a central cavity is formed. In most cases, a small blood vessel forms the hub at the center.

Medulloblastoma

Medulloblastoma is a rapidly growing embryonic neuroectodermal tumor that arises in the neuroepithelial roof of the fourth ventricle and posterior part of the cerebellar vermis (Allen, Bloom, Ertel, et al., 1986). Seedings of the tumor may be seen on the walls of the third and lateral ventricles and on the meningeal surfaces and may metastasize into the spinal canal or supratentorial region.

It occurs most frequently in chidlren aged 4–8, with males outnumbering females

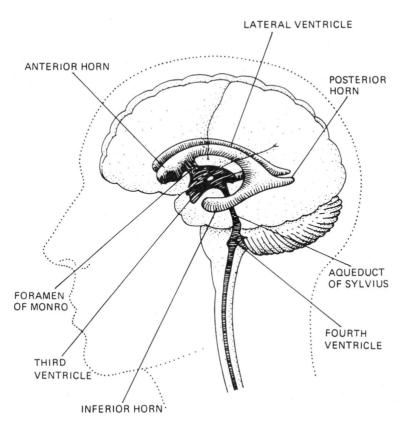

FIGURE 71. Schematic diagram of the ventricles, lateral view. Reproduced, with permission, from *Correlative neuroanatomy,* 20th Ed., by J. DeGroot & J. G. Chusid, copyright Appleton & Lange, E. Norwalk, CT, 1988.

3 : 2. Symptoms associated with medulloblastomas, however, may not become manifest until patients reach their early 20s. Symptoms are usually present for 1–5 months before diagnosis.

Children with these tumors characteristically become listless, vomit repeatedly, and suffer early-morning headache. Because of cerebellar involvement, patients develop a stumbling gait and frequently fall. Examination will demonstrate papilledema.

If the tumor grows unchecked, there is a danger of cerebellar herniation. As this develops, patients may tend to hold their head tilted at an angle, the occiput being tilted back away from the side of tumor. The 5-year survival of patients who have been treated is about 50% (Allen *et al.*, 1986; Berry, Keen, *et al.*, 1981) The risk of recurrence is limited to the first 3 years after treatment (Bloom, 1979).

Tumors of the Pineal Gland: Pinealmomas

The germinoma that makes up more than one half of all pineal tumors is a firm discrete mass that reaches ≤3–4 cm in diameter. Although its effects on the pineal body are benign, it tends to compress the superior colliculi (causing visual and visual attentional disturbances); sometimes the superior surface of the cerebellum and narrows the aqueduct of Sylvius. When these later regions are involved, gait and brainstem abnormalities may arise, as well as hydrocephalus. Moreover, often these tumors expand into the third ventricle and may compress the hypothalamus. This can give rise to extreme changes in emotionality as well as exert profound disturbances on neuroendocrine and hormonal functioning. Children, adolescents, and young adult males are most often affected, as these tumors rarely develop after age 30. Most characteristic localizing symptoms are an inability to look upward (Parinaud's syndrome) and slighty dilated pupils that react to accommodation but not to light.

Midbrain Tumors

Tumors of the midbrain usually cause internal hydrocephalus due to cerebral aqueduct obstruction and may lead to headache, papilledema, and vomiting. Ocular abnormalities are prominent, including weakness of upward conjugate deviation. Pupils are unequal and tend to be dilated, and reactions to light and convergence–accommodation may be lost. Corticospinal tracts are involved on both sides, although asymmetrically, such that the extremities become weak and possibly paralyzed.

Pituitary Tumors

Pituitary tumors (e.g., pituitary adenomas) typically produce a variety of symptoms, as abnormalities of this gland frequently cause hyper- or hyposecretion and other endocrine changes. These include acromegaly, pituitary giantism, depression of sexual functioning, personality changes, and hypercortisolism. Overgrowth of bones may be evident in the skull, face, and mandible, and the hands may become broad and spadelike. The patient (particularly men) may also experience changes in the texture of the skin such that it becomes soft and pliable. There may also be a loss of hair over the body such that in the extreme patients may no longer need to shave (Adams & Victor, 1981).

As the optic nerves and chiasm pass directly beneath the pituitary, tumors in this vicinity often disrupt visual functioning through compression. These visual changes may range from a loss of visual acuity to progressive narrowing of the visual fields, i.e., tunnel vision. As these tumors expand, they can also displace and compress the carotid arteries, causing ischemic conditions throughout the brain. Frequently, these tumors hemorrhage spontaneously and in fact carry the highest risk of hemorrhage of all intracranial neoplasms.

Nevertheless, there are a variety of pituitary tumors, each of which give rise to specific hypersecretory products. These include prolactin-secreting adenomas, which in turn can cause amenorrhea and infertility: growth hormone-secreting adenomas, which give rise to giantism and acromegaly; adrenocorticorticotropic hormone (ACTH)-secreting adenomas, which are responsible for producing Cushing's syndrome; and oncocytomas, which are nonsecreting pituitary tumors (Salcman, 1986). Oncocytomas make their presence known via pituitary hypofunction.

The annual incidence of pituitary tumor is 1.0 per 100,000 persons. However, there is an increased risk of developing a pituitary adenomas as patients grow older, and women are more at risk than men. For example, among women between the ages of 15 and 44, the incidence is 7.1 per 100,000 (Salcman, 1986). These tumors are also associated with "ice cream cone" headaches in which the apex of pain points downward toward the center of the head.

Tumors of the Meninges: Meningioma

Meningiomas are tumors of the dura mater and/or arachnoid, and arise from abnormal arachonoidal cells of the arachnoid villae. They comprise 15% of all extracranial tumors. However, the risk for developing a meningioma increases with age. People in their 70s have the highest incidence of all age groups. They also occur twice as often among women as men. Indeed, portions of these tumors actually contain estrogen and progesterone receptors (Salcman & Kaplan, 1986). Women with breast cancer appear to have the highest risk of all.

These tumors are very slow growing and can become extremely immense before giving rise to symptoms. Although considered benign, they can kill and cause extensive damage through pressure effects. They also can form metastatic deposits, which infiltrate and invade other organs such as the liver and lungs. Indeed, they may invade the sagittal sinus, envelop the carotid arteries, or even erode through the skull (Salcman & Kaplan, 1986).

Nevertheless, although originating within the meninges, through compression and infiltration, they exert their predominant disruptive effects on the surface of the cerebral hemispheres, the base of the skull, as well as regions in which the dura forms tentorial compartments. These tumors occur most often along the Sylvian region, superior parasagittal surface of the frontal and parietal lobes, the olfactory grooves, sphenoid bones, superior surface of the cerebellum, and spinal canal.

Like many tumors, their initial development may not cause any symptoms, particularly in that they are very slow growing. Nevertheless, focal seizures are often an early sign. Patients may also develop focal neurological deficits, such as motor weakness with frontal involvement, gait disturbances if the cerebellum is involved, or somesthetic abnormalities with parietal invasion.

Prognosis and Recovery

The survival of patients with meningeal tumors tends to be directly correlated with the extent of surgical resection. Unfortunately, incompletely removed meningiomas tend to regrow over a period of 5–10 years. In fact, they may reconstitute from what seem to be very tiny amounts of residual tumor. Nevertheless, 90% of those who have had the tumor surgically resected (and who survived the initial surgery) are alive after 5 years (Salcman & Kaplan, 1986).

Acoustic Neuromas and Schwannomas

Schwannomas and neuromas are tumors of the cranial nerves, usually the eighth, fifth, ninth, and first. They are thought to be benign and develop from the Schwann cells that cover the cranial nerves. Acoustic (eighth nerve) neuromas (which are essentially a schwannoma) are the most common type. These tumors usually have their onset at an early age. However, the highest incidence is during the fifth decade of life.

Acoustic neuroma occurs occasionally as part of neurofibromatosis; it may be bilateral and combined with multiple meningiomas. It originates in the junction between the nerve root and medulla, i.e., at the point where axons become enveloped in Schwann cells. Acoustic neuromas also attack the vestibular division of the eighth nerve just within the internal auditory canal. As it grows, it increasingly occupies the angle between the cerebellum and pons, i.e, the posterior fossa; and may compress the fifth, seventh, and ninth or tenth nerves. With increased growth, these tumors come to compress the pons and lateral medula and obstruct CSF circulation. The earliest signs are loss of hearing, headache, disturbed sense of balance, unsteadiness of gait, and facial pain. Approximately one third of affected patients are troubled by vertigo associated with nausea, vomiting, and pressure in the ear.

ASTROCYTOMA AND GLIOBLASTOMA MULTIFORME

Astrocytomas

Astrocytomas are the most frequently occurring type of tumor and arise from the dedifferentiation of astrocytes that have lost their ability to limit their own replication (Salcman & Kaplan, 1986). Although the abnormal cells themselves are not as numerous as what constitutes a higher-grade glioblastoma, these tumors tend to be evenly distributed and to infiltrate a wide zone of tissue. Indeed, they frequently infiltrate and entrap normal neurons and glia (Burger, 1986) and may occur anywhere in the brain or spinal cord. Astrocytomas are slow-growing tumors that infiltrate and form large cavities in the regions occupied. Some are noncavitating and form in the white matter. Sometimes these tumors form microcysts (Kepes, 1987). If several tumors are adjacent, these microcysts can coalesce to form larger cysts.

Grading

These tumors are usually graded on a four-point scale, depending on the degree of differentiation, grade 1 being the most benign and the smallest. Typically, grade 1 astrocytomas contain normal as well as abnormal astrocytes, and they tend to be well differentiated. They are apparently quite difficult to detect on gross inspection. Grade 2 represents an increased density of abnormal cells as well as reduced differentiation. Both grade 1 and 2 astrocytomas are often referred to as low grade gliomas.

Preferential Regions of Formation

In general, astrocytomas occur most frequently along the frontal–temporal convexity (Salcman & Kaplan, 1986)—areas that are most susceptible to contusion following head injury or acceleration–rotational traumas. In fact, both structurally and metabolically, grade 1 astrocytomas resemble a normal astrocytic reaction to an injury (Salcman & Kaplan, 1986). Indeed, it appears that some patients develop these tumors only after a head injury. Presumably the head injury acts as the environmental event, interacting with a genetic predisposition to trigger tumor formation. Nevertheless, astrocytomas also tend to grow almost anywhere within the cerebrum, including the cerebellum, hypothalamus, pons, optic nerve, and chiasm.

Although considered relatively benign, as these tumors grow they can initially give rise to focal neurological deficits and may distort the lateral and third ventricle and displace the anterior and cerebral arteries and give rise to seizures; 50% of patients present with initial focal or generalized seizure. Many of these patients continue to experience recurrent seizures throughout the illness. Headache and signs of increased ICP occur late. Age of onset is 20–60 years.

Mortality and Malignancy

Astrocytomas are relatively dangerous and are associated with a high mortality rate, with 50% of patients dying over the course of the first 5 years (Salcman & Kaplan, 1986). In addition, although initially a grade 1 or 2, it appears that as patients age these initially slow-growing astrocytomas become less well differentiated and possibly progress to a more rapidly growing grade 3 or 4 tumor (Burger, 1986). Grade 3 and 4 astrocytomas are also referred to as gliomas. For example, the probability that an astrocytoma is malignant is less than .35, among individuals below age 45, whereas after age 60 it increases to .85. In this regard, as age increases, the likelihood of suffering a malignant astrocytoma (i.e., glioma) increases. Moreover, many malignant gliomas contain fields of benign tumor, further suggesting that astrocytomas progress from a slow-growing benign neoplasm to a rapidly growing malignant tumor (W. R. Shapiro & Shapiro, 1986).

Gliomas

Grade 3 lesions are very densely packed, are less well differentiated, contain necrotic tissue, and are very malignant. Sometimes they are accompanied by small areas of hemorrhage. These cells also tend to develop and divide much more rapidly than normal cells (Nelson, Urtasum, Saunders, et al., 1986). Patients who develop higher-grade gliomas are older than those with the lower-grade astrocytoma and typically become or have been symptomatic for a shorter period before coming to the attention of a physician, i.e., on the average of 5.4 months versus 15.7 months (Burger, 1986). Glioblastomas grow at a much more rapid pace.

They have their peak incidence between the ages of 40–60 and occur among males more frequently than among females (Ransohoff, Kelly, & Laws, 1986). The 18-month survival of patients with glioblastoma is anywhere from 15 to 30% (Burger, 1986; W. R. Shapiro, 1986). In part, the grim outlook for these patients is attributable to the development of local disease (Gaya, 1979; Nelson et al., 1986), as well as their potential for rapidly infiltrating wide regions of the cerebrum.

Glioblastoma Multiforme

Grade 4 astrocytomas are an extremely malignant form of neoplasm, commonly referred to as glioblastoma multiforme. Some have argued, however, that grade 3 and 4 gliomas should be considered one and the same (Burger, 1986) and that grading should be based on a three-point rather than a four-point scale. Glioblastoma multiforme accounts for about 20% of all intracranial neoplasms, for about 55% of all glioma tumors, and for 90% of gliomas of the adult cerebral hemisphere.

As the name implies, a glioblastoma multiforme is highly dedifferentiated, consisting of multiple cells intermingled among others of various consistencies, cytoplasmic contents, colors, textures, and atypical nuclei (Shapiro, Young, & Shapiro, 1981). These tumors also contain large areas of necrosis (surrounded in a picket-fence manner by astrocytic nuclei). In addition, they are heavily vascularized and exhibit considerable abnormal capillary proliferation. Many of these capillaries also have vessel walls that demonstrate endothelial hyperplasia, hence the tendency for these tumors to hemorrhage spontaneously (Laurent, Bruce, & Schut, 1981).

These tumors also have a tendency to develop predominantly within the frontal–temporal regions (Burger, 1986; Salcman & Kaplan, 1986). However, they are very rapidly growing and tend to be multifocal. If allowed to run their course, they will freely infiltrate the cerebrum, brainstem, spinal cord, and cerebellum and will extend into the opposite cerebral hemisphere. About 50% are bilateral or occupy more than one lobe of a hemisphere. Even when unilateral, midline structures are often compressed and the lateral ventricles distorted and displaced contralaterally. In addition, they may attain enormous size before attracting medical attention.

Grade 4 glioblastoma multiforme are thus very dangerous as well as very resistant to treatment because of their cellular, metabolic, vascular and chromosomal diversity (Shapiro & Shapiro, 1986). Indeed, the central portion of the tumor (which contains areas of necrosis and cells that are hypoxic but viable) is highly resistant to radiation and chemotherapy (Salcman, Kaplan, Ducker, et al., 1982). This is because of their reduced blood flow, which in turn impedes the ability to treat them chemically. Moreover, because they are hypoxic, they are more resistant to radiation than well-oxygenated cells (Nelson et al., 1986). Because the tumor is multicentric, it is impossible to remove completely.

In addition, even following resection and chemoradiation therapy, recurrence usually occurs within 1 year (Burger, 1986). It will often revert back to its original size and distribution. Unfortunately, even among patients who survive, the long-term effects of treatment are associated with progressive cerebral atrophy and deterioration of cognitive ability (Burger, 1986; Ransohoff et al., 1986). Thus the outlook for patients with this form of tumor is extremely grim. Less than 20% of adults will survive beyond 1 year. Among children, 50% will die within 18 months, and only 25% survive 5 years (Allen et al., 1986). Peak incidence, however, is during middle life.

Oligodendroglioma

Oligodendrogliomas are said to have a fried egg appearance and are not typically graded. They arise due to the dedifferentiation of oliogodendrocytes—the cells that form myelin. Oligodendrogliomas occur most commonly in the deep white matter of the frontal and temporal lobes, with little or no surrounding edema. The tumor is slow growing, and the first symptom in 50% of patients is a focal or generalized seizure. These have a tendency to calcify.

LYMPHOMAS, SARCOMAS, NEUROBLASTOMAS, CYSTS

Lymphomas

Lymphomas are tumors composed of cells that reside in the lymph nodes, i.e., lymphocytes, lymphoblasts, histocytes, and reticulum cells. These tumors often develop preferentially within the adventitial spaces of the blood vessels (Kepes, 1987); they have also been referred to as reticulum cell sarcomas (Portlock, 1979).

Lymphomas also develop within the meninges (Lister, Sutcliffe, Brearley, & Cullen, 1979; Portlock, 1979) and are sometimes caused by bone marrow disease (Young, Howser, Anderson, Jaffe & De Vita, 1979). However, lesions are often multifocal and may extend into the basal ganglia, thalamus, and corpus callosum (Portlock, 1979).

Lymphomas occur most commonly among persons in their 50s. However, they have been known to affect infants as young as 16 days of age (Portlock, 1979). Symptoms develop quite rapidly, and death ensues quickly, many people dying during the first 13 months but a few living as long as $3\frac{1}{2}$ years (Portlock, 1979).

Sarcomas

Sarcomas are malignant tumors composed of cells derived from mesenchymal tissues (fibroblasts, lipocytes, osteoblasts) and are rare. Many occur within the cranial cavity or the temporal–frontal–basal regions during the fifth to sixth decade of life.

Neuroblastomas

Neuroblastomas are tumors that occur predominantly among young children, infants, and even neonates (Pochedly, 1976). They arise from sympathetic nervous tissue from any region of the body. Within the brain, they originate in the sympathetic ganglia or the adrenal medulla. Their effects on the brain are primarily the result of compression, although they have a tendency to infiltrate the meninges and venous sinus. Usually, however, they infiltrate the cranium, causing destruction and widening of the sutures, as well as the meninges, particularly the dura behind the orbit of the eyes and at the base of the brain (Pochedly, 1976). The major effects of neuroblastomas involve compression and increased ICP.

Cysts

Cysts are pseudotumors that simulate intracranial neoplasm. They are usually found overlying the Sylvian fissure or the cerebral convexity and may develop within the ventricular system. Sometimes, however, tumors will either calcify or coalesce, or both, forming cysts. Colloid cysts are congenital but do not generally exert significant effects until adulthood, when they begin to compress or obstruct the third ventricle, producing obstructive hydrocephalus.

UNILATERAL TUMORS AND BILATERAL DYSFUNCTION

In general, as a tumor grows, it exerts pressure on underlying structures; with sufficient development, it will not only compress but cause shifting of the brain, such that subcortical and contralateral brain tissue becomes dysfunctional. In some cases, during the early stages of tumor growth, patients may complain of or demonstrate symptoms that suggest bilateral lesions. If the tumor is too small to be visualized by computed tomography (CT) scan, the bilateral nature of the patient's deficits (which might be detected only by a competent neuropsychologist) may seem paradoxical.

Neoplasms use less oxygen and have a lower blood flow as compared with normal tissue. However, possibly because of the effects of compression or bilateral arterial adjustments to localized blood flow reductions, cerebral tissue contralateral to the tumor also demonstrates lower than normal oxygen utilization and blood flow (Beaney, Brooks, Leenders, *et al.*, 1985). This in turn depresses the functioning of this otherwise normal tissue. However, with treatment of the tumor, blood flow returns to normal in this contralateral region (Brooks *et al.*, 1986).

Thus, in some respects, a tumor can exert both localized as well as seemingly paradoxical contralateral disruptive influences. A patient with a tumor of the right motor strip may display not only unilateral left-sided weakness or paresis, but clouding of consciousness, confusion, depressive-like emotional changes, and expressive language difficulties (the result of contralateral compression and hypoxia).

HERNIATION

With the formation of a neoplasmic growth, local tissue becomes depressed, the development of edema is incited, the brain begins to swell, and the volume of the intracranial contents is increased. When brain tissue swells, midline structures shift and become compressed, the lumen of the affected veins and capillaries collapses, as do the ventricles, sulci, and subarachnoid space of the swollen hemisphere. If ICP is raised sufficiently, the brain not only shifts, but the brainstem may become compressed, interfering with life-sustaining functions of respiration, blood pressure control, and temperature regulation.

The first compensation for increased ICP depends on the two rapidly mobile intracranial fluid pools: the CSF and intravascular blood. If the hemispheric swelling exceeds the compensatory mechanisms, the only escape for the displaced hemisphere is to herniate. The manner in which herniation occurs depends on the location of the tumor. For example, frontal or parietal tumors tend to induce herniation medially under the falx cerebri, which separates the two hemispheres (subfalcial herniation). With subfalcial herniation, the medial part of one frontal or parietal lobe is pushed under the falx, damaging not only these regions but the cingulate gyrus as well.

Temporal lobe tumors induce downward herniation over the edge of the tentorial notch surrounding the mesencephalon (transtentorial or temporal lobe herniation). That is, the medial portion of the temporal lobe is forced into the oval-shaped tentorial opening through which the midbrain and subthalamus pass, pushing these structures to the opposite side and exerting great pressure on them and their vessels. This results in a hemiparesis caused by compression of the cerebral peduncle, which is ipsilateral to the lesion. In addition, the medial aspects of the temporal lobe, including the amygdala and hippocampus, become seriously compromised. Transtentorial herniation may be bilateral if there are multiple neoplasms. Tumors that have invaded the cerebellum are likely to cause cerebellar herniation. This also results in brainstem compression as the cerebellum is forced down in the foramen magnum.

After subfacial or transtentorial herniation, the diencephalon and mesencephalon become compressed and torqued, and the brainstem becomes seriously damaged. Interference not only with vital centers but with the reticular activating system leads to rapid changes in conscious-awareness, descending into somnolence, semicoma, coma, and then death. Many patients, however, experience a transient phase of elevated consciousness, with excitement and delirium before gradually descending through lower levels of consciousness.

As transtentorial herniation increases, the uncus displaces the posterior cerebral artery and the third nerve which in turn causes the pupil to constrict. Eventually both third nerves may cease to function, and both pupils become dilated and fixed—no longer responding to light.

Decerebrate rigidity is a postural syndrome of transtentorial herniation. The mouth is closed, and the wrists, fingers, and toes are flexed; the head, trunk, arms, and legs are extended, with hands and feet internally rotated. Breathing also becomes irregular and shallow. Appearance of this syndrome requires transection/compression of the mesencephalon and sparing of the vestibulospinal tract and dorsal/ventral roots as well as brainstem compression.

Tumors most likely to cause increased ICP without conspicuous focal or lateralizing signs are medullablastoma, ependymoma of the fourth ventricle, glioblastoma of the cerebellum, and colloid cysts of the third ventricle.

PROGNOSIS

Major prognostic indicators regarding so-called malignant neoplasms are the age at diagnosis, Karnofsky performance score (a measure of quality of life), the presence of seizures, tumor pathology (e.g., anaplastic astrocytoma versus glioblastoma multiforme), and even blood type (Green, Bayer, Walker, et al. 1983; Shapiro, 1986b). Hence, young patients live longer than older persons—the death rate for those under 45 being one third that of those over age 65; those with type B or O blood have a better prognosis than do those with A or B; and patients who have developed seizures are more likely to survive than those who have not. In fact, the longer they have had seizures, the longer the survival time (W. R. Shapiro, 1986b).

Some researchers have noted that preoperative tumor size is strongly related to survival (Andreou, George, Wise, et al., 1983), whereas others have not noted a strong relationship. Nevertheless, it has been noted consistently that the smaller the residual tumor following surgery, the longer the patient will live (Andreou et al., 1983; Salcman, 1986; Wood, Green, & Shapiro, 1988).

Unfortunately, total resection is quite difficult in that it is neither practical nor ethical to remove a sufficient quantity of normal tissue to ensure total removal, and thereby total elimination. Given the infiltrative and regenerative abilities of most tumors, recurrence is likely. Moreover, combined resection and chemotherapy is not always successful because of the protective influences of the blood–brain barrier (Blasberg & Groothuis, 1986; Shapiro & Shapiro, 1986). It is this same blood–brain barrier that protects the tumor from the antigens of the immune system—a functional result of the relative absence of vesicular transport across the endothelial cytoplasm between the tightly spaced capillary endothelial cells.

Nevertheless, I have had the opportunity of examining patients who have lived (and/or are still living) 10–15 years after the initial discovery and treatment of cerebral neoplasm. As new methods of therapy are discovered and employed, and with early detection, the prognosis for many patients should only improve.

REFERENCES

Adams, R. D. & Victor, M. (1981). *Principles of Neurology*. New York: McGraw-Hill.

Allen, J. C., Bloom, J., Ertel, I., *et al.*, (1986). Brain tumors in children. *Seminars in Oncology, 13,* 110–122.

Andreou, J., George, A. E., Wise, A., *et al.*, (1983). CT prognostic criteria of survival after malignant glioma surgery. *American Journal of Neuroradiology, 4,* 488–490.

Alitalo, K., Schwab, M., Lin, C. C., *et al.* (1983). Homogeneously staining chromosomal regions contain amplified copies of an abundantly expressed cellular oncogene in malignant neuroendocrine cells from a human. *Proceedings of the national Academy of Sciences, 80,* 1701–1711.

Beaney, R. P., Brooks, D. J., Leenders, K. L., *et al.* (1985). Blood flow and oxygen utilisation in the contralateral cortex of patients with untreated intracranial tumors as studied by positron emission tomography with observations on the effect of decompressive surgery. *Journal of Neurology, Neurosurgery and Psychiatry, 48,* 310–319.

Berry, M., Jenkin, R., Keen, C., *et al.* (1981). Radiation therapy for medulloblastoma. A 21 year review. *Journal of Neurosurgery, 55,* 43–51.

Blasberg, R. G., & Groothuis, D. R. (1986). Chemotherapy of brain tumors. *Seminars in Oncology, 13,* 70–82.

Blasberg, R. G., Groothuis, D. R., & Molnar, P. (1981). Application of quantitative autoradiographic measurements in experimental brain tumor models. *Seminars in Neurology, 1,* 203–221.

Bloom, H. J. M. (1979). Intracranial secondary carcinomas and disseminating gliomas. Treatment and prognosis. In J. M. A. Whitehouse & H. E. M. Kay (Eds.), *CNS complications of malignant disease* (pp. 331–350). Baltimore: University Park Press.

Brooks, D. J., Beaney, R. P., & Thomas, D. G. T. (1986). The role of positron emission tomography in the study of cerebral tumors. *Seminars in Oncology, 13,* 83–93.

Burger, P. C. (1986). Malignant astrocytic neoplasms. *Seminars in Oncology, 13,* 16–25.

Gaya, H. (1979). Central nervous system infections in neoplastic disease. In J. M. A. Whitehouse & H. E. M. Kay (Eds.), *CNS complications of malignant disease*. Baltimore: University Park Press.

Gilbert, F., Feder, M., Balaban, G., et al. (1984). Human neuroblastomas and abnormalties of chromoses 1 and 17. *Cancer Research, 44,* 5444–5449.

Green, S. B., Bayer, D. B., Walker, M. D., *et al.* (1983). Comparisons of carmustine, procarbazine, and high-dose methylprednisolone as additons to surgery and radiotherapy for the treatment of malignant glioma. *Cancer Treatment Reports, 67,* 121–132.

Hirsh, F. R., Hansen, H. H. M., Paulson, O. B., & Vraa-Jensen, J. (1979). Development of brain metastases in small-cell anaplastic carcinoma of the lung. In J. M. A. Whitehouse & H. E. M. Kay (Eds.), *CNS complications of malignant disease*. Baltimore: University Park Press.

Ito, M., Lammserstman, A. A., Wise, J. R. S., *et al.* (1982). Measurement of regional cerebral blood flow and oxygen utilization in patients with cerebral tumours using positron emission tomography, *Neuroradiology, 23,* 63–74.

Kepes, J. J. (1987). Astrocytomas: Old and newly reconized variants, their spectrum of morphology and antigen expression. *Canadian Journal of Neurological Science, 14,* 109–121.

Laurent, J., Bruce, D., & Schut, L. (1981). Hemorrhagic brain tumors in pediatric patients. *Child's Brain, 8,* 263–270.

Lister, T. A., Sutcliffe, S. B. J., Brearley, R. L., & Cullen, M. H. (1979). Patterns of CNS involvement in malignant lymphoma. In J. M. A. Whitehouse & H. E. M. Kay (Eds.), *CNS complications of malignant disease.* Baltimore: University Park Press.

Nelson, D. F., Urtasum, R. C., Saunders, W. M., *et al.* (1986). Recent and current investigations of radiation therapy of malignant gliomas. *Seminars in Oncology, 13,* 46–55.

Pochedly, C. (1976). Neuroblastomas in the head and central nervous system. In C. Pochedly (Ed.), *Neuroblastoma* (pp. 1–23). Acton, MA: Publishing Sciences Group.

Portlock, C. S. (1979). Lymphomatous involvement of the central nervous system. In J. M. A. Whitehouse & H. E. M. Kay (Eds.), *CNS complications of malignant disease* (pp. 77–92). Baltimore: University Park Press.

Ransohoff, J., Kelly, P., & Laws, E. (1986). *The role of intracranial surgery for the treatment of malignant gliomas. Seminars in Oncology, 13,* 27–37.

Rowley, J. D. (1983). Human oncogene locations and chromosome aberrations. *Nature (London) 301,* 290–291.

Salcman, M. (1986). Tumors of the pituitary gland. In A. R. Moossa, M. C. Robson, & S. C. Schimpff (Eds.), *Oncology.* Los Angeles: Williams & Wilkins.

Salcman, M., & Kaplan, R. S. (1986). Intracranial tumors in adults. In A. R. Moossa, M. C. Robson, & S. C. Schimpff (Eds.), *Oncology.* Los Angeles: Williams & Wilkins.

Salcman, M., Kaplan, R. S., Ducker, T. B., *et al.* (1982). Effects of age and reoperation on survival in the combined modality treatment of malignant astrocytoma. *Neurosurgery, 10,* 454–463.

Shapiro, J. R. (1986). Biology of gliomas: Heterogeneity, oncogenes, growth factors. *Seminars in Oncology, 13,* 4–15.

Shapiro, J. R., Young, W.-K. A., & Shapiro, W. R. (1981). Isolation, karyotyupe and clonal growth of heterogenous subpopulations of human malignant gliomas. *Cancer Research, 41,* 2349–2359.

Shapiro, W. R. (1986). Therapy of adult malignant brain tumors. *Seminars in Oncology, 13,* 38–45.

Shapiro, W. .R, & Shapiro, J. R. (1986). Principles of brain tumor chemotherapy. *Seminars in Oncology, 13,* 56–69.

Sherbet, G. V. (1982). *The biology of tumour malignancy.* New York: Academic press.

Williams, C. J. (1979). The prevention of CNS metastases in small-cell carcinoma of the bronchus. In J. M. A. Whitehouse & H. E. M. Kay (Eds.), *CNS complications of malignant disease.* Baltimore: University Park Press.

Wood, J. R., Green, S. B., & Shapiro, W. R. (1988). The prognostic importance of tumor size in malignant gliomas. *Journal of Clinical Oncology, 6,* 338–343.

Young, R. C., Howser, D. M., Anderson, T., Jaffe, E., & DeVita, V. T. (1979). CNS infiltration: A complication of diffuse lymphomas. In J. M. A. Whitehouse & H. E. M. Kay (Eds.), *CNS complications of malignant disease.* Baltimore: University Park Press.

Yunis, J. J. (1983). The chromosomal basis of human neoplasia. *Science, 221,* 227–236.

Index